PDE AND LEVEL SETS

Algorithmic Approaches to Static and Motion Imagery

TOPICS IN BIOMEDICAL ENGINEERING
INTERNATIONAL BOOK SERIES

Series Editor: Evangelia Micheli-Tzanakou
Rutgers University
Piscataway, New Jersey

Signals and Systems in Biomedical Engineering:
Signal Processing and Physiological Systems Modeling
Suresh R. Devasahayam

Models of the Visual System
Edited by George K. Hung and Kenneth J. Ciuffreda

PDE and Level Sets: Algorithmic Approaches to Static and Motion Imagery
Edited by Jasjit S. Suri and Swamy Laxminarayan

A Continuation Order Plan is available for this series. A continuation order will bring delivery of each new volume immediately upon publication. Volumes are billed only upon actual shipment. For further information please contact the publisher.

PDE AND LEVEL SETS

Algorithmic Approaches to Static and Motion Imagery

Edited by

Jasjit S. Suri, Ph.D.
Philips Medical Systems, Inc.
Cleveland, Ohio, USA

and

Swamy Laxminarayan, Ph.D.
New Jersey Institute of Technology
Newark, New Jersey, USA

Kluwer Academic / Plenum Publishers
New York, Boston, Dordrecht, London, Moscow

ISBN 0-306-47353-4

233 Spring Street, New York, NY 10013

http://www.wkap.nl/

10 9 8 7 6 5 4 3 2 1

A C.I.P. record for this book is available from the Library of Congress

Printed in the United States of America

Jasjit Suri would like to dedicate this book
to his parents and especially to his late mother
for her immortal softness and encouragements.

Swamy Laxminarayan would like to dedicate this book
to his late sister, Ramaa, whose death at the tender age of 16
inspired his long career in biomedical engineering.

Contributors

Jasjit S. Suri, Ph.D. Philips Medical Systems, Inc., Cleveland, Ohio, USA

Jianbo Gao, Ph.D. KLA-Tencor, Milpitas, California, USA

Jun Zhang, Ph.D. University of Wisconsin, Milwaukee, Wisconsin, USA

Weison Liu, Ph.D. University of Wisconsin, Milwaukee, Wisconsin, USA

Alessandro Sarti, Ph.D. University of Bologna, Bologna, Italy

Xioaping Shen, Ph.D. University of California, Davis, California, USA

Laura Reden, B.S. Philips Medical Systems, Inc., Cleveland, Ohio, USA

David Chopp, Ph.D. Northwestern University, Chicago, Illinois, USA

Swamy Laxminarayan, Ph.D. New Jersey Institute of Technology, Newark, New Jersey, USA

The Editors

Dr. Jasjit S. Suri received his B.S. in computer engineering with distinction from MACT, Bhopal, M.S. in computer sciences from the University of Illinois, and Ph.D. in electrical engineering from the University of Washington, Seattle. He has been working in the field of computer engineering/imaging sciences for more than 18 years, and has published more than 85 papers on image processing. He is a lifetime member of various research engineering societies, including Tau Beta Pi and Eta Kappa Nu, Sigma Xi, the New York Academy of Sciences, EMBS, SPIE, ACM and is also a senior member of IEEE. He is also on the editorial board/reviewer of several international journals, including *Real-Time Imaging*, *Pattern Analysis and Applications*, *Engineering in Medicine and Biology Society*, *Radiology*, *JCAT*, *IEEE-ITB* and *IASTED*. He has chaired image processing sessions at several international conferences and has given more than 30 international presentations. Dr. Suri has written a book on medical imaging covering cardiology, neurology, pathology, and mammography imaging. He also holds and has filed several US patents. Dr. Suri has been listed in *Who's Who* five times (World, Executive and Mid-West), is a recipient of President's Gold Medal in 1980, and has been awarded more than 50 scholarly and extra-curricular awards during his career. Dr. Suri's major interest are: computer vision, graphics and image processing (CVGIP), object-oriented programming, and image guided surgery. Dr. Suri has been with Picker/Marconi/Philips Medical Systems Inc., Cleveland since December 1998.

Dr. Swamy Laxminarayan is currently the Chief Information Officer at the National Louis University (NLU) in Chicago. Prior to coming to NLU, he was an adjunct Professor of Biomedical Engineering at the New Jersey Institute of Technology, Newark, New Jersey and a Clinical Associate Professor of Medical Informatics and Director and Chair of VocalTec University. Until recently, he was the Director of Health Care Information Services as well as Director of Bay Networks, authorized educational center at NextJen Internet, Princeton, New Jersey. He also serves as a visiting Professor of Biomedical Information Technology at the University of Brno, Slovak Republic, and an Honorary Professor at Tsinghua University, China. He is an internationally recognized scientist, engineer, and educator with over 200 technical publications in areas as wide ranging as biomedical information technology, computation biology, signal and image processing, biotechnology, and physiological system modeling. He has been involved in Internet and information technology application for well over a decade with significant contributions in the applications of the disciplines in medicine and health care. Dr. Laxminaryan has won numerous international awards and has lectured widely as an invited speaker in over 35 countries. He has been closely associated with the IEEE Engineering and Medicine and Biology Society in various administrative and executive committee roles, including his previous appointments as a Vice President of the society and currently as Editor-in-Chief of IEEE *Transactions on Information Technology and Biomedicine*. Among the many awards and honors he has received, he is one of the 1995 recipients of the Purkynje Award, one of Europe's highest forms of recognition, given for pioneering contributions in cardiac and neurophysiological modeling work and his international bioengineering leadership. In 1994, he was inducted into the College of Fellows of the American Institute of Medical and Biological Engineering (AIMBE) for "outstanding contributions to advanced computing and high performance communication applications in biomedical research and education." He recently became the recipient of the IEEE 3rd Millennium Medal.

Preface

Chapter 1 is for readers who have less background in partial differential equations (PDEs). It contains materials which will be useful in understanding some of the jargon related to the rest of the chapters in this book. A discussion about the classification of the PDEs is presented. Here, we outline the major analytical methods. Later in the chapter, we introduce the most important numerical techniques, namely the finite difference method and finite element method. In the last section we briefly introduce the level set method. We hope the reader will be able to extrapolate the elements presented here to initiate an understanding of the subject on his or her own.

Chapter 2 presents a brief survey of the modern implementation of the level set method beginning with its roots in hyperbolic conservation laws and Hamilton-Jacobi equations. Extensions to the level set method, which enable the method to solve a broad range of interface motion problems, are also detailed including reinitialization, velocity extensions, and coupling with finite element methods. Several examples showing different implementation issues and ways to exploit the level set representation framework are described.

Level sets have made a tremendous impact on medical imagery due to its ability to perform topology preservation and fast shape recovery. In chapter 3, we introduce a class of geometric deformable models, also known as level sets. In an effort to facilitate a clear and full understanding of these powerful state-of-the-art applied mathematical tools, this chapter attempts to explore these geometric methods, their implementations, and integration of regularizers to improve the robustness of these topologically independent propagating curves and surfaces. This chapter first presents the origination of level sets, followed by the taxonomy of level sets. We then derive the fundamental equation of curve/surface evolution and zero-level curves/surfaces. The chapter then focuses on the first core class of level sets, known as "level sets without regularizers." This class presents five prototypes: gradient, edge, area-minimization, curvature-dependent and application driven. The next section is devoted to second core class of level sets, known as "level sets with regularizers." In this class, we present four kinds: clustering-based, Bayesian bi-directional classifier-based, shape-based, and coupled constrained-based. An entire section is dedicated to optimization and quantification techniques for shape recovery when used in the level-set framework.

Finally, the chapter concludes with the general merits and demerits on level sets, and the future of level sets in medical image segmentation.

Chapter 4 focuses on the partial differential equations (PDEs), as these have dominated image processing research recently. The three main reasons for their success are: (1) their ability to transform a segmentation modeling problem into a partial differential equation framework and their ability to embed and integrate different regularizers into these models; (2) their ability to solve PDEs in the level set framework using finite difference methods; and (3) their easy extension to a higher dimensional space. This chapter is an attempt to understand the power of PDEs to incorporate into geometric deformable models for segmentation of objects in 2-D and 3-D in *static* and *motion* imagery. The chapter first presents PDEs and their solutions applied to image diffusion. The main concentration of this chapter is to demonstrate the usage of regularizers, PDEs and level sets to achieve image segmentation in *static* and *motion* imagery. Lastly, we cover miscellaneous applications such as mathematical morphology, computation of missing boundaries for shape recovery, and low pass filtering, all under the PDE framework. The chapter concludes with the merits and the demerits of PDE and level set-based framework techniques for segmentation modeling. The chapter presents a variety of examples covering both synthetic and real world images.

In chapter 5, we describe a new algorithm for color image segmentation and a novel approach for image sequence segmentation using PDE framework. The color image segmentation algorithm can be used for image sequence intraframe segmentation, and it gives accurate region boundaries. Because this method produces accurate boundaries, the accuracy of motion boundaries of the image sequence segmentation algorithms may be improved when it is integrated in the sequence segmentation framework. To implement this algorithm, we have also developed a new multi-resolution technique, called the "Narrow Band", which is significantly faster than both single resolution and traditional multi-resolution methods. As a color image segmentation technique, it is unsupervised, and its segmentation is accurate at the object boundaries. Since it uses the Markov Random Field (MRF) and mean field theory, the segmentation results are smooth and robust. This is then demonstrated by showing good results obtained in dermatoscopic images and image sequence frames. We then present a new approach to the image sequence segmentation that contains three parts: (i) global motion compensation, (ii) robust frame differencing and (iii) curve evolution. In the global motion compensation, we adopt a fast method, which needs only a sparse set of pixels evenly distributed in the image frames. Block-matching and regression are used to classify the sparse set of pixels into inliers and outliers according to the affine model. With the regression, the inliers of the sparse set, which are related to the global motion, is determined iteratively. For the robust frame differencing, we used a local structure tensor field, which robustly represents the object motion characteristics. With the level set curve evolution, the algorithm can detect all the moving objects and circle out the objects' outside contours. The approach discussed in this chapter is computationally efficient, does not require a dense motion field and is insensitive to global/background motion and to noise. Its efficacy is demonstrated on both TV and surveillance video.

In chapter 6, we describe a novel approach to image sequence segmentation and its real-time implementation. This approach uses the 3-D structure tensor to produce a more robust frame difference and uses curve evolution to extract whole (moving) objects. The algorithm is implemented on a standard PC running the MS Windows operating system with a video camera that supports USB connection and Windows standard multi-media interface. Using the Windows standard video I/O functionalities, our segmentation software is highly portable and easy to maintain and upgrade. In its current implementation, the system can segment 5 frames per second with a frame resolution of 100 × 100.

In chapter 7, we present a fast region-based level set approach for extraction of white matter, gray matter, and cerebrospinal fluid boundaries from two dimensional magnetic resonance slices of the human brain. The raw contour is placed inside the image which is later pushed or pulled towards the convoluted brain topology. The forces applied in the level set approach utilized three kinds of speed control functions based on region, edge, and curvature. Regional speed functions were determined based on a fuzzy membership function computed using the fuzzy clustering technique while edge and curvature speed functions are based on gradient and signed distance transform functions, respectively. The level set algorithm is implemented to run in the "narrow band" using a "fast marching method". The system was tested on synthetic convoluted shapes and real magnetic resonance images of the human head. The entire system took approximately one minute to estimate the white and gray matter boundaries on an XP1000 running Linux Operating System when the raw contour was placed half way from the goal, and took only a few seconds if the raw contour was placed close to the goal boundary with close to one hundred percent accuracy.

In chapter 8, a geometric model for segmentation of images with missing boundaries is presented. Some classical problems of boundary completion in cognitive images, like the pop-up of subjective contours in the famous triangle of Kanizsa, are faced from a surface evolution point of view. The method is based on the mean curvature evolution of a graph with respect to the Riemannian metric induced by the image. Existence, uniqueness and maximum principle of the parabolic partial differential equation are proved. A numerical scheme introduced by Osher and Sethian for evolution of fronts by curvature motion is adopted. Results are presented for modal completion of cognitive objects with missing boundaries.

The last chapter discusses the future on level sets and PDEs. It presents some of the challenging problems in medical imaging using level sets and PDEs. The chapter concludes on the future aspects on coupling of the level set method with other established numerical methods followed by the future on the subjective surfaces.

Jasjit S. Suri
Laxminarayan Swamy

Acknowledgements

This book is the result of collective endeavours from several noted engineering and computer scientists, mathematicans, physicists, and radiologists. The authors are indebted to all of their efforts and outstanding scientific contributions. The editors are particularly grateful to Drs. Xioping Shen, Jianbo Gao, David Chopp, Weisong Liu, Jun Zhang, Alexander Sarti, and Laura Reden for working with us so closely in meeting all of the deadlines of the book.

We would like to express our appreciation to Kluwer Academic / Plenum Publishers for helping create this invitational book. We are particularly thankful to Aaron Johnson, Anthony Fulgieri, and Jennifer Stevens for their excellent coordination of the book at every stage.

Dr. Suri would like to thank Philips Medical Systems, Inc., for the MR data sets and encouragements during his experiments and research. Special thanks are due to Dr. Larry Kasuboski and Dr. Elaine Keeler from Philips Medical Systems, Inc., for their support and motivations. Thanks are also due to my past Ph.D. committee research professors, particularly Professors Linda Shapiro, Robert M. Haralick, Dean Lytle and Arun Somani, for their encouragements.

We extend our appreciations to Dr. George Thoma, Chief Imaging Science Division from National Institutes of Health, Dr. Sameer Singh, University of Exeter, UK for his motivations. Special thanks go to the Book Series Editor, Professor Evangelia Tzanakou for advising us on all aspects of the book.

We thank the IEEE Press, Academic Press, Springer Verlag Publishers, and several medical and engineering journals for permitting us to use some of the images previously published in these journals.

Finally, Jasjit Suri would like to thank his beautiful wife Malvika Suri for all the love and support she has showered over the years and to our cute baby Harman whose presence is always a constant source of pride and joy. I also express my gratitude to my father, a mathematician, who inspired me throughout my life and career, and to my late mother, who most unfortunately passed away a few days before my Ph.D. graduation, and who so much wanted to see me write this book. I love you, Mom. I would like to also thank my in-laws who have a special place for me in their hearts and have shown lots of love and care for me.

Swamy Laxminarayan would like to express his loving acknowledgements to his wife

Marijke and to his kids, Malini and Vinod, for always giving the strength of mind amidst all life frustrations. The book kindles fondest memories of my late parents who made many personal sacrifices that helped shape our careers and the support of my family members who were always there for me when I needed them most. I have shared many ideas and thoughts on the book with numerous of my colleagues in the discipline. I acknowledge their friendship, feedbacks and discussions with particular thanks to Prof. David Kristol of the New Jersey Institute of Technology for his constant support over the past two decades.

Contents

Chapter 1

Basics of PDEs and Level Sets

Xiaoping Shen[1], *Jasjit S. Suri*[2] *and Swamy Laxminarayan*[3]

1.1 Introduction

Why should anyone but mathematicians care about Partial Differential Equations ? To laymen, the answer is far from obvious. A major virtue of this Chapter is that it provides answers laymen can understand.

As the basis of almost all areas of applied sciences, the Partial Differential Equation (PDE) is one of the richest branches in mathematics. A tremendous number of the greatest advances in modern science have been based on the discovery of the underlying partial differential equations which describe various natural phenomena. Without exception, the implications for this subject on image processing are profound; however, to reflect all the facets of this huge subject in such a short Chapter seems impossible. We apologize in advance for the bias in materials selected.

As a "service Chapter", this Chapter has been written for readers who have less background in partial differential equations (PDEs). It contains materials which will be found useful in understanding some of the jargons related to the rest of the Chapters in this book.

The Chapter is organized as follows: in section 1.2, we begin with a brief classification of PDEs. In section 1.3, we outline the major analytical methods. In section 1.4, we introduce the most important numerical techniques, namely the finite difference method and finite element method. In the last section,

[1]Department of Mathematics, Univ. of California, Davis, CA, USA
[2]Marconi Medical Systems, Inc., Cleveland, OH, USA
[3]New Jersey Institute of Technology, Newark, NJ, USA

PDE & Level Sets: Algorithmic Approaches to Static & Motion Imagery
Edited by Jasjit Suri and Swamy Laxminarayan, Kluwer Academic/Plenum Publishers, 2002

we introduce the level set method. Finally, we have included some references to supplement whatever important aspects the authors have indeed hardly touched upon in this short introduction. Hopefully, the reader will be able to extrapolate the elements presented here to initiate an understanding of the subject on his or her own.

1.2 Classification of PDEs

We begin with defining the concept of PDE: this is a functional equation in which the partial derivatives of the unknown function occur. To be worth serious attention, the classification of PDEs is important. In fact, an analytical method or a numerical approach may work for only one type of PDE.

In general, PDEs are classified in several different ways:

- Order of the differential equation (order of the highest derivative)
- Number of independent variables
- Linearity
- Homogeneity
- Types of coefficients

However, in most of mathematics literature, PDEs are classified on the basis of their characteristics, or curves of information propagation. They are grouped into three categories:

- elliptic equation (Laplace equation)
- hyperbolic equation (wave equation)
- parabolic equation (diffusion equation).

Many problems of mathematical physics lead to PDEs. PDEs of the second order are the type that occurs most frequently. A general linear equation of the second order in two dimensional space is:

$$Lu = a\frac{\partial^2 u}{\partial x^2} + 2b\frac{\partial^2 u}{\partial x \partial y} + c\frac{\partial^2 u}{\partial y^2} + p\frac{\partial u}{\partial x} + q\frac{\partial u}{\partial y} + ru = f\,, \tag{1.1}$$

where the coefficients may be functions of x and y. We will restrict ourselves in this class of PDEs in this Chapter.

If we denote $I = b^2 - ac$, then Eq. (1.1) is:

$$\begin{array}{ll} \textit{elliptic} & \textit{if } I < 0 \\ \textit{parabolic} & \textit{if } I = 0 \\ \textit{hyperbolic} & \textit{if } I > 0 \,. \end{array}$$

To this end, it is helpful to take concrete examples.

The Poisson equation

$$\frac{\partial^2 u}{\partial x^2} + \frac{\partial^2 u}{\partial y^2} = f(x, y) \tag{1.2}$$

is the most well known example of an elliptic equation. By using "*Laplacian*", $\nabla^2 = \frac{\partial^2}{\partial x^2} + \frac{\partial^2}{\partial y^2}$, we can re-write Eq. (1.2) as $\nabla^2 u = f$.

A typical example for a hyperbolic equation is the one dimensional wave equation:

$$\frac{\partial^2 u}{\partial t^2} = \alpha \frac{\partial^2 u}{\partial x^2} \,, \tag{1.3}$$

where α is the velocity of the wave propagation.

A prototypical parabolic equation is the diffusion equation

$$\frac{\partial u}{\partial t} = -\frac{\partial}{\partial x}(\rho \frac{\partial u}{\partial t}) \,, \tag{1.4}$$

where ρ is the diffusion coefficient.

The Laplace equation for the uncharged space

$$\nabla^2 u = 0 \tag{1.5}$$

is linear and homogeneous.

The Poisson equation for a given charged distribution is inhomogeneous:

$$\nabla^2 u = f \,. \tag{1.6}$$

In practical applications, it is not very common that the general solution of an equation is required. What is more interesting is a particular solution satisfying certain conditions. The PDEs together with additional conditions are then classified into two different groups:

- boundary value problem (static solution)

- initial value problem (time evolution).

As a simple example of a boundary value problem, we consider the steady-state equation for heat conduction

$$\nabla(K\nabla u) = f, \text{ in } \Omega, \tag{1.7}$$

where Ω is a closed region with the boundary curve C, k (given) is the conductivity and f is the source term:

$$\begin{cases} u & = & g_1 \\ K\frac{\partial u}{\partial n} & = & g_2 \end{cases}, \text{ on } C, \tag{1.8}$$

where $\frac{\partial u}{\partial n}$ is the directed derivative along the normal of C. Eq. (1.7) together with its boundary condition in Eq. (1.7) is a boundary value problem of an elliptic equation. The Cauchy problem is an example of an initial value problem:

$$\begin{array}{lll} \text{PDE} & \frac{\partial u}{\partial t} = \alpha^2 u_{xx}, & -\infty < x < \infty,\ 0 < t < \infty \\ \text{IC} & u(x,0) = \phi(x), & -\infty < x < \infty\,. \end{array} \tag{1.9}$$

Still another way to classify PDEs is according to whether or not the derivatives of an unknown function are occurring in the boundary or initial conditions.

As an example, we consider a region Ω of space which is bounded by a surface Σ. The problem of the stationary temperature distribution leads to:

$$\nabla^2 u = -f(x,y,z)\,,$$

and one of the following boundary conditions:

1. First boundary value problem (Dirichlet problem):

$$u = \phi_1,\ (x,y,z) \in \Sigma\,. \tag{1.10}$$

2. Second boundary value problem (Neumann problem):

$$\frac{\partial u}{\partial n} = \phi_2,\ (x,y,z) \in \Sigma\,. \tag{1.11}$$

3. Third boundary value problem:

$$\frac{\partial u}{\partial n} + h(u - \phi_3) = 0,\ (x,y,z) \in \Sigma\,. \tag{1.12}$$

Similarly, we can have first, second and third initial value problems.

In closing this section, we should like to call the reader's attention to notice the following:

1. There is a very practical distinction to be made between elliptic equations on the one hand and hyperbolic and parabolic equations on the other hand. Generally speaking, elliptic equations have boundary conditions which are specified around a closed boundary. Usually all the derivatives are with respect to spatial variables, such as in Laplace's or Poisson's Equation. Hyperbolic and parabolic equations, by contrast, have at least one open boundary. The boundary conditions for at least one variable, usually time, are specified at one end and the system is integrated indefinitely. Thus, the wave equation and the diffusion equation contain a time variable and there is a set of initial conditions at a particular time. These properties are, of course, related to the fact that an ellipse is a closed object, whereas hyperbolic and parabolic are open objects (see http://www.sst.ph.ic.ac.uk/angus/Lectures/compphys/node24.html).

2. With respect to solving PDEs by numerical methods or principal computational methods, there is a concern for stability. In contrast, for a boundary value problem, the efficiency of the algorithms, both in computational load and storage requirements, becomes the principal concern.

1.3 Analytical Methods to Solve PDEs

For most scientists and engineers, the analytical techniques for solving linear PDEs involve the separation of the variables and Transform Methods. Rather than show the method in general, we will demonstrate the idea by using examples. References found in Chester [5], Evans *et al.* [10], Farlow [11], Tikhonov *et al.* [21] and Zwillinger [23] provide introductory and advanced discussions.

1.3.1 Separation of the Variables

Consider the linear homogeneous wave equation:

$$\frac{\partial^2 u}{\partial t^2} = a^2 \frac{\partial^2 u}{\partial x^2} \tag{1.13}$$

with boundary value and initial value conditions:

$$u(0,t) = 0, \; u(l,t) = 0 \tag{1.14}$$

and

$$u(x,0) = \phi(x), \; u_t(x,0) = \phi(x). \tag{1.15}$$

Separation of the variables looks for the solutions in the form

$$u_n(x,t) = X_n(x)T_n(t). \tag{1.16}$$

Because of the linearity and homogeneity of the given problem, the sum

$$u(x,t) = \sum_{n=1}^{\infty} c_n u_n(x,t) = \sum_{n=1}^{\infty} c_n X_n(x)T_n(t) \tag{1.17}$$

is a general solution. We should like to point out that the idea of superposition, demonstrated by this example, is the backbone of linear systems analysis.

If the coefficients c_n are chosen in such a way that Eq. (1.16) satisfies the initial and boundary value conditions (see Eq. (1.14) and (1.15)), then we have a solution to the given problem.

To begin with, we write $u(x,t) = X(x)Y(y)$ and plug in Eq. (1.13). A simple calculation reveals that

$$\frac{X''(x)}{X(x)} = \frac{1}{a^2}\frac{T''(t)}{T(t)}. \tag{1.18}$$

We observe that the right hand side of Eq. (1.18) is independent of variable t, while the left hand side is independent of x, therefore both sides must be constant! That is,

$$\frac{X''(x)}{X(x)} = \frac{1}{a^2}\frac{T''(t)}{T(t)} = -\lambda, \tag{1.19}$$

where λ is a constant. Eq. (1.19) can be rewritten as

$$X''(x) + \lambda X(x) = 0, \tag{1.20}$$

$$T''(t) + \lambda T(t) = 0. \tag{1.21}$$

The boundary value condition yields

$$u(0,t) = X(0)T(t) = 0 \tag{1.22}$$

$$u(l,t) = X(l)T(t) = 0. \tag{1.23}$$

Combining Eq. (1.20) and Eq. (1.22), we get the simple eigenvalue problem

$$X''(x) + \lambda X(x) = 0, \; X(0) = X(l) = 0 \,. \tag{1.24}$$

The general solution to Eq. (1.20) is:

$$X(x) = C_1 e^{\sqrt{-\lambda}x} + C_2 e^{-\sqrt{-\lambda}x} \,.$$

We then consider three different cases: $\lambda < 0$, $\lambda = 0$, and $\lambda > 0$.

For the first two cases, the problem does not have any non-trivial solution. For the last case, we have

$$X(x) = D_1 \cos \sqrt{\lambda}x + D_2 \sin \sqrt{\lambda}x$$

with boundary condition

$$X(0) = D_1 = 0, \; X(l) = D_2 \sin \sqrt{\lambda}l = 0 \,. \tag{1.25}$$

A non-trivial solution is only for the values

$$\lambda_n = (\frac{\pi n}{l})^2$$

with associate eigenfunctions

$$X_n(x) = \sin \frac{\pi n}{l} x \,.$$

The solution to Eq. (1.21) corresponding to these eigenvalues is

$$T_n(t) = A_n \cos \frac{\pi n}{l} at + B_n \sin \frac{\pi n}{l} at \,, \tag{1.26}$$

where A_n and B_n are coefficients to be defined. Formally, we can write the general solution as

$$u(x,t) = \sum_{n=1}^{\infty} u_n(x,t) = \sum_{n=1}^{\infty} (A_n \cos \frac{\pi n}{l} at + B_n \sin \frac{\pi n}{l} at) \sin \frac{\pi n}{l} ax \,. \tag{1.27}$$

The last step is to determine A_n and B_n such that Eq. (1.27) satisfies the initial condition Eq. (1.14).

The ability to change coordinates is a very important technique in PDEs. By looking at physical systems with different coordinates, the equations are sometimes simplified. More importantly, a PDE that is separable in one coordinate system is not necessarily separable in another coordinate system.

1.3.2 Integral Transforms

There are a number of methods based on integral transforms used to obtain analytical solutions of PDEs. The greatest difficulty with the integral transform methods is the inversion. We can not find the inversion formulae in general. However, the theory of using integral transform lays a foundation for the numerical method. To convert an integral transform numerically is possible in most cases. For example, in the case of Fourier Transform, the Fast Fourier Transform (FFT) and Inverse Fourier Transform (IFFT) methods are available.

The most popular methods are the Laplace Transform method and the Fourier Transform method. Others, such as Hankel Transforms and Mellin Transforms, are also used on ocassion. We will take the Laplace Transform method as an example to sketch the basic idea of the Integral Transform method.

1.3.2.1 The Method Using the Laplace Transform

To begin with, we recall the definition of the Laplace Transform.

Definition 1 Let a function $f(t)$ be defined for $t \geq 0$. The Laplace Transform is given by the integral operation:

$$\mathcal{L}[f](s) = \overline{f}(s) = \int_0^{\infty} f(t)e^{-st}dt,$$

which provides that the integral converges.

The sufficient conditions for the Laplace Transform to existence for $s > a$ are:

1. $f(x)$ is piecewise continuous on the interval $0 \leq x \leq X$, for any $X > 0$, and

2. $|f(x)| \leq Ae^{a_0 x}$ for $X \geq X_0$, where $A > 0, a_0 \leq a$, and $X_0 > 0$ are real constants.

A wide range of functions possesses Laplace Transforms. As the simplest example, we consider the Heaviside function

$$H(x) = \begin{cases} 1 & , \quad x > 0 \\ 0 & , \quad x < 0. \end{cases}$$

The Laplace Transform of H is then

$$\overline{H}(t) = \int_0^\infty H(t)e^{-st}dt = \int_0^\infty e^{-st}dt = \frac{1}{s}.$$

The Laplace Transform possesses many elegant properties. We will list the most important properties below.

Assume all functions are defined on the half real line ($x > 0$) and that their Laplace Transforms exist.

1. **Linearity**

   $\mathcal{L}[af_1 + bf_2] = a\mathcal{L}[f_1] + b\mathcal{L}[f_2]$ (a, b are constants).

2. **Translation**

   $\mathcal{L}[e^{-ks}f](s) = \mathcal{L}[f](s + k)$.

3. **Scaling**

   $\mathcal{L}[kf(kt)](s) = \mathcal{L}[f](s/k)$.

4. **Convolution** (Borel's theorem)

   $\mathcal{L}[f * g] = \mathcal{L}[f]\ \mathcal{L}[g]$, where $f * g$ is the convolution of f and g defined by

   $$f * g(t) = \int_0^t g(t - x)f(x)dx = \int_0^t f(t - x)g(x)dx\,.$$

5. **Limit**

   $\lim_{s\to 0} \mathcal{L}[f](s) = f(0)$.

6. **Derivatives**

   $\mathcal{L}[f'] = s\mathcal{L}[f] - f(0^+)$, where $f(0+) = \lim_{x\to 0+} f(x)\,.$

   $\mathcal{L}[f^{(n)}] = s^n\mathcal{L}[f] - \sum_{k=1}^n s^{n-k} f^{(k-1)}(0^+)\,.$

7. **Integration**

   $\mathcal{L}[\int_0^t f(x)dx] = \frac{\mathcal{L}[f']}{s}\,.$

8. **Inversion** (T. J. Bromwich)

   Let f be a piecewise differentiable function. The inverse of a Laplace Transform of f can be expressed as the contour integral

   $$f(t) = \frac{1}{2\pi i}\int_{c-\infty i}^{c+\infty i} \mathcal{L}[f](z)e^{tz}dz\,. \tag{1.28}$$

   Eq. (1.28) is called the Bromwich integral.

9. **Asymptotic Properties** (Watson's lemma)

   Suppose that $f(t)$ has the asymptotic expansion

$$f(t) \sim \sum_{i=1}^{\infty} a_i t^{\lambda_i}, \ t \to 0,$$

   where $-1 < Re(\lambda_1) < Re(\lambda_2) < \ldots < Re(\lambda_n) < \ldots$

   Then the Laplace Transform of f, $\mathcal{L}[f]$ has the corresponding asymptotic expansion

$$\mathcal{L}[f] \sim \sum_{i=1}^{\infty} \frac{a_i \lambda_i!}{\lambda_i + 1}, |s| \to \infty, \ -\frac{\pi}{2} < \arg(s) < \frac{\pi}{2}.$$

Properties 4 and 5 above indicate that the Laplace Transform converts differentiation and integration to algebraic operations. Properties 1, 2, 3 and 6 are used to find Laplace Transforms and their inverse. Watson's lemma gives information about the behavior of $\mathcal{L}[f]$ for large s, which is derived from the behavior of $f(t)$ for small t. The major tool is the Bromwich integral, which can deal with the contour integration technique in complex analysis. However, it is difficult in general to do this. Luckily, we can find most of the transforms in the Laplace Transform table (see Oberhettinger *et al.* [16]).

Now we are ready to describe the integral transform method. In general, the procedure consists of the following:

1. Apply the integral transform to the given PDE in n variables to get an equation in $n-1$ variables.

2. Solve the lower dimensional equation to obtain the integral transform of the solution of the given equation if it is possible; otherwise, repeat step 1.

3. Take the inverse transform to get the desired solution.

The following simple example will demonstrate this idea.

Example (A model problem) Assume we have a diffusion equation

$$\frac{\partial u}{\partial t} = a^2 \frac{\partial^2 u}{\partial x^2}, \ 0 < x < l, \ 0 < t < \infty \tag{1.29}$$

together with the boundary value condition

$$\begin{cases} u(0,t) = 0 \\ u(l,t) = f(t) \end{cases} ,0 < t < \infty \tag{1.30}$$

and the initial value condition

$$u(x,0) = 0, \ 0 \leq x \leq l. \tag{1.31}$$

We then proceed with the three steps given above.

1. Take the Laplace Transform on both sides of the PDE to get an ordinary differential equation (ODE):

$$\frac{d^2\overline{u}(x,s)}{dx^2} = \frac{1}{a^2} s\overline{u}(x,s)\,. \tag{1.32}$$

   Here we have used linearity, differentiate property and the boundary condition (see Eq. (1.29)).

2. Solve ODE, (i.e., Eq. (1.32))

$$\overline{u}(x,s) = \frac{1}{s}\frac{\sinh(x\sqrt{s})}{\sinh(\sqrt{s})}\,.$$

   where

$$\sinh(x) = \frac{1}{2}(e^x - e^{-x})$$

   is the hyperbolic sine function.

3. Find the inverse Laplace Transform of $\overline{u}(x,s)$ to get

$$u(x,t) = x + \frac{2}{\pi}\sum_{n=1}^{\infty}\frac{(-1)^n}{n}e^{-(n\pi)^2 t}\sin n\pi x\,.$$

   Next, we use the Laplace Transform table and the initial value condition.

Example Wave Propagation - Semi infinite string

The simplest continuous vibrational system is a uniform flexible string of mass ρ per unit length, stretched to a tension T. If the string executes small transverse vibrations in a plane, then the displacement $u(x,t)$ must satisfy the partial differential equation

$$\frac{\partial^2 u}{\partial t^2} = a^2\frac{\partial^2 u}{\partial x^2} + \frac{f(x,t)}{\rho}\,, \tag{1.33}$$

where $a^2 = T/\rho$ and $f(x,t)$ is the external force per unit length. In the case of a semi-infinite string, we have $f(x,t) \equiv 0$, for $x \geq 0$, and Eq. (1.33) is associated with the following initial and boundary value conditions:

$$u(x,0) = \frac{\partial u}{\partial t}(x,0) = 0, \; x \geq 0 \tag{1.34}$$

$$u(0,t) = \phi(t), \; t \geq 0 \,. \tag{1.35}$$

Applying Laplace Transform to Eq. (1.33) and using Eq. (1.34), we have

$$\begin{aligned} a^2 \frac{\partial^2 U}{\partial x^2} - s^2 U &= 0 \\ U(0,s) &= \Phi(s)\,, \end{aligned} \tag{1.36}$$

where U and Φ are the Laplace Transform of u and ϕ, respectively.

We then solve the ordinary differential Eq. (1.36) to get

$$U(x,s) = \Phi(s)e^{-sx/a}\,,$$

where we have used the requirement that the solution u is bounded for $x \to \infty$.

By using the translation property 2, the inverse Laplace Transform is easily to be found as

$$u(x,t) = \begin{cases} \phi(t - x/a) & , \quad x < at \\ 0 & , \quad x > at \end{cases}$$

As you may recognize, this problem can be solved by D'Alembert's method as well.

1.3.2.2 The Method Using Fourier Transform

In the case of having the initial value condition as the example in the previous sub-section, we used Laplace Transforms to reduce the order of a PDE, then solve the derived equation. Since the Laplace Transform is defined on the half line, it is not suitable for the problem defined in the whole space.

The Fourier Transform can be considered as a generalized Laplace Transform:

$$\widehat{f}(w) = \mathcal{F}[f](w) = \int_{-\infty}^{\infty} f(x)e^{-iwx}dx$$

with the inverse transform given by

$$f(x) = \frac{1}{2\pi}\int_{-\infty}^{\infty} \widehat{f}(w)e^{-iwx}dw\,,$$

presume that the integrals are convergent.

Similarly to the Laplace Transform, Fourier Transform and its inverse are linear transforms and have the following properties:

1. **Translations**

   $\mathcal{F}[f(t-a)](w) = e^{-iwa}\mathcal{F}[f](w).$

2. **Scalings**

   $\mathcal{F}[f(bt)](w) = \frac{1}{b}\mathcal{F}[f](\frac{w}{b})\,.$

3. **Derivatives**

   $\mathcal{F}[f^{(n)}](w) = (iw)^n\mathcal{F}[f](w)\ \mathcal{F}^{-1}[f^{(n)}](t) = (-it)^n\mathcal{F}^{-1}[f](t)\,.$

4. **Moments**

   $\mathcal{F}[x^n f(x)](w) = i^n \frac{d^n}{dw^n}\{\mathcal{F}[f](w)\}$

   $\mathcal{F}^{-1}[w^n f(w)](x) = (-i)^n \frac{d^n}{dt^n}\mathcal{F}^{-1}[f](x)\,.$

5. **Convolutions**

   $\mathcal{F}[f * g](w) = \mathcal{F}[f](w)\cdot\mathcal{F}[g](w)$, where the convolution is defined as $f * g(t) = \int_{-\infty}^{\infty} g(t-x)f(x)dx = \int_{-\infty}^{\infty} f(t-x)g(x)dx.$

6. **Relation to Laplace Transform**

   If $f(t) = 0$, $t < 0$, then

   $$\mathcal{L}[f](s) = \int_0^\infty f(t)e^{-ts}dt\,.$$

7. **Parseval Relations**

   $\int_{-\infty}^{\infty} f(t)g^*(t)dt = \frac{1}{2\pi}\int_{\infty}^{\infty}\widehat{f}(w)\cdot\widehat{g}^*(w)dw$, where * is the complex conjugate.

8. **Product**

   $\mathcal{F}[f(t)g(t)] = \frac{1}{2\pi}\int_{\infty}^{\infty}\widehat{f}(\xi)\cdot\widehat{g}(w-\xi)d\xi.$

Now we are ready to take a specific example.

Example (Potential problem): A simple choice is the PDE raised in electrostatics, which involves the Laplace equation with the initial value condition:

$$\nabla^2 u = 0, -\infty < x < \infty,\ y \geq 0 \tag{1.37}$$

$$u(x,0) = \phi(x). \tag{1.38}$$

In addition, we assume that the solution function u is bounded as $y \to \infty$.

Taking the Fourier Transform of Eq. (1.37) with respect to the variable x, we obtain

$$\begin{aligned} \frac{d^2}{dy^2}\widehat{u}(w,y) - w^2\widehat{u}(w,y) &= 0 \\ \widehat{u}(w,0) &= \widehat{\phi}(w). \end{aligned} \tag{1.39}$$

Next, we solve the ordinary differential equation (Eq. 1.39) to get

$$u(w,y) = A(w)e^{wy} + B(w)e^{-wy},$$

where A and B are constant functions to be determined. Using the constrain that the solution u is bounded as $y \to \infty$, we have

$$\widehat{u}(w,y) = \begin{cases} \widehat{\phi}(w)e^{-wy}, & Re(w) > 0 \\ \widehat{\phi}(w)e^{wy}, & Re(w) < 0. \end{cases}$$

Notice that $\widehat{u}$ is a product of two functions, so we use the convolution property (shown above) to obtain its inverse Fourier Transform

$$u(x,y) = \frac{y}{\pi}\int_{-\infty}^{\infty} \frac{\phi(s)}{y^2 + (x-s)^2} ds$$

as the desired solution.

We will now summarize this section:

1. A procedure using integral transforms reduces a PDE in n independent variables to a $n-1$ variables. In the two dimensional case, the given PDE is reduced to an ordinary differential equation as we demonstrated in the examples given. Consequently, many techniques in solving ODE can be applied to solve the problem.

2. The mathematics behind the integral transform is very rich and complicated. The more interested reader can find detailed information in see Davies [6], Debnath [7] and Duffy [9]. For transform tables, readers can see Oberhettinger *et al.* [15], [16] and Roberts *et al.* [20].

3. There are many other transforms used in solving PDEs, such as Hankel transforms, which are related to cylindrical coordinates and Bessel functions.

1.4 Numerical Methods

A numerical technique is employed to solve problems in which an analytical solution is either very difficult or impossible to obtain. However, in practice, even with greatly simplified initial and boundary conditions, the analytical solution is too difficult to obtain or not in a closed form. In this sense, it is more useful to know of such numerical methods which provide us such a technique to be actually used in everyday life.

On the other hand, it may not as obvious that it is even more important to comprehend the convergence, stability and error bounds of each method used in calculation (see Chatelin [3], [4] and Gautschi [13] for advanced discussions). As we know, every numerical method provides a formalism for generating discrete algorithms for approximating the solution of a PDE. Such a task could be done automatically by a computer if there were no mathematical skills that required human involvement. Consequently, it is necessary to understand the mathematics in this "black box" which you put your PDE into for processing. The latter, however, is beyond the scope of this introductory Chapter. We do hope the loose ends we left here will stimulate your curiosity and further motivate your deepening interest in this subject (see Zwillinger [23]).

1.4.1 Finite Difference Method (FDM)

The finite difference method (FDM) consists in replacing the (partial) derivatives by some convergent numerical differentiation formulas. In other words, we approximate a derivative by "difference". The PDE is then approximated by a finite matrix equation.

Taylor polynomials and the intermediate value theorem can be used to generate numerical differentiation formulas. For example, we have the centered-difference formula:

$$g'(x) = \frac{1}{2h}(g_{i+1} - g_{i-1}).$$

The second derivative is then given by:

$$g''(x) = \frac{1}{h^2}(g_{i+1} - 2g_i + g_{i-1}).$$

As an example, we consider using FDM to solve the Poisson Eq. (1.2) on a rectangular domain (see Press [17] for more details):

$$R = \{(x,y),\ a < x < b,\ c < y < d\},$$

with the boundary value condition given by

$$u(x,y)|_{(x,y)\in\Omega} = g(x,y)\,,$$

where Ω is the boundary of R and g is a given function. We discretize the domain of the equation by the grid:

$$\begin{aligned} x_j &= x_0 + jh,\ j = 0,1,...,J \\ y_l &= y_0 + lh,\ l = 0,1,...,L\,, \end{aligned}$$

where h is the grid spacing. For simplicity, we will write $u_{j,l}$ for $u(x_j, y_l)$, and $f_{j,l}$ for $f(x_j, y_l)$. Using the centered-difference formula above, the Poisson equation is discretized as

$$\frac{u_{j+1,l} - 2u_{j,l} + u_{j-1,l}}{h^2} + \frac{u_{j,l+1} - 2u_{j,l} + u_{j,l-1}}{h^2} = f_{j,l}\,,$$

or equivalently

$$u_{j+1,l} + u_{j-1,l} + u_{j,l+1} + u_{j,l-1} - 4u_{j,l} = h^2 f_{j,l}\,, \tag{1.40}$$

for $j = 1,...,J-1$ and $l = 1,...,L-1$. The associated boundary value conditions are

$$\begin{aligned} u_{0,l} &= g_{0,l},\ u_{J,l} = g_{J,l},\ \text{for } l = 0,1,...,L \\ u_{j,L} &= g_{j,L},\ u_{j,L} = g_{j,L},\ \text{for } j = 0,1,...,J\,. \end{aligned} \tag{1.41}$$

To be more specific, if we further assume that the domain $\Omega = \{(x,y), 0 < x < 1, 0 < y < 1\}$ together with the boundary value conditions:

$$\begin{aligned} u(0,y) &= 0,\ u(1,y) = y,\ 0 \le y \le 1 \\ u(x,0) &= x,\ u(x,1) = 1,\ 0 \le x \le 1. \end{aligned}$$

We partition Ω by the mesh with grid spacing $h = 0.25$, or $J = L = 4$ (see Figure 1.1).

Each node is associated with a linear equation. We relabel the interior grid points to change the two dimensional sequence to a one dimensional sequence. To do this, we set $i = j(L+1) + l$, or equivalently $l = i - j(L+1)$ and denote $w_i = u_{j,l} = u(x_j, y_l)$, for $j = 0,...,J$ and $l = 0,...,L$. In this way, we can rewrite the deference equation as

$$w_{i+L+1} + w_{i-(L+1)} + w_{i+1} + w_{i-1} - 4w_i = h^2 f_i\,, \tag{1.42}$$

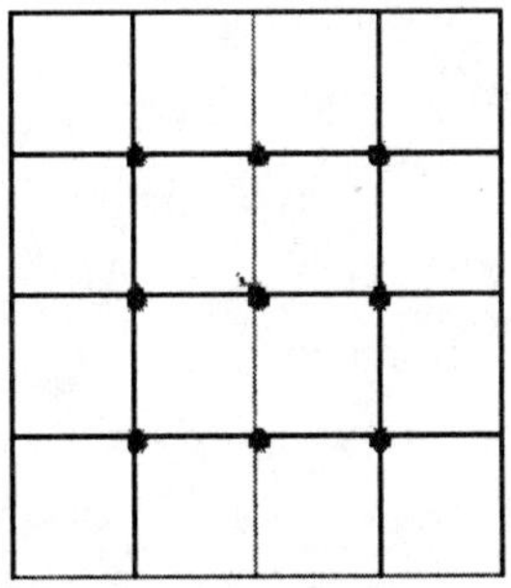

Figure 1.1: The grid mesh with grid spacing h=0.25.

where the right hand side of the equation can be obtained from the boundary value conditions:

$$\left\{ \begin{array}{lcl} u(0,y) & = & 0,\ u(1,y) = y,\ 0 \le y \le 1 . \end{array} \right. \tag{1.43}$$

We can re-write the linear system as matrix format:

$$\mathbf{A}\mathbf{w} = \mathbf{f} . \tag{1.44}$$

where $\mathbf{A}$ is a 9 by 9 matrix:

$$\mathbf{A} = \begin{bmatrix} -4 & 1 & 0 & 1 & 0 & 0 & 0 & 0 & 0 \\ 1 & -4 & 1 & 0 & 1 & 0 & 0 & 0 & 0 \\ 0 & 1 & -4 & 0 & 0 & 1 & 0 & 0 & 0 \\ 1 & 0 & 0 & -4 & 1 & 0 & 1 & 0 & 0 \\ 0 & 1 & 0 & 1 & -4 & 0 & 0 & 1 & 0 \\ 0 & 0 & 1 & 0 & 1 & -4 & 0 & 0 & 1 \\ 0 & 0 & 0 & 1 & 0 & 0 & -4 & 1 & 0 \\ 0 & 0 & 0 & 0 & 1 & 0 & 1 & -4 & 1 \\ 0 & 0 & 0 & 0 & 0 & 1 & 0 & 1 & -4 \end{bmatrix}$$

$\mathbf{w} = [w_1, w_2, w_3, ..., w_8, w_9]^T$ and $\mathbf{f} = [f_1, f_2, f_3, ..., f_8, f_9]^T$.

The linear system is then solved by a numerical method, such as the Gauss-Seidel method (see Gautschi [13]).

In closing this sub-section, we will say a few words about the error analysis and stability of FDM.

When the right hand side function f and any corresponding functions in the boundary conditions and the shape of the boundary of the problem are all sufficiently smooth, then we can expect the true solution $u(x, y)$ to have similar smoothness. In this case, the error bound is $O(h^2)$.

If the difference method is used to solve a diffusion equation, the stability needs to be tested. In practice, the knowledge of whether the difference schemes are stable can be achieved by using the *Von Neumann test.* For the difference schemes with constant coefficients, the test consists of examining all exponential solutions to determine whether they grow exponentially in the time variable, even when the initial values are bounded functions of the space variable. If any of them do increase without limit, then the method is unstable. Otherwise, it is stable. For the hyperbolic equation, the Courant-Friedrichs-Lewy consistency criterion using characteristic values can be used in the test (see Zwillinger [23]).

1.4.2 Finite Element Method (FEM)

The finite element method (FEM) is one of the most widely used techniques for engineering design and analysis. In particular, it is appreciated by engineers and numerical analysts because of the flexibility in handling irregular domains (compared to FDM) (see Axelsson *et al.* [1], Brenner *et al.* [2] and Gladwell *et al.* [12]).

The FEM method provides a global approximation based on very simple local representations. The basic idea of FEM can be described as follows:

1. Partition the given region Ω into a large number of small sub-domains, which are called by element. Associated with the partition, we define a finite element space, which is a collection of the elements.

2. Choose an appropriate basis for the finite element space. The basis functions should have small supports so that the resulting linear system is sparse. Then, represent the global approximation solution by using basis functions.

3. Use the variational principle to formulate the associated discrete problem and then choose "test functions" to derive the matrix system.

4. Solve the resulting linear system to obtain local approximation solutions which are pieced together to obtain a global approximation.

There are many different ways to partition a given domain. Each partition will relate to one type of finite element. The most popular ones are the triangular finite elements and rectangular elements. Depending on the method to approximate the local solution on each individual element, the finite element spaces are classified as different groups. For example, we can have a linear Lagrange triangular element, quadratic Lagrange triangular element, cubic Lagrange triangular element (see Figure 1.2) on which we approximate the solution by linear, quadratic, cubic Lagrange interpolation polynomial, respectively. Similarly, we have tensor product elements, such as bilinear Lagrange rectangular element and biquadratic Lagrange rectangular elements. The reader may be able to guess the associated local basis functions from their names. For a detailed discussion, see Ciarlet [8].

Let us demonstrate the idea by using a simple example. Suppose we are given an elliptic equation, say the Poisson Eq. (1.2) in a domain Ω with boundary condition

$$\begin{cases} u &= g_1 \\ K\frac{\partial u}{\partial n} &= g_2 \end{cases}, \text{on } C. \tag{1.45}$$

We proceed with the procedures step by step.

To be more specific, let us take that Ω is a polygonal domain in Figure 1.3. We partition this domain into two small pieces in a triangular shape, E_1, E_2.

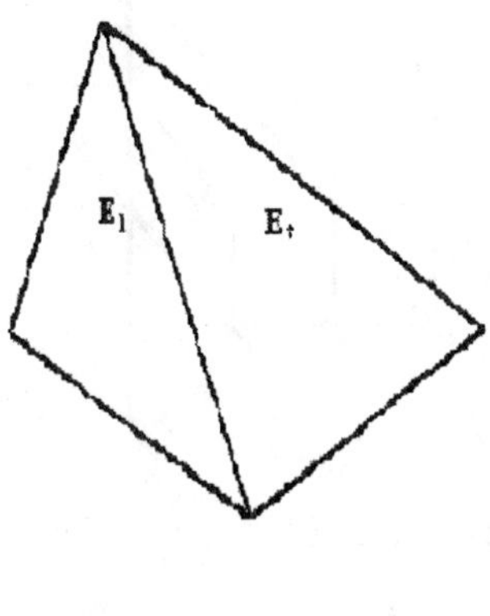

Figure 1.2: Support of basis functions.

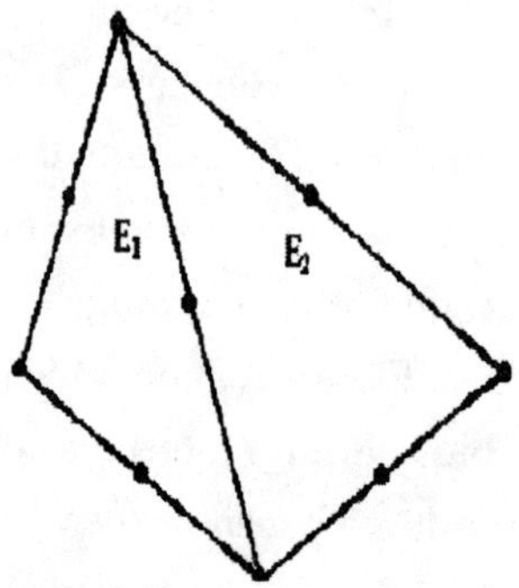

Figure 1.3: A simple triangular partition with two elements.

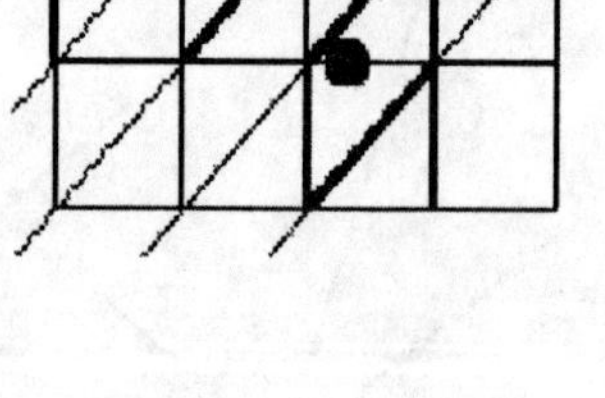

Figure 1.4: Placement of nodes.

1. Now, say we decide to use piecewise quadratic polynomials to approximate the solution of Eq. (1.2), that is, place the restriction of the global solution on each individual element that has the format:

$$u_E(x,y) = a + bx + cy + dx^2 + exy + fy^2. \tag{1.46}$$

In this case, we need to determine six coefficients, namely, a, b, c, d, e, f. Thus we choose six points (x_i, y_i), $i = 1, ..., 6$. The nodes (x_i, y_i) should be selected carefully to provide the global continuity and guarantee the existence of basis functions. Then we apply the idea of Lagrange interpolation to define the basis functions as quadratic polynomials with interpolating property:

$$\phi_E^k(x_i, y_i) = \begin{cases} 1, & k = i \\ 0, & k \neq i \end{cases} \quad 1 \leq i, k \leq 6\,. \tag{1.47}$$

Eq. (1.46) is then rewritten as

$$u_E(x,y) = \sum_{k=1}^{6} u_E^k \phi_E^k(x,y). \tag{1.48}$$

Notice that $u_{E_1}(x,y) = u_{E_2}(x,y)$ along the interface, so the global solution is continuous. To this end, we can construct a global piecewise quadratic polynomial basis as

$$\phi_k(x,y) = \begin{cases} \phi_E^k(x,y), & \text{if } (x_k, y_k) \in E \\ 0, & \text{if } (x_k, y_k) \notin E \end{cases} \quad \text{when } (x,y) \in E. \tag{1.49}$$

The union of elements in which $\phi_k \neq 0$ is called "support" of the global basis. Clearly, the finite element basis functions have local support (see Figure 1.4). Now we can write the global approximation solution as

$$U(x,y) = \sum_{i=1}^{N} U_i \phi_k(x,y)\,. \tag{1.50}$$

$N = 12$ in this case.

2. We now use the variational principle and Eq. (1.50) to formulate discretization of Eq. (1.2). We choose N linearly independent test functions ψ_j, such that

$$(\nabla^2 U - f, \psi_j) = 0, \; j = 1, ..., N. \tag{1.51}$$

Clearly, there are many different ways to do this. A criterion has to be adopted to decide in which way the test functions are to be chosen. The different criteria to choose the testing functions result in a different linear system and associated numerical solution. The popular methods are:

- Galerkin method
- Collocation method
- Least - Square method.

We take the Galerkin method as an example. The Galerkin method is to take $\psi_j = \phi_j$, $j = 1, ..., N$. Using Eq. (1.51), the approximation problem is reduced to the linear system

$$\mathbf{KU} = \mathbf{F}, \tag{1.52}$$

where $\mathbf{K} = [k_{ij}]$, $k_{ij} = (\nabla^2\phi_i, \phi_j)$, $i,j = 1, ..., N$, $\mathbf{U} = [U_1, ..., U_N]^T$, and $\mathbf{F} = [(f, \phi_1), ..., (f, \phi_N)]^T$.

3. Now we reach the final step, which is to solve the linear system Eq. (1.52). The matrix $\mathbf{K}$ is often referred to as the stiffness matrix, a name coming from corresponding matrices in the context of structural problems. It is clear that $\mathbf{K}$ is symmetric, since the energy inner product is symmetric. It is, in fact, also positive definite. In solving the linear system, the properties of the coefficient matrix are important. If the condition number of $\mathbf{K}$ is too large, then $\mathbf{K}$ is not invertible from a practical perspective. The number of non-zero elements in any row of $\mathbf{K}$ depends on the support of the basis functions.

It is difficult to give an error bound in general, because it is dependent on the smoothness of the solution and the regularity of the boundary. Very roughly speaking, the error bound for elliptic second-order problems, such as our example, is $O(h^2)$, if linear triangular elements are used, where h is the maximum diameter of the triangular elements. This is $O(h^4)$ if the bilinear rectangular elements are used. The complexity of the construction is increased.

FEM can also be used in solving diffusion and wave equations. Interested readers can find an excellent introduction in Brenner *et al.* [2].

1.4.3 Software Packages

The numerical solution of partial differential equations (PDEs) was one of the earliest applications of electronic digital computers, and it remains the source of many challenging computational problems today. Such problems can be found in every scientific discipline. In practice, mathematical models based on PDEs are found in almost every area; however, analytical treatment for these models is extremely difficult, if not impossible. The numerical solution of PDEs has been the focus of a great deal of research over the years. Many problems were solved by using software packages. When a numerical approximate solution to a PDE is required, it is best to use existing software whenever possible. Unfortunately, very few general-purpose software packages for solving PDEs have appeared due to the large range of the variety of PDEs; however, there are specialized packages available. Some of the popular software libraries for PDEs include:

- **ELLPACK** and **DEQSOL**

  ELLPACK is an American project, while DEQSOL is a Japanese project. Both are preprocessor-based packages; they read very-high-level descriptions of PDE problems and solution algorithms and produce a Fortran 77 program as an output. When linked with their respective run-time libraries and executed, the generated programs will solve the given PDE problem. Both support graphical output. Linear second-order steady-state PDE problems in fairly general domains in two or three spatial dimensions are the most straightforward to solve using each system.

- **NASTRAN**

  NASTRAN is **NASA** Structural Analysis software package for Orbital analysis and structural analysis using finite element methods.

- **PDECOL**

  The software package PDECOL is a popular code among scientists who desire to solve systems of non-linear partial differential equations. The code is based on a method-of-lines approach, with collocation in the space variable to reduce the problem to a system of ordinary differential equations.

- **FISHPACK**

  FISHPACK is a collection of FORTRAN sub-programs which utilize cyclic reduction to directly solve second- and fourth-order finite difference approximations into separable elliptic Partial Differential Equations (PDEs) in a variety of forms. More information can be found at: http://www.scd.ucar.edu/css/software/fishpack

- **PDELIB**

  PDELIB is a collection of software components which is useful to create simulators based on partial differential equations. The main idea of the package is modularity, based on a pattern-oriented bottom-up design.

- **CLAWPACK**

  CLAWPACK is a software package designed to compute numerical solutions to hyperbolic partial differential equations using a wave propagation approach. The software package can be retrieved at: http://www.netlib.org.

- **PETSc**

  PETSc is a suite of data structures and routines for the scalable (parallel) solution of scientific applications modeled by partial differential equations. More information can be found at: http://www-fp.mcs.anl.gov/petsc/.

For programming, readers can find sample codes in Press [17], [18] and Roberts *et al.* [20] (in three different languages). Book Chapters can be reterived at: http://www.nr.com.

In this section, we have considered numerical methods to solve PDEs. We restricted our attention to the two most popular methods, the finite difference method and the finite element method. For simplicity, we took the Poisson equation as a model problem to demonstrate this idea. We should like to point out that the difference method and the finite element method can be applied to diffusion equations and hyperbolic equations as well. There are many facets of the subject which we have been omitted. Among them, spline-based methods are very important both in theory and in practice.

In considering computing efficiency, there is a class of methods on the acceleration of numerical methods. For example, multigrid, multilevel, multiscale, aggregation, defect correction, and domain decomposition methods are used primarily by scientists and engineers to solve partial differential equations on serial or parallel computers.

Having discussed the basics of PDEs, we will very briefly discuss the definition of level sets and the zero level surface concept in the next section before going to applications of these.

1.5 Definition of Zero Level Surface

Let $\Gamma(t)$ be the closed interface or front propagating along its normal direction (see Figure 1.5, bottom). This closed interface $\Gamma(t)$: $[0, \infty) \rightarrow \Re^N$, can either be a curve in 2-D space or a surface in 3-D space. The main idea is to represent the front $\Gamma(t)$ as the *zero level set* of a higher dimensional function ϕ.

Let $\phi(x, t = 0)$, where $x \in \Re^N$ be defined by $\phi(x, t = 0) = d$, where d is the signed distance from position x to $\Gamma(0)$ and the plus (minus) sign is chosen if the point x is outside (inside) the initial front $\Gamma(0)$. Thus an initial function is: $\phi(x, t = 0) = \Re^N \rightarrow \Re$ with the property: $\Gamma(t = 0) = (x \mid \phi(x, t = 0) = 0)$. The goal now is to produce an equation for the evolving function $\phi(x, t)$ so that ϕ always remains zero on the propagating interface. Let $x(t)$, $t \in [0, \infty)$ be the path of a point on the propagation front (see Figure 1.5, bottom), i.e., $x(t = 0)$ is a point on the initial front $\Gamma(t = 0)$ and $x_t = V(x(t))$ with the vector x_t normal to the front at $x(t)$. Since the evolving function ϕ is always zero on the propagating front, thus $\phi(x(t), t) = 0$. By chain rule:

$$\phi_t + \sum_{i=1}^{N} \phi_{x_i} x_{i_t} = 0, \tag{1.53}$$

where x_i is the ith component of x. Since

$$\sum_{i=1}^{N} \phi_{x_i} x_{i_t} = (\phi_{x_1}, \phi_{x_2}, \phi_{x_3} ... \phi_{x_N}) \cdot (x_{1_t}, x_{2_t}, x_{3_t} ... x_{N_t}) = V(x(t)) \, |\nabla\phi|, \tag{1.54}$$

hence, using Equations 1.53 and ??, the final curve evolution equation is given as:

$$\frac{\partial \phi}{\partial t} = V(\kappa) \,|\, \nabla \phi \,|, \tag{1.55}$$

where ϕ is the level set function and $V(\kappa)$ is the speed with which the front (or *zero level curve*) propagates. This fundamental[4] equation describes the time evolution of the level set function (ϕ) in such a way that the *zero level curve* of this evolving function is always identified with the propagating interface. The term "level set function" will be interchangeably used with the term "flow field" or simply "field" during the course of this Chapter. The above equation is also called an Eulerian representation of evolution due to the work of Osher and Sethian [25]. Equation (1.55) for 2-D and 3-D cases can be generalized as: $\frac{\partial \phi}{\partial t} = V_\kappa(x,y)\,|\,\nabla\phi\,|$ and $\frac{\partial \phi}{\partial t} = V_\kappa(x,y,z)\,|\,\nabla\phi\,|$, respectively, where $V_\kappa(x,y)$ and $V_\kappa(x,y,z)$ are curvature dependent speed functions in 2-D and 3-D, respectively.

$$\left\{ \begin{array}{lcl} \frac{\partial \phi}{\partial t} & = & V_\kappa(x,y)\,|\,\nabla\phi\,| \\ \frac{\partial \phi}{\partial t} & = & V_\kappa(x,y,z)\,|\,\nabla\phi\,|, \end{array} \right\} \tag{1.57}$$

where $V_\kappa(x,y)$ and $V_\kappa(x,y,z)$ are curvature dependent speed functions in 2-D and 3-D. *Three Analogies of the Curve Evolution Equation:* (**1**) Note that these equations can be compared with the Euclidean geometric heat equation (see Grayson [26]), given as: $\frac{\partial \mathcal{C}}{\partial t} = \kappa \mathcal{N}$, where κ is the curvature and $\mathcal{N}$ is the inward unit normal and $\mathcal{C}$ is the curve coordinates. (**2**) Equation (1.55) is also called the curvature motion equation, since the rate of change of the length of the curve is a function of $\frac{\partial \mathcal{C}}{\partial t}$. (**3**) The above equations can be written in terms of differential geometry using divergence as: $\frac{\partial \phi}{\partial t} = \nabla \cdot (\frac{\nabla\phi}{|\nabla\phi|})\,|\,\nabla\phi\,|$, where geometrical properties such as normal curvature ($\mathcal{N}$) and mean curvature ($\mathcal{H}$) are given as: $\mathcal{N} = \frac{\nabla\phi}{|\nabla\phi|}$ and $\mathcal{H} = \nabla \cdot (\frac{\nabla\phi}{|\nabla\phi|})$.

We will be covering in greater detail the applications of level sets and PDE in the subsequent Chapters.

---

[4] Recently, Faugeras and his coworkers from INRIA (see Gomes *et al.* [24]) modified Eq. (1.55) into the "preserving distance function" as:

$$\frac{\partial \phi}{\partial t} = V(\mathbf{x})\,(\mathbf{x} - \phi\,\nabla\phi), \tag{1.56}$$

where $\mathbf{x}$ was the vector of x and y coordinates, ϕ is the signed distance function. The main characteristic of this equation was that ϕ and V are orthogonal to each other (see details by Gomes *et al.* [24]).

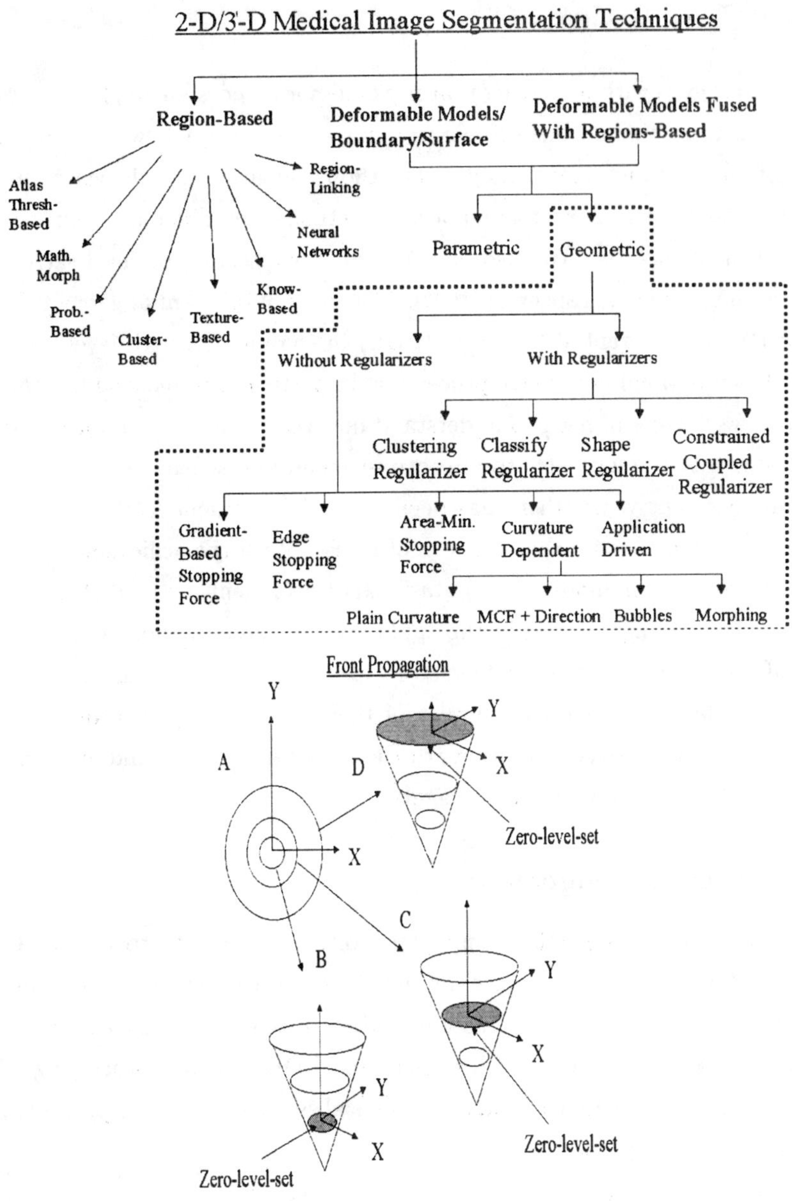

Figure 1.5: **Top**: The place of level sets in the medical segmentation tree. Note the classification sub-tree of geometric deformable models or level sets (shown in dotted line area). **Bottom**: Front propagation of the *zero level set.* Filled circles in figures (B), (C) and (D) show the position of the *zero level curve* as the front propagates. These three projected circles are seen in figure (A).

1.6 Conclusions

Although it goes without saying that it would not be possible to give a comprehensive introduction on this subject in a single chapter, we do wish to highlight some of the most important analytical methods: separation of the variables and integral transforms, as well as numerical methods, the difference method and finite element method. We also have included one section on level set to emphasize the geometric aspect of PDEs. The class of differential geometry, also called Partial Differential Equation (PDE) in conjunction with level sets, has been shown to dominate image processing, in particular in medical imaging, in a major way. We still need to understand how the regularization terms can be integrated into the level sets to improve segmentation schemes.

During recent years, there has been rapid development in theoretical and numerical techniques for the solutions of PDEs. With the achievement of software development in modern computational environment, we predict that there will be an increasing interest in the application of these methods to significant scientific and technological problems. In fact, the rest of the chapters of this book provide readers with a sampler of these practical applications. In the next chapter, we discuss extentions to the level set methods and applications to the level sets such as crack propagation.

1.6.1 Acknowledgements

The first author was partially supported by Dr. Naoki Saito's grant ONR YIP N00014-00-1-0469 while completing this Chapter. Dr. Suri would like to give thanks to IEEE Transactions and EMBS review boards for accepting his research work in application of level sets and PDE in image processing. The authors thank Laura Reden, Marconi Medical Systems, Inc. for proofreading the Chapter.

Bibliography

[1] Axelsson, O. and Barker, V. A., Finite element solution of boundary value problems, Academic Press, Inc., 1984.

[2] Brenner, S. and Scott, R., The mathematical theory of finite element methods, Springer-Verlag, 1994.

[3] Chatelin, F., Lectures on finite precision computations, Soc. for Industry and Applied Mathematics (SIAM), 1996.

[4] Chatelin, F., Spectral approximation of linear operators, Academic Press, 1983.

[5] Chester, C. R., Techniques in partial differential equations, McGraw-Hill, 1971.

[6] Davies, B., Integral transforms and their applications, Springer-Verlag Inc., New York, 1985.

[7] Debnath, L., Integral transforms and their applications, CRC Press, Boca Raton, p. 457, 1995.

[8] Ciarlet, Philippe G., The finite element method for elliptic problems, Elsevier, North-Holland, 1978.

[9] Duffy, D. G., Transform methods for solving partial differential equations, CRC Press, 1994.

[10] Evans, G., Blackledge, J. M. and Yardley, P. D., Analytic Methods for Partial Differential Equations, Springer-Verlag, New York, 1999.

[11] Farlow, S. J., Partial differential equations for scientists and engineers, John Wiley & Sons, New York, 1982.

[12] Gladwell, I. and Wait, R., A Survey of numerical methods for partial differential equations, Clarendon Press, 1979.

[13] Gautschi, W., Numerical Analysis, Birkhauser, 1997.

[14] Harris, J. W. and Sttocker, H., Handbook of mathematics and computational science, Springer-Verlag, 1998.

[15] Oberhettinger, F., Tables of Fourier Transforms and Fourier Transforms of distributions, Springer-Verlag, 1990.

[16] Oberhettinger, F. and Badii, L., Tables of Laplace Transforms, Springer-Verlag, 1973.

[17] Press, W. H., Numerical recipes in FORTRAN: the art of scientific computing, 2nd ed., Cambridge University Press, 1992.

[18] Press, W. H., Numerical recipes in C: the art of scientific computing, Cambridge University Press, 1988.

[19] Press, W. H., Numerical recipes in fortran 90 : the art of parallel scientific computing, 2nd ed, Cambridge University Press, 1996.

[20] Roberts, G. E. and Kaufman, H., Table of Laplace Transforms, Saunders, Philadelphia, 1966.

[21] Tikhonov, A. N. and Samariskii, Equations of mathematical physics, Macmillan, 765 pp., 1963,

[22] Weinberger, H., A first course in PDE, Ginn and Co., 1965.

[23] Zwillinger, D., Handbook of differential equations, Academic Press, Inc., 1989.

[24] Gomes, J. and Faugeras, O., Level sets and distance functions, In Proc. of the 6th European Conference on Computer Vision (ECCV), pp. 588-602, 2000.

[25] Osher, S. and Sethian, J., Fronts propagating with curvature-dependent speed: algorithms based on Hamiltons-Jacobi formulations, J. Comput. Physics, Vol. 79, No. 1, pp. 12-49, 1988.

[26] Grayson, M., The heat equation shrinks embedded plane curves to round points, J. of Differential Geometry, Vol. 26, pp. 285-314, 1987.

Chapter 2

Level Set Extentions, Flows and Crack Propagation

David Chopp[1]

2.1 Introduction

Since its introduction, the level set method, by Osher and Sethian [37] has become a popular numerical method for the purpose of capturing the evolution of moving interfaces. In its simplest form, the method is very elegant and offers some significant advantages over other interface tracking/capturing methods. Probably the most appealing feature of the method is its ability to handle changes in topology without complicated mesh generation, surface reconstruction, or collision detection. Particularly when considering applications in three dimensions or higher, this becomes a significant advantage: some other methods do not generalize so easily to higher dimensions.

Another appealing feature of the level set method, which is often overlooked, is its ties to numerical methods derived for hyperbolic conservation laws. This connection allows the method to capture corners and cusps in the interface properly without non-physical loops and oscillations. In this context, the corners play the role of shocks in hyperbolic conservation laws, and the numerical methods from hyperbolic conservation laws are designed for maintaining sharp shocks. Therefore, the level set method is also able to maintain sharp corners in an interface. These methods also contribute to the stability of the level set method in the presence of corners in the interface.

[1]Northwestern University, Evanston, IL, USA

PDE & Level Sets: Algorithmic Approaches to Static & Motion Imagery
Edited by Jasjit Suri and Swamy Laxminarayan, Kluwer Academic/Plenum Publishers, 2002

The level set approach to front propagation has been employed in a wide variety of investigations. Examples include flame propagation [60], crystal growth and dendrite simulation [41], fluid dynamics [58, 39, 47, 14], granular flow [20], image processing [17, 16, 57], material science [19, 29, 3], solid mechanics [49], and optimization [38]. This list barely scratches the surface of the variety of implementations found in the literature.

In this chapter, the details of the level set method are laid out beginning with the underlying hyperbolic conservation laws, describing implementation details of the full state-of-the-art method, and concluding with examples of how the level set method can be used in various applications.

2.2 Background Numerical Methods

2.2.1 Hyperbolic Conservation Laws

A scalar hyperbolic conservation law in one dimension is an equation of the form

$$\frac{\partial u}{\partial t} + \frac{\partial}{\partial x} f(u) = 0 \tag{2.1}$$

where $u(x,t)$ is a conserved quantity or state variable. It is helpful to think of u as a density function so that

$$\int_{x_1}^{x_2} u(x,t)\, dx$$

is the total quantity of u in the interval $[x_1, x_2]$ at time t.

Hyperbolic conservation laws do not always have classical solutions, but can be solved using weak solutions. Weak solutions are solutions which solve an associated integral equation. Integrating (2.1) in time and space gives the equation

$$\int_{x_1}^{x_2} u(x,t_2)\, dx = \int_{x_1}^{x_2} u(x,t_1)\, dx - \int_{t_1}^{t_2} f(u(x_2,t)) - f(u(x_1,t))\, dt \tag{2.2}$$

The weak formulation (2.2) suggests the form of an appropriate numerical method. If we define

$$u_j^n = \int_{x_{j-1/2}}^{x_{j+1/2}} u(x,t_n)\, dx, \tag{2.3}$$

and approximate the flux function by

$$F(u(x_{j+1/2},t_n)) \approx f(u_{j-p}^n, u_{j-p+1}^n, \ldots, u_{j+q}^n), \tag{2.4}$$

then (2.2) can be approximated by

$$u_j^{n+1} = u_j^n - \frac{\Delta t}{\Delta x}(F(u_{j-p}^n, u_{j-p+1}^n, \ldots, u_{j+q}^n) - F(u_{j-p-1}^n, u_{j-p}^n, \ldots, u_{j+q-1}^n)) \tag{2.5}$$

A method which can be put in the form of (2.5) is called a conservative method, and if the method converges, it will converge to a solution of (2.2).

An example of a conservative method is the Lax-Friedrichs method which is given by

$$\begin{aligned} u_j^{n+1} &= \frac{1}{2}(u_{j-1}^n + u_{j+1}^n) - \frac{\Delta t}{2\Delta x}(f(u_{j+1}^n) - f(u_{j-1}^n)) \\ &= u_j^n - \frac{\Delta t}{\Delta x}(F(u_j^n, u_{j+1}^n) - F(u_{j-1}^n, u_j^n)) \end{aligned} \tag{2.6}$$

where

$$F(\mathbf{v}, \mathbf{w}) = \frac{\Delta x}{2\Delta t}(\mathbf{v} - \mathbf{w}) + \frac{1}{2}(f(\mathbf{v}) + f(\mathbf{w})) \tag{2.7}$$

For the conservative method to work, the numerical flux function F must be consistent with the conservation law. The flux function is consistent if for some constant $\tilde{u}$,

$$F(\tilde{u}, \tilde{u}, \ldots, \tilde{u}) = f(\tilde{u})$$

The Lax-Friedrichs method is first order accurate, and contains a significant amount of artificial diffusion which smears out any discontinuities in the solution. Other conservative methods which are also first order, but with much less artificial diffusion include the upwind method

$$\begin{aligned} F_U(u_j, u_{j+1}) = \frac{1}{2}\frac{f(u_{j+1}) - f(u_j)}{u_{j+1} - u_j}(u_j + u_{j+1}) \\ - \frac{1}{2}\left|\frac{f(u_{j+1}) - f(u_j)}{u_{j+1} - u_j}\right|(u_{j+1} - u_j), \end{aligned} \tag{2.8}$$

and Godunov's method

$$F_G(u_j, u_{j+1}) = \begin{cases} \min_{u_j \le u \le u_{j+1}} f(u) & u_j \le u_{j+1} \\ \max_{u_j \ge u \ge u_{j+1}} f(u) & u_j > u_{j+1} \end{cases}. \tag{2.9}$$

Higher order methods exist such as slope-limiter methods [31] and essentially non-oscillatory methods [26].

For a more complete treatment of the numerical methods for hyperbolic conservation laws, an excellent text is [31].

2.2.2 Hamilton-Jacobi Equations

An evolution equation of the form

$$\phi_t + H(\nabla\phi) = 0 \tag{2.10}$$

is a Hamilton-Jacobi equation, and H is called the Hamiltonian. We use the theory from hyperbolic conservation laws to approximate this equation by a numerical Hamiltonian (flux function).

$$H(\nabla\phi) \approx G(D_{-x}\phi, D_{+x}\phi, D_{-y}\phi, D_{+y}\phi) \tag{2.11}$$

where the finite difference operators $D_{\pm x}$, $D_{\pm y}$ are defined by

$$D_{+x}\phi_{i,j} = \frac{\phi_{i+1,j} - \phi_{i,j}}{\Delta x}, \quad D_{-x}\phi_{i,j} = \frac{\phi_{i,j} - \phi_{i-1,j}}{\Delta x} \tag{2.12}$$

and similarly for $D_{\pm y}$. In a sense, we have integrated the numerical method itself, where H is playing the role of the integral of the flux function for f for the hyperbolic conservation laws.

For example, consider the equation

$$\phi_t + F\|\nabla\phi\| = 0. \tag{2.13}$$

This is a Hamilton-Jacobi equation and $H(\nabla\phi) = F\|\nabla\phi\|$ is the Hamiltonian. If we apply Godunov's method to (2.13), then we get the following first order method:

$$\begin{aligned}\phi_{ij}^{n+1} = \phi_{ij}^n - \Delta t(&\max(\operatorname{sign}(F_{ij})D_{-x}\phi_{ij}^n, -\operatorname{sign}(F_{ij})D_{+x}\phi_{ij}^n, 0)^2 \\ &+ \max(\operatorname{sign}(F_{ij})D_{-y}\phi_{ij}^n, -\operatorname{sign}(F_{ij})D_{+y}\phi_{ij}^n, 0)^2)^{1/2}\end{aligned} \tag{2.14}$$

Notice that we must look in the appropriate directions depending upon the sign of F.

A second order method based upon the ENO conservation law method [26] is given by

$$\begin{aligned}\phi_{ij}^{n+1} = \phi_{ij}^n - \Delta t(&\max(\operatorname{sign}(F_{ij})A, -\operatorname{sign}(F_{ij})B, 0)^2 \\ &+ \max(\operatorname{sign}(F_{ij})C, -\operatorname{sign}(F_{ij})D, 0)^2)^{1/2}\end{aligned} \tag{2.15}$$

where

$$A = D_{-x}\phi_{ij}^n + \frac{\Delta x}{2}\,\mathrm{minmod}(D_{-x}D_{-x}\phi_{ij}^n, D_{-x}D_{+x}\phi_{ij}^n) \tag{2.16}$$

$$B = D_{+x}\phi_{ij}^n + \frac{\Delta x}{2}\,\mathrm{minmod}(D_{+x}D_{-x}\phi_{ij}^n, D_{+x}D_{+x}\phi_{ij}^n) \tag{2.17}$$

$$C = D_{-y}\phi_{ij}^n + \frac{\Delta y}{2}\,\mathrm{minmod}(D_{-y}D_{-y}\phi_{ij}^n, D_{-y}D_{+y}\phi_{ij}^n) \tag{2.18}$$

$$D = D_{+y}\phi_{ij}^n + \frac{\Delta y}{2}\,\mathrm{minmod}(D_{+y}D_{-y}\phi_{ij}^n, D_{+y}D_{+y}\phi_{ij}^n) \tag{2.19}$$

and where

$$\mathrm{minmod}(a, b) = \frac{1}{2}(\mathrm{sign}(a) + \mathrm{sign}(b))\min(|a|, |b|) \tag{2.20}$$

2.2.3 The Fast Marching Method

The fast marching method is an optimal method for solving an equation of the form

$$||\nabla\phi|| = 1/F(\mathbf{x}) \tag{2.21}$$

where $F(\mathbf{x})$ is a monotonic speed function for an advancing interface. If $\phi^{-1}(0)$ represents the initial interface, and ϕ solves (2.21), then $\phi^{-1}(t)$ gives the location of the interface evolving with normal velocity $F(\mathbf{x}) > 0$ at time t. The advantage of this method over traditional iterative methods is that the entire evolution of the front is computed in one pass over the mesh with an operation count of $O(N \log N)$ for N mesh points. It is also advantageous over other front tracking algorithms in that it uses techniques borrowed from hyperbolic conservation laws to properly advance fronts with sharp corners and cusps. We present here a basic description of the method, the interested reader is referred to [42, 43, 44, 7].

In the fast marching method, (2.21) is solved numerically by using upwind finite differences to approximate $\nabla\phi$. The use of upwind finite differences indicates a causality, or a direction for the flow of information propagating from the initial contour $\phi^{-1}(0)$ outwards to larger values of ϕ. This causality means that the value of $\phi(\mathbf{x})$ depends only on values of $\phi(\mathbf{y})$ for which $\phi(\mathbf{y}) \leq \phi(\mathbf{x})$. Thus, if we solve for the values of ϕ in a monotonically increasing fashion, then the upwind differences are always valid and all the mesh points are eventually computed. This sequential procession through the mesh points is maintained by a heap sort which controls the order in which the mesh points are computed.

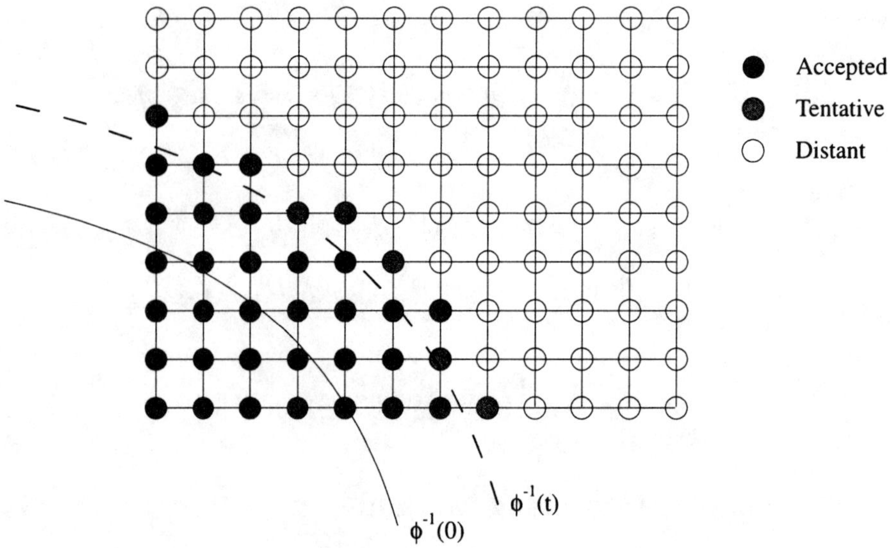

Figure 2.1: Illustration of the sets A, T, and D

To begin, the mesh points are separated into three disjoint sets, the set of *accepted* points A, the set of *tentative* points T, and the set of *distant* points D. The mesh points in the set A are considered computed and are always closer to the initial interface than any of the remaining mesh points. The mesh points in T are all potential candidates to be the next mesh point to be added to the set A. The mesh points in T are always kept sorted in a heap sort so that the best candidate is always easily found. The mesh points in D are considered too far from the initial interface to be possible candidates for inclusion in A. Thus, if $\mathbf{x} \in A$, $\mathbf{y} \in T$, and $\mathbf{z} \in D$, then $\phi(\mathbf{x}) < \phi(\mathbf{y}) < \phi(\mathbf{z})$. Figure 2.1 shows the relationship between the different sets of mesh points.

One of the key components in the fast marching method is the computation of the estimate of ϕ for points in T. Suppose, for example, mesh points $\mathbf{x}_{i-1,j}$, $\mathbf{x}_{i,j+1} \in A$, and $\mathbf{x}_{i,j} \in T$. Given the values of $\phi_{i-1,j}$, $\phi_{i,j+1}$, we must estimate the value of $\phi_{i,j}$. This is accomplished by looking at the discretization of (2.21) given by

$$(D_{-x}\phi_{i,j})^2 + (D_{+y}\phi_{i,j})^2 = \frac{1}{F_{i,j}^2}. \tag{2.22}$$

(2.22) reduces to a quadratic equation in $\phi_{i,j}$ given by

$$\left(\frac{1}{\Delta x^2}+\frac{1}{\Delta y^2}\right)\phi_{i,j}^2-2\left(\frac{\phi_{i-1,j}}{\Delta x^2}+\frac{\phi_{i,j+1}}{\Delta y^2}\right)\phi_{i,j}+\frac{\phi_{i-1,j}^2}{\Delta x^2}+\frac{\phi_{i,j+1}^2}{\Delta y^2}-\frac{1}{F^2}=0. \tag{2.23}$$

The new estimate for $\phi_{i,j}$ is given by the largest of the two roots of (2.23). The remaining configurations and the resulting quadratic equations can be derived in a similar fashion.

Note that (2.22) is a first order approximation of (2.21). The general second and third order approximations of (2.21) requires the use of switches determined by which points are in A:

$$\begin{aligned}
&(\max(D_{-x}\phi_{i,j}+s_{x,-1}\frac{\Delta x}{2}D_{-x}D_{-x}\phi_{i,j}+s_{x,-1}s_{x,-2}\frac{\Delta x^2}{6}D_{-x}D_{-x}D_{-x}\phi_{i,j},\\
&\quad -D_{+x}\phi_{i,j}+s_{x,1}\frac{\Delta x}{2}D_{+x}D_{+x}\phi_{i,j}+s_{x,1}s_{x,2}\frac{\Delta x^2}{6}D_{+x}D_{+x}D_{+x}\phi_{i,j},0)^2\\
&+\max(D_{-y}\phi_{i,j}+s_{y,-1}\frac{\Delta y}{2}D_{-y}D_{-y}\phi_{i,j}+s_{y,-1}s_{y,-2}\frac{\Delta y^2}{6}D_{-y}D_{-y}D_{-y}\phi_{i,j},\\
&\quad -D_{+y}\phi_{i,j}+s_{y,1}\frac{\Delta y}{2}D_{+y}D_{+y}\phi_{i,j}+s_{y,1}s_{y,2}\frac{\Delta y^2}{6}D_{+y}D_{+y}D_{+y}\phi_{i,j},0)^2\\
&=\frac{1}{F_{i,j}^2}
\end{aligned} \tag{2.24}$$

where the switches are

$$s_{x,k}=\begin{cases}1 & \mathbf{x}_{i+k,j}\in A\\ 0 & \text{otherwise}\end{cases}$$

$$s_{y,k}=\begin{cases}1 & \mathbf{x}_{i,j+k}\in A\\ 0 & \text{otherwise}\end{cases}$$

Now the fast marching method can be assembled as an algorithm:

1. Initialize all the points adjacent to the initial interface with an initial value, put those points in A. A discussion about initialization follows in § 2.2.3.1. All points $\mathbf{x}_{i,j}\notin A$, but are adjacent to a point in A are given initial estimates for $\phi_{i,j}$ by solving (2.24). These points are tentative points and put in the set T. All remaining points unaccounted for are placed in D and given initial value of $\phi_{i,j}=+\infty$.

2. Choose the point $\mathbf{x}_{i,j}\in T$ which has the smallest value of $\phi_{i,j}$ and move it into A. Any point which is adjacent to $\mathbf{x}_{i,j}$ (i.e. the points $\mathbf{x}_{i-1,j}$, $\mathbf{x}_{i,j-1}$,

$\mathbf{x}_{i+1,j}$, $\mathbf{x}_{i,j+1}$) which is in T has its value $\phi_{i,j}$ recalculated using (2.24). Any point adjacent to $\mathbf{x}_{i,j}$ and in D has its value $\phi_{i,j}$ computed using (2.24) and is moved into the set T.

3. If $T \neq \emptyset$, go to step 2.

The fast marching method algorithm presented in [43], is first order accurate and can be recovered from (2.24) by taking all the switches $s_{*,*} = 0$. The second order accurate method presented in [44] can also be recovered from (2.24) by taking all the switches $s_{*,\pm 2} = 0$.

2.2.3.1 Locally Second Order Approximation of the Level Set Function

In [44], it is shown that the fast marching method behaves as a globally second order accurate method. However, it is also noted that the method is only first order accurate in the set of nodes immediately adjacent to the initial front. This does not destroy the global accuracy because as the mesh shrinks, so too does the size of the region of first order accuracy. To achieve a fully second order accurate fast marching method, we must ensure that the initial data is at least second order accurate. Furthermore, we can also get a globally third order accurate fast marching method by virtue of having at least second order initial data.

The underpinning of this higher degree of accuracy around the initial front is the use of a bicubic interpolation function p which is a second order accurate local representation of a level set function ϕ, (i.e. $p(\mathbf{x}) \approx \phi(\mathbf{x})$). The interpolation function $p(\mathbf{x})$ can serve many purposes including second order accuracy for the distance to the zero level set, subgrid resolution of the shape of the interface, as well as subgrid resolution of the level set function $\phi(\mathbf{x})$ itself.

We begin with a description of the bicubic interpolation for a level set function given on a rectangular mesh. The approximation is done locally in a box of the mesh bounded by grid points, call them $\mathbf{x}_{i,j}$, $\mathbf{x}_{i+1,j}$, $\mathbf{x}_{i,j+1}$, and $\mathbf{x}_{i+1,j+1}$, as in Figure 2.2.

A bicubic interpolation $p(\mathbf{x})$ of a function $\phi(\mathbf{x})$ is a function

$$p(\mathbf{x}) = p(x, y) = \sum_{m=0}^{3} \sum_{n=0}^{3} a_{m,n} x^m y^n \tag{2.25}$$

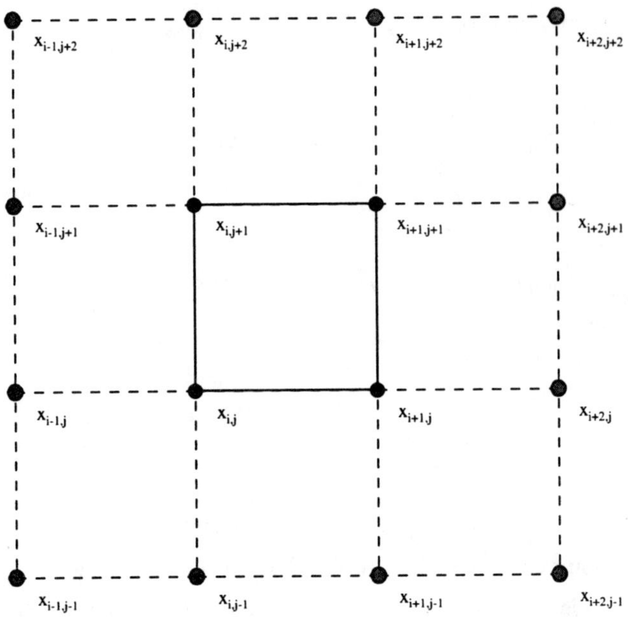

Figure 2.2: Sample portion of the mesh where a bicubic interpolation is used

which solves the following set of equations:

$$\begin{aligned}
p(\mathbf{x}_{k,\ell}) &= \phi(\mathbf{x}_{k,\ell}) \\
\frac{\partial p}{\partial x}(\mathbf{x}_{k,\ell}) &= \frac{\partial \phi}{\partial x}(\mathbf{x}_{k,\ell}) \\
\frac{\partial p}{\partial y}(\mathbf{x}_{k,\ell}) &= \frac{\partial \phi}{\partial y}(\mathbf{x}_{k,\ell}) \\
\frac{\partial^2 p}{\partial x \partial y}(\mathbf{x}_{k,\ell}) &= \frac{\partial^2 \phi}{\partial x \partial y}(\mathbf{x}_{k,\ell})
\end{aligned}$$

for $k = i, i+1$; $\ell = j, j+1$. This gives sixteen equations for the sixteen unknown coefficients $a_{m,n}$. Solving for the $a_{m,n}$ makes $p(x, y)$ a bicubic interpolating function of $\phi(x, y)$ on the rectangle bounded by the corners $\mathbf{x}_{i,j}$, $\mathbf{x}_{i+1,j}$, $\mathbf{x}_{i,j+1}$, and $\mathbf{x}_{i+1,j+1}$.

Since ϕ is only known on the mesh points, then the values for the derivatives of ϕ must be approximated. We use second order finite difference approximations for the derivatives of ϕ:

$$\begin{aligned}
\frac{\partial \phi}{\partial x}(\mathbf{x}_{m,n}) &\approx \frac{1}{2\Delta x}(\phi(\mathbf{x}_{m+1,n}) - \phi(\mathbf{x}_{m-1,n})) \\
\frac{\partial \phi}{\partial y}(\mathbf{x}_{m,n}) &\approx \frac{1}{2\Delta y}(\phi(\mathbf{x}_{m,n+1}) - \phi(x_{m,n-1})) \\
\frac{\partial^2 \phi}{\partial x \partial y}(\mathbf{x}_{m,n}) &\approx \frac{1}{4\Delta x \Delta y}(\phi(\mathbf{x}_{m+1,n+1}) - \phi(\mathbf{x}_{m-1,n+1}) \\
&\qquad - \phi(\mathbf{x}_{m+1,n-1}) + \phi(\mathbf{x}_{m-1,n-1}))
\end{aligned}$$

for $m = i, i+1$ and $n = j, j+1$. Thus, construction of the interpolant p requires all the points shown in Figure 2.2. The observant reader will note that the accuracy of this method is restricted to second order by our use of second order approximations for the derivatives of ϕ. In principle, higher order local approximations can be made using higher order finite difference approximations and using a larger set of grid points around the box where the interpolant is used.

Now, given the interpolating function $p(x, y)$ in the domain $[x_i, x_{i+1}] \times [y_j, y_{j+1}]$, and given a point (x_0, y_0) in that domain, we compute the distance between (x_0, y_0) and the zero level curve of $p(x, y)$. The point (x_1, y_1) on the zero level curve closest to (x_0, y_0) must satisfy two conditions:

$$p(x_1, y_1) = 0 \tag{2.26}$$

$$\nabla p(x_1, y_1) \times ((x_0, y_0) - (x_1, y_1)) = 0 \tag{2.27}$$

Equation (2.26) is a requirement that (x_1, y_1) must be on the zero contour of $p(x, y)$. Equation (2.27) is a requirement that the normal to the zero contour, given by $\nabla p(x_1, y_1)$ must be aligned with the line through the points (x_0, y_0) and (x_1, y_1).

We employ Newton's method to solve the simultaneous pair of conditions (2.26), (2.27). Thus, we compute a sequence of iterates (x_k, y_k) with initial point (x_0, y_0). The update for the iterates is given by

$$\delta x = \frac{(x_k - x_0)(p_y^2 - pp_{yy}) + (y_k - y_0)(pp_{xy} - p_x p_y) + pp_x}{(p_x p_{yy} - p_y p_{xy})(x_k - x_0) + (p_y p_{xx} - p_x p_{xy})(y_k - y_0) - p_x^2 - p_y^2}$$

$$\delta y = \frac{(y_k - y_0)(p_x^2 - pp_{xx}) + (x_k - x_0)(pp_{xy} - p_x p_y) + pp_y}{(p_x p_{yy} - p_y p_{xy})(x_k - x_0) + (p_y p_{xx} - p_x p_{xy})(y_k - y_0) - p_x^2 - p_y^2}$$

$$x_{k+1} = x_k + \delta x$$

$$y_{k+1} = y_k + \delta y$$

where all the p functions are evaluated at (x_k, y_k). Typically, less than five iterations are necessary in order to achieve reasonable accuracy.

The approximation $p(x, y)$ is now a local subgrid representation of the level set function ϕ inside the box, and can be used as an initializer for the fast marching method. Given the front speed F and the initial distance to the front as determined from $p(x, y)$, the initial value for a point adjacent to the initial front for the general fast marching method solving (2.21) is ϕ/F.

2.3 Basic Level Set Method

The level set method [37] is based upon representing an interface as the zero level set of some higher dimensional function ϕ. Typically, the level set function ϕ is the signed distance function to the interface γ, where $\phi > 0$ on one side of the interface and $\phi < 0$ on the other side. A diagram relating the level set function to the interface is shown in Figure 2.3.

At all times, the interface is given by the equation $\phi(x, y, t) = 0$. In order to move the interface, we need to describe the evolution equation of the whole function ϕ.

Let $\mathbf{x}(t) = (x(t), y(t))$ be a point on the interface. We are given that $\frac{d}{dt}\mathbf{x}(t) = F\mathbf{n}$ for some normal speed function F. Since $\mathbf{x}(t)$ is on the interface at all times, then it must be that $\phi(\mathbf{x}(t), t) \equiv 0$ for all t. If we differentiate with respect to t, we get

$$\phi_t + \nabla\phi \cdot \frac{d}{dt}\mathbf{x}(t) = 0 \tag{2.28}$$

$$\phi_t + \nabla\phi \cdot F\mathbf{n} = 0 \tag{2.29}$$

Now, the normal to the interface is the normal to the zero level set, and hence

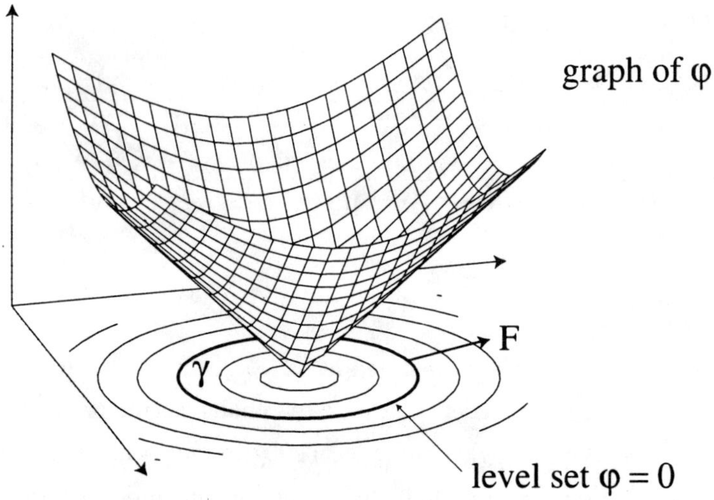

Figure 2.3: Level set function for a circle

we have

$$\mathbf{n} = \frac{\nabla \phi}{||\nabla \phi||}$$

Using this, (2.29) becomes

$$\phi_t + F||\nabla \phi|| = 0 \tag{2.30}$$

This is the basic evolution equation for the level set method.

There are still a host of difficulties that are yet to be tackled, however.

1. What do we do if F is only defined on the interface? In this formulation, we expect F to be defined not only on the front itself, but everywhere ϕ is defined. We will need to have the ability to extend the velocity field to the entire domain.

2. How do we take advantage of the conservation law methods? We have seen that conservation laws play an important role in the evolution of fronts, how can we take advantage of those methods so that our evolution produces the correct weak solution when appropriate.

3. The function ϕ is now defined on some domain which contains the original interface. In order to evolve ϕ, we will need to know what the appropriate boundary conditions are so that we can build a stable numerical method.

Let us apply this method to some model problems. The first model problem is speed $F = 1$. Using the approximation in (2.14), the method is fairly simple, namely

$$\phi_{ij}^{n+1} = \phi_{ij}^n - \Delta t(\max(D_{-x}\phi_{ij}^n, -D_{+x}\phi_{ij}^n, 0)^2 + \max(D_{-y}\phi_{ij}^n, -D_{+y}\phi_{ij}^n, 0)^2)^{1/2}$$

It is important to remember that the direction of the normal to the interface is implicitly chosen by the sign of ϕ. In other words, given an initial circle, there are two different ways the interface can be represented, $\phi < 0$ inside or $\phi > 0$ inside. If $\phi < 0$ inside, then $\mathbf{n} = \frac{\nabla\phi}{\|\nabla\phi\|}$ points outward and $F = 1$ means that the circle expands. If $\phi > 0$ inside, then $\mathbf{n}$ changes direction and the circle shrinks.

Another important point about this method is that we have nowhere computed the velocity of the front itself. This is a very subtle, but crucial, point to understand. What is happening is that we are really evolving a continuous family of interfaces simultaneously, and that each interface corresponding to $\phi(x,t) = C$ for some C is moving according to the speed law $F = 1$. We are then relying on the fact that the speed function F varies continuously in the normal direction $\nabla\phi$.

What is really happening is that at each grid point x_{ij}, we look at the level curve which passes through x_{ij}, then apply the speed function for that level set to find how to change ϕ_{ij}. This view of how the method works will come in handy when we discuss velocity extensions later on.

The second model problem involves the curvature of the interface. Fortunately, we can derive an expression for the curvature in terms of ϕ.

$$\kappa = \nabla \cdot \frac{\nabla\phi}{\|\nabla\phi\|} = \frac{\phi_{xx}\phi_y^2 + \phi_{yy}\phi_x^2 - 2\phi_{xy}\phi_x\phi_y}{(\phi_x^2 + \phi_y^2)^{3/2}} \tag{2.31}$$

For the model problem $F = 1 - \epsilon\kappa$, it is important to notice that $\epsilon\kappa$ is a diffusive term and is not directional as compared to speed $F = 1$ which travels only in the direction of the normal. Thus, we want to use upwind differencing for terms such as $F = 1$, and central differences for diffusive terms. In general, we break F into two parts, $F = F_{\text{adv}} + F_{\text{diff}}$ where F_{adv} is advective velocity such as $F = 1$ and F_{diff} is the diffusive velocity which is not directional. The basic evolution equation is then broken down into

$$\phi_t + F_{\text{adv}}\|\nabla\phi\| = -F_{\text{diff}}\|\nabla\phi\| \tag{2.32}$$

This is a Hamilton-Jacobi equation with viscosity. The left hand side of the equation is computed using a conservative method for Hamilton-Jacobi equations, and the right hand side is computed using central differences.

The last model problem is where F is determined by an independently generated velocity field $\mathbf{V}$. Frequently, $\mathbf{V}$ is generated by solving a fluid velocity problem and then the front is advected according to the resulting fluid velocity field.

Given a velocity field $\mathbf{V}$, only the part of $\mathbf{V}$ which is orthogonal to the interface affects the motion of the interface. Using the level set formulation, the normal component of $\mathbf{V}$ is

$$\mathbf{V}^{\perp} = (\mathbf{V} \cdot \mathbf{n})\mathbf{n} = \left(\mathbf{V} \cdot \frac{\nabla \phi}{||\nabla \phi||}\right)\mathbf{n}$$

Thus, the interface speed is $F = \mathbf{V} \cdot \frac{\nabla \phi}{||\nabla \phi||}$ and the equation of motion becomes

$$\begin{aligned} \phi_t + F||\nabla \phi|| &= 0 \\ \phi_t + \mathbf{V} \cdot \nabla \phi &= 0 \end{aligned}$$

Notice that this is an advective velocity, hence we would use upwind differences to compute $\nabla \phi$. For upwind differencing, we get

$$\begin{aligned} \mathbf{V} \cdot \nabla \phi = \max(V_x, 0) D_{-x} \phi_{ij}^n + \min(V_x, 0) D_{+x} \phi_{ij}^n \\ + \max(V_y, 0) D_{-y} \phi_{ij}^n + \min(V_y, 0) D_{+y} \phi_{ij}^n \end{aligned} \quad (2.33)$$

There is one note of caution about this model problem. For the level set method to work properly, $|\frac{\partial F}{\partial \mathbf{n}}|$ needs to be small. In many problems, this condition is not satisfied when $\mathbf{V}$ is an independently generated velocity (and often even when it only depends upon ϕ). A large variation in $\frac{\partial F}{\partial \mathbf{n}}$ can cause a breakdown in stability. Without this condition, the level set function ϕ can develop large gradients and/or small gradients and consequently go unstable. For stability purposes, the function ϕ will ideally maintain constant length gradients $||\nabla \phi|| \approx 1$ for all time, but that is generally not possible if the evolution of ϕ is controlled by $\mathbf{V}$. To provide stability, a means of enforcing $||\nabla \phi|| \approx 1$ while not changing the location of $\phi = 0$ is needed. This process is called reinitialization, and it will be discussed in the next section.

2.4 Extensions to the Level Set Method

While the basic level set method is very elegant, it is not so elegant in practice. Except for very special cases, the typical velocity field does not permit a very stable calculation. Difficulties arise when the level set function ϕ develops large or small gradients [4]. The remedy for this problem presented in [4] has been significantly refined by a number of researchers since that time, e.g. [56, 1, 7]. But the underlying principle remains the same: The ideal level set function is the signed distance function. The introduction of this remedy set the stage for an explosion of level set method applications. Since then, a number of important extensions to the level set method have emerged which further broaden the utility and impact of the level set method.

2.4.1 Reinitialization and Velocity Extensions

Reinitialization was first conceived while trying to compute minimal surfaces using the level set method [4]. It was observed that while advancing to steady state, an initially well behaved solution would eventually go unstable, but if the position of the front was set just before instability and the level set function was reconstructed so as to look like an initial condition, then the computation could proceed further. The instability in the method came from the development of large and small gradients in the level set function ϕ. The solution is to notice that the function ϕ should be reconstructed to be the signed distance function. So reinitialization is the process by which ϕ is reconstructed to be the signed distance function to the set $\phi^{-1}(0)$.

A straightforward, naive approach to reinitialization is to explicitly calculate the signed distance function. The algorithm proceeds by using a concept similar to the Marching Cubes algorithm used in computer graphics. Consider the mesh as a collection of "voxels" which have grid points at each corner. If all the corner points have the same sign, then the interface does not pass through this voxel. If there are mixed signs on the corners, then the interface must pass through this voxel. Using interpolation, a linear approximation of the interface can be constructed. Now for each grid point in the domain, the distance to the linear approximate is computed. The new value of ϕ at each grid point is then the minimum of all distances computed and having the same sign as the original ϕ function. This method is exceedingly costly, and should not be used.

An alternative approach is to not find the front at all [56]. Consider the partial differential equation

$$\phi_t = \text{sign}(\phi)(1 - ||\nabla\phi||)$$

Notice that steady state is achieved when $||\nabla\phi|| = 1$ which is the goal. The sign function is there to control the flow of information. We want information to travel outwards from $\phi = 0$. Thus, if ϕ is too steep, i.e. $||\nabla\phi|| > 1$ and $\phi > 0$, then $\phi_t < 0$. But if $\phi < 0$, then $\phi_t > 0$ which is what we want so that $\phi = 0$ is preserved. This is an iterative procedure and can be used to rebuild the distance function without specifically locating the front. The drawback to this method is that the interface $\phi = 0$ is not held stationery. This is a highly diffusive process resulting in sharp features of the interface such as corners getting badly smeared, and convex parts of an interface will tend to recede leading to poor mass conservation.

A third way of doing reinitialization is by using the fast marching method. In this case, reinitialization corresponds to solving $||\nabla\phi|| = 1$ with the given initial condition $\phi^{-1}(0)$. To rebuild the entire signed distance function, the fast marching method will require two passes: one to compute values of $\phi > 0$ and one to compute values of $\phi < 0$. If the bicubic interpolation process is used to initialize the fast marching method, this technique produces excellent reinitializations with much less mass error and at a cheaper computational cost than the iterative method.

Reinitialization is not the only way in which the level set function can be made to maintain the signed distance function. A different way is to essentially pre-condition the velocity field in such a way as to preserve the signed distance function. This is called a velocity extension, and it was introduced in [2]. To see how this works, start with the assumption that $||\nabla\phi|| = 1$ while solving the level set evolution equation

$$\phi_t + F||\nabla\phi|| = 0. \tag{2.34}$$

Differentiating the equation $\nabla\phi \cdot \nabla\phi = 1$ gives

$$\begin{aligned} \frac{\partial}{\partial t}(\nabla\phi \cdot \nabla\phi) &= 0 \\ 2\left(\nabla\frac{\partial\phi}{\partial t} \cdot \nabla\phi\right) &= 0 \\ 2\nabla(-F\|\nabla\phi\|) \cdot \nabla\phi &= 0 \\ \nabla F \cdot \nabla\phi &= 0. \end{aligned} \tag{2.35}$$

Thus, if the speed function F has the property that it solves (2.35), then $\|\nabla\phi\| = 1$ will be preserved.

In general, (2.35) does not hold. However, a technique similar to the fast marching method can be employed to construct such a speed function. This time, the function ϕ is known at all the gridpoints, and the speed function F is to be constructed in such a way that (2.35) is satisfied while not altering the value of F on the zero level set. This time, (2.35) is discretized to give

$$\begin{aligned} &\min(D_{+x}\phi_{i,j}, 0)D_{+x}F_{i,j} + \max(D_{-x}\phi_{i,j}, 0)D_{-x}F_{i,j} \\ &\qquad + \min(D_{+y}\phi_{i,j}, 0)D_{+y}F_{i,j} + \max(D_{-y}\phi_{i,j}, 0)D_{-y}F_{i,j} = 0. \end{aligned} \tag{2.36}$$

This is a linear equation in terms of $F_{i,j}$, and by computing values of $F_{i,j}$ in order of the magnitude of the $\phi_{i,j}$, (2.35) can be solved in one pass just like the fast marching method.

The velocity extension construction also enables the level set method to solve a much larger collection of problems. In many physical applications, the speed function is not known everywhere, but is known only on the interface. A velocity extension will take that locally defined speed function and extend it to the rest of the level set function domain so that the level set method can proceed. Here too, the bicubic interpolation process can be used to improve the accuracy of the starting values for the velocity extension calculation by associating grid points with the nearest point on the zero level set.

2.4.2 Narrow Band Method

Note that the embedding of the interface as the zero level set of a higher dimensional function means that calculations are performed over the entire computational domain; which is wasteful. Instead, an efficient modification is to perform work only in a neighborhood of the zero level set; this is known as

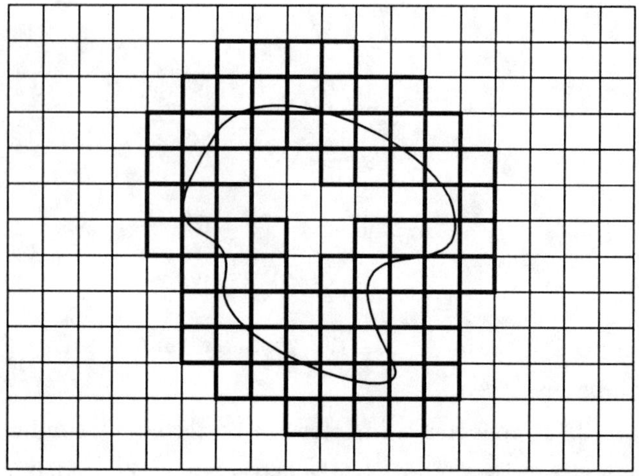

Figure 2.4: Grid points in the narrow band

the *Narrow Band Approach.* This results in an optimal technique which has a much lower operation count. The strategy was introduced in Chopp [13], used in recovering shapes from images in Malladi, Sethian and Vemuri [32], and analyzed extensively by Adalsteinsson and Sethian in [1]. Briefly, the interface propagates until it reaches the edge of its narrow band, at which a new narrow band is built by re-initializing a new narrow band around the current front's position. An illustration of a narrow band is shown in Figure 2.4. The width of the narrow band is a balance between the labor involved in re-initializing vs. calculations performed on far away points. A narrow band one or two grid cells large requires re-initialization every time step; an infinitely large narrow band requires no re-initialization, but defaults to the regular level set method. For details, see [1].

2.4.3 Triple Junctions

Representing the surface implicitly also restricts the types of surfaces which can be represented, namely orientable manifolds. It also effectively excludes the construction of surfaces which have triple junctions such as for multi-phase fluid problems. For example, the spreading of a liquid droplet on a solid surface involves air, liquid, and solid phases all joined together at a contact line. Consider the problem of three phases in $\mathbf{R}^2$. The level set method breaks down at triple-junctions, points where all three phases meet because it is not possible to

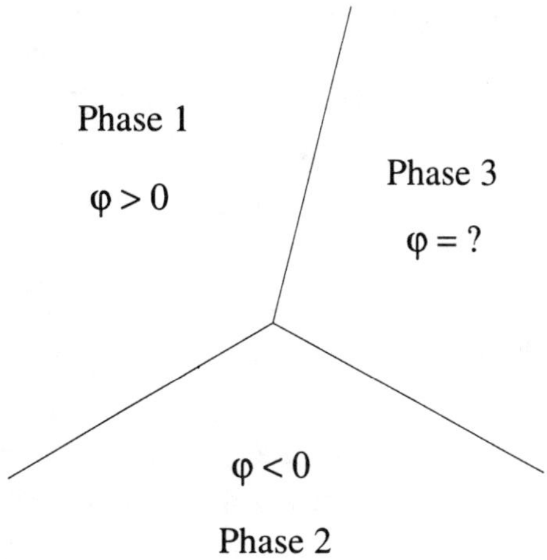

Figure 2.5: Triple junction requires more than one level set function.

build a single smooth function ϕ which can simultaneously represent all three interfaces between phases (See Figure 2.5). One obvious choice to correct this is to use three separate level set functions ϕ_i, with $\phi_i > 0$ in phase i, and $\phi_i < 0$ in the other phases.

While the use of multiple level set functions solves the problem of representation, additional constraints to couple the ϕ_i are required or else non-physical results can arise. One such problem occurs in interface flows where the motion of the interface is driven solely by surface tension. Without an additional constraint at the triple junction, the three level set functions will pull away from the triple junction leaving a middle region in which all three level set functions are negative indicating no phase exists. For more complicated flows, it is also possible, sometimes simply through numerical error, for multiple level set functions to be positive at a point indicating more than one phase at a single point.

Neither of these non-physical situations is acceptable, so attempts to apply the level set method to multi-phase flows have led to modifications that try to account for these problems. The key to a better scheme for handling multiphase flows using level set methods is to establish a mapping between the physical domain and the set of phases, where each point maps onto exactly one of the phases. The resulting mapping must then be coupled to the equations of motion so it is preserved during evolution in time.

2.4.3.1 Projection Method

Consider the problem of three phases lying in $\mathbf{R^d}$. For each phase i, define $\Omega_i \subset \mathbf{R^d}$ to be the region occupied by phase i, and define $\Gamma_i = \partial\Omega_i$, its boundary. The interface between phase i and phase j, $\Gamma_{ij} = \Gamma_i \cap \Gamma_j$ has dimension $d-1$, while a triple junction $\Gamma_{123} = \Gamma_1 \cap \Gamma_2 \cap \Gamma_3$, the intersection of three interfaces, has dimension, $d-2$.

At any given point $\mathbf{x}$, we define the vector $\boldsymbol{\phi}(\mathbf{x}) = (\phi_1(\mathbf{x}), \phi_2(\mathbf{x}), \phi_3(\mathbf{x})) \in \mathbf{R^3}$. where $\phi_i(\mathbf{x})$ is the signed distance to the interface Γ_i. From this construction, if $\mathbf{x}$ is in the ith phase, and letting $\mathbf{y} \in \Gamma_{ij}$ be the nearest boundary point to $\mathbf{x}$, then $\phi_i(\mathbf{x}) = -\phi_j(\mathbf{x}) = |\mathbf{x}-\mathbf{y}|$. The distances to boundaries of all phases other than i and j must be equal to or greater than $|\phi_i(\mathbf{x})|$, so that at any point $\mathbf{x}$ in the ith phase there is some $j \neq k$ such that,

$$\phi_i(\mathbf{x}) \geq 0 \tag{2.37}$$

$$\phi_j(\mathbf{x}) = -\phi_i(\mathbf{x}) \tag{2.38}$$

$$\phi_k(\mathbf{x}) \leq \phi_j(\mathbf{x}), \quad \text{for } k \neq i, j \tag{2.39}$$

These conditions were also identified in [34, 59, 45].

Equations (2.37)–(2.39) restrict the set of permissible values of $\boldsymbol{\phi}$ to points that lie in a two-dimensional manifold Π embedded in $\mathbf{R^3}$. This manifold consists of the union of three different pieces $\Pi_{ij} \subset \mathbf{R^3}$ that are sectors of two-hyperplanes, each labeled by a pair of distinct indices i, j and with $\Pi_{ij} \equiv \Pi_{ji}$. If $\boldsymbol{\phi}(\mathbf{x})$ satisfies (2.37)–(2.39) for some $i \neq j$, then $\boldsymbol{\phi}(\mathbf{x}) \in \Pi_{ij}$.

Ideally, the level set evolution equation would be rewritten to work with functions defined on the manifold Π. However, the manifold is not smooth, and it is difficult to remain on the manifold. Instead, a one-to-one relationship is established between Π and a two-dimensional plane. This two-dimensional plane will serve to connect the triples (ϕ_1, ϕ_2, ϕ_3) with points on the surface of Π.

There are many well defined maps from Π onto $\mathbf{R^2}$. The map described in [45] is piecewise linear, and treats all phases symmetrically. The three phase version is described here. To construct a map $\Psi : \Pi \to \mathbf{R^2}$, define the vector

$$\mathbf{n} = (1/\sqrt{n})(1, 1, \ldots, 1)_e, \tag{2.40}$$

and the hyperplane H orthogonal to $\mathbf{n}$. A basis $\{\mathbf{h}_1, \mathbf{h}_2\}$ for the hyperplane H

can be generated by projecting the first two basis functions in $\mathbf{R}^3$:

$$\mathbf{h}_1 = \frac{1}{\sqrt{6}}(2,-1,-1)^T \tag{2.41}$$

$$\mathbf{h}_2 = \frac{1}{\sqrt{2}}(0,1,-1)^T \tag{2.42}$$

Using this basis for elements $\psi \in H$, then a one-to-one mapping is established where the transformation from ϕ to ψ is:

$$\psi_1 = (2\phi_1 - \phi_2 - \phi_3)/\sqrt{6} \tag{2.43}$$

$$\psi_2 = (\phi_2 - \phi_3)/\sqrt{2} \tag{2.44}$$

and the inverse transformation is:

$$\theta_1 = 2\psi_1/\sqrt{6} \tag{2.45}$$

$$\theta_2 = -\psi_1/\sqrt{6} + \psi_2/\sqrt{2} \tag{2.46}$$

$$\theta_3 = -\psi_1/\sqrt{6} - \psi_2/\sqrt{2} \tag{2.47}$$

$$\phi_1 = (\theta_1 - \theta_2 - \theta_3 + \min(\theta_1,\theta_2,\theta_3))/2 \tag{2.48}$$

$$\phi_2 = (-\theta_1 + \theta_2 - \theta_3 + \min(\theta_1,\theta_2,\theta_3))/2 \tag{2.49}$$

$$\phi_3 = (-\theta_1 - \theta_2 + \theta_3 + \min(\theta_1,\theta_2,\theta_3))/2 \tag{2.50}$$

Note that the zero contour of ψ_2 contains Γ_{23}. By rotating the triple (ϕ_1,ϕ_2,ϕ_3), ψ_2 can also represent Γ_{ij} for any pair i, j. Thus, the level set method evolution can be written in terms of ψ_2 for each of the interfaces Γ_{ij}, and ψ_2 is a single level set function as is used for the basic level set method.

The modified level set method is now clear. Given a triple $\phi = (\phi_1,\phi_2,\phi_3)$, project ϕ onto H using (2.43), (2.44). Use the speed function for the Γ_{23} to evolve ψ_2 in time, then reverse the projection back into a triple ϕ using (2.45)–(2.50). In principle this projection procedure could be done at every grid point, but in practice it is only necessary for the grid points near the triple junction where the finite difference approximations would be affected. Further details about this method can be found in [45].

2.4.4 Elliptic Equations and the Extended Finite Element Method

The eXtended Finite Element Method (X-FEM) [35, 15, 54] is a numerical method to model internal (or external) boundaries without the need for the mesh to conform to these boundaries. The X-FEM is based on a standard Galerkin procedure, and uses the concept of partition of unity [33] to accommodate the internal boundaries in the discrete model. The partition of unity method [33] generalized finite element approximations by presenting a means to embed local solutions of boundary-value problems into the finite element approximation.

For a standard finite element approximation, consider a point $\mathbf{x}$ of $\mathbf{R^d}$ (d = 1, 2, 3) that lies inside a finite element e. Denote the nodal set $\mathbf{N} = \{n_1, n_2, \ldots, n_m\}$, where m is the number of nodes of element e. ($m = 2$ for a linear one-dimensional finite element, $m = 3$ for a constant-strain triangle, $m = 8$ for a tri-linear hexahedral element, etc.) The approximation for a vector-valued function $\mathbf{u}(\mathbf{x}) : \mathbf{R^d} \to \mathbf{R^d}$ assumes the form:

$$\mathbf{u}^h(\mathbf{x}) = \sum_{\substack{I \\ n_I \in \mathbf{N}}} \phi_I(\mathbf{x})\mathbf{u}_I, \quad (\mathbf{u}_I \in \mathbf{R^d}) \tag{2.51}$$

where the functions $\phi_I(\mathbf{x})$ are the finite element basis functions and the $\mathbf{u}_I$ are the weights.

The extended finite element method uses enrichment functions, extra basis functions which are sensitive to prescribed boundaries to capture the boundary conditions and improve the solution in the neighborhood of regions which would otherwise require greater spatial resolution. Considering again a point $\mathbf{x}$ of $\mathbf{R^d}$ (d = 1, 2, 3) that lies inside a finite element e. The enriched approximation for the function $\mathbf{u}(\mathbf{x}) : \mathbf{R^d} \to \mathbf{R^d}$ becomes

$$\mathbf{u}^h(\mathbf{x}) = \underbrace{\sum_{\substack{I \\ n_I \in \mathbf{N}}} \phi_I(\mathbf{x})\mathbf{u}_I}_{classical} + \underbrace{\sum_{\substack{J \\ n_J \in \mathbf{N}^g}} \phi_J(\mathbf{x})\psi(\mathbf{x})\mathbf{a}_J}_{enriched}, \quad (\mathbf{u}_I, \mathbf{a}_J \in \mathbf{R^d}) \tag{2.52}$$

where the nodal set $\mathbf{N}^g$ is defined as:

$$\mathbf{N}^g = \{n_J : n_J \in \mathbf{N},\ \omega_J \cap \Omega_g \neq \emptyset\}. \tag{2.53}$$

In the above equation, $\omega_J = \text{supp}(n_J)$ is the support of the nodal shape function $\phi_J(\mathbf{x})$, which consists of the union of all elements with n_J as one of its vertices, or in other words the union of elements in which $\phi_J(\mathbf{x})$ is non-zero. In addition, Ω_g is the domain associated with a geometric entity such as crack-tip [35], crack surface in 3-dimensions [54], or material interface [50, 28]. In general, the choice of the enrichment function $\psi(\mathbf{x})$ that appears in (2.52) depends on the geometry and the elliptic equation being solved.

To illustrate the effectiveness of this approach, consider the following simple example. Suppose we wish to solve the radial heat equation on an annulus given by

$$u_{rr} + \frac{1}{r}u_r = 0, \quad 0 < \epsilon \leq r < L \tag{2.54}$$

$$u_r(\epsilon) = -10, \quad u(L) = 0. \tag{2.55}$$

The exact solution is given by

$$u(r) = -10\epsilon \ln(r) + 10\epsilon \ln(L). \tag{2.56}$$

If we solve this equation for $\epsilon = 0.01$, $L = 9$ using a standard finite element method with linear elements and with nodes at $r = 0, \ldots, 9$, the solution for $\epsilon \leq r < 1$ is very unsatisfactory as shown in Fig. 2.6. However, by using a simple enrichment function $\psi_1(r) = \ln(r)$, and using this enrichment function on the first two nodes (located at $r = 0,\ 1$), dramatically better results are achieved (Fig. 2.6). Of course, refining the finite element mesh would also improve the results, but this requires remeshing as the interface (in this example the left boundary) moves. The X-FEM achieves this accuracy without remeshing.

The merits of coupling level sets to the extended finite element method was first explored in [50], and subsequently its advantages further realized in [52, 48, 36, 24, 28, 11]. The two methods make a natural pair of methods where:

1. Level sets provide greater ease and simplification in the representation of geometric interfaces.

2. The X-FEM, given the right enrichment functions, can very accurately compute solutions of elliptic equations which are often required for computing the interface velocity.

3. Geometric computations required for evaluating the enrichment functions (such as the normal or the distance to the interface) are readily computed from the level set function [52].

4. The nodes to be enriched are easily identified using the signed distance construction of the level set function[52, 48, 50].

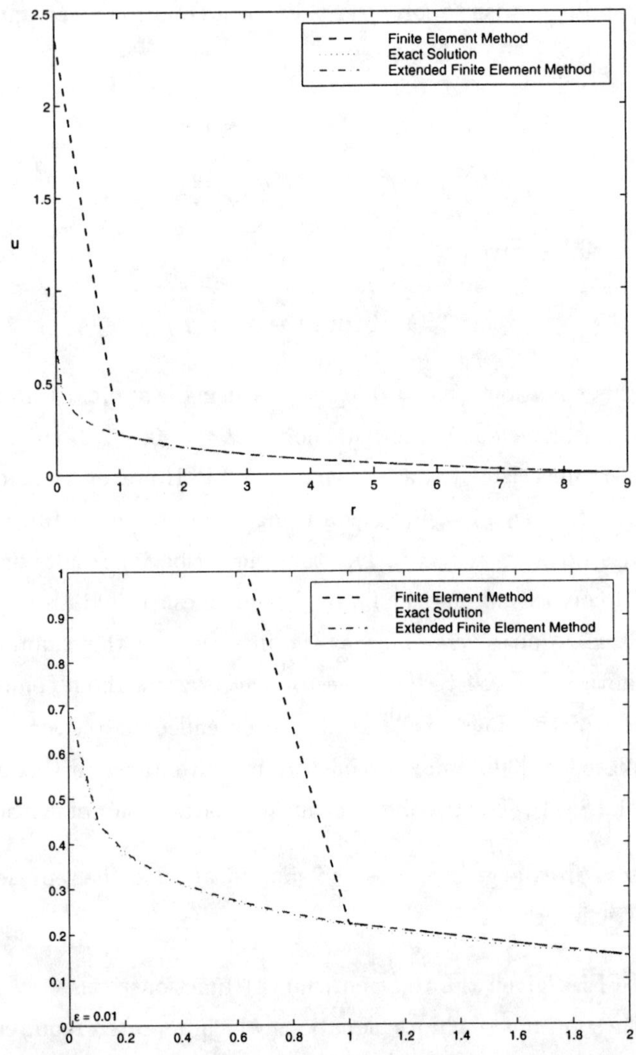

Figure 2.6: Solutions of the radial heat equation. (a) whole domain $\epsilon \leq r \leq L$; and (b) across first three nodes.

2.5 Applications of the Level Set Method

Once the basic level set method is assembled, there are many ways that the level set method can be applied to handle different applications. In this section, a number of different adaptations are described which illustrate the flexibility and power of the level set method.

2.5.1 Differential Geometry

The first applications of the level set method were directed primarily towards solving flows derived from the local geometry of the interface. These applications are the easiest for the level set method because the speed function F can be defined locally at any point of the domain, and curvature based flows are special in that they require no reinitialization or velocity extensions to remain stable.

2.5.1.1 Mean Curvature Flow

For speed $F = -\kappa$, we get the equation for mean curvature flow. The curvature κ may be determined from the level set function ϕ. For example, in three space dimensions the mean curvature is given by

$$\kappa = \frac{\begin{array}{r}\phi_{xx}(\phi_y^2+\phi_z^2)+\phi_{yy}(\phi_x^2+\phi_z^2)+\phi_{zz}(\phi_x^2+\phi_y^2)\\ -2(\phi_x\phi_y\phi_{xy}+\phi_y\phi_z\phi_{xz}+\phi_x\phi_z\phi_{xz})\end{array}}{2(\phi_x^2+\phi_y^2+\phi_z^2)^{3/2}} \tag{2.57}$$

Grayson [25] has shown that any non-intersecting closed curve must collapse smoothly to a circle; see also [21, 22, 23]. Consider the wound spiral traced out by

$$\gamma(0) = (0.1e^{(-10y(s))} - (0.1 - x(s))/20)(\cos(a(s)), \sin(a(s))) \tag{2.58}$$

$$a(s) = 25\tan^{-1}(10y(s)) \tag{2.59}$$

$$(x(s), y(s)) = ((0.1)\cos(2\pi s) + 0.1, (.05)\sin(2\pi s) + 0.1), s \in [0, 1]. \tag{2.60}$$

Figure 2.7 verifies Grayson's result with spiral unwrapping and eventually disappearing. The propagating curve vanishes when $\phi(x, y) > 0$ everywhere.

Grayson's Theorem does not hold for two-dimensional surfaces in $\mathbf{R}^3$. A well-known example is the collapse of a dumbbell, studied in [40]. A more dramatic and pronounced version is shown in Figure 2.8, which shows the

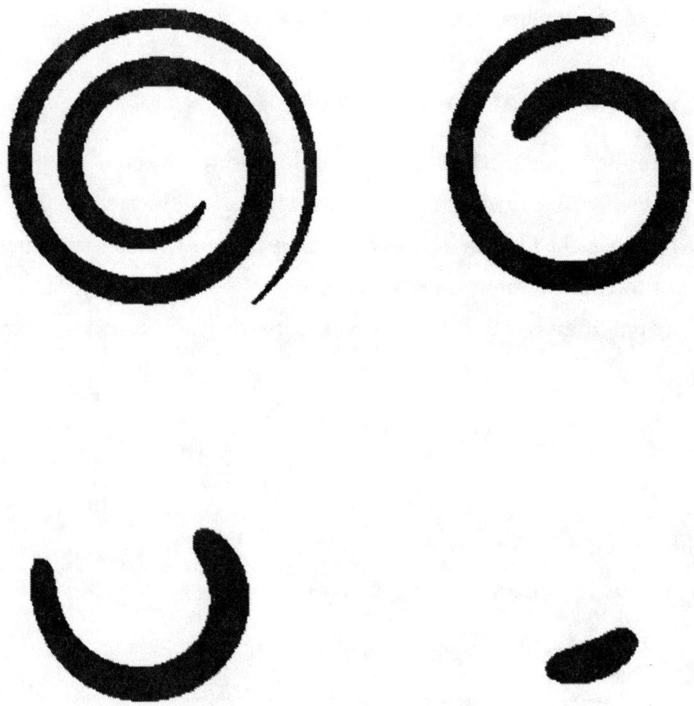

Figure 2.7: Collapsing 2-dimensional spiral

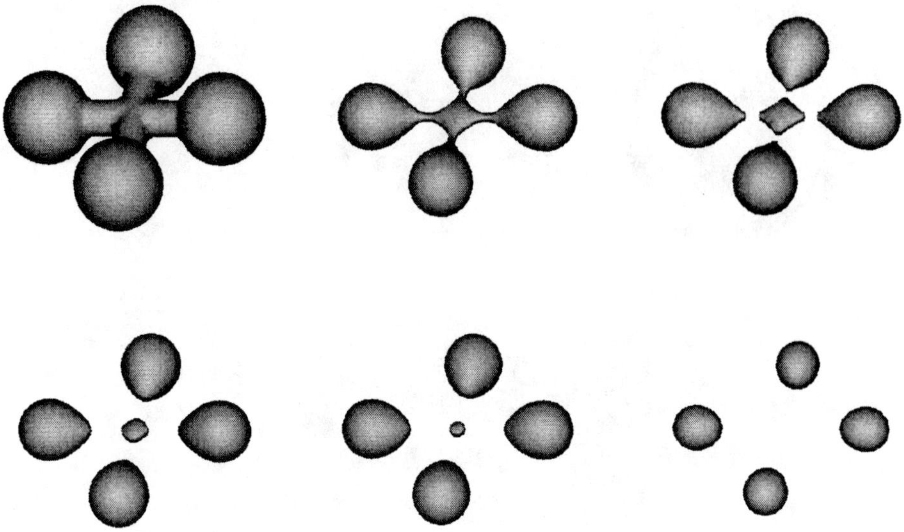

Figure 2.8: Collapse of a four-armed dumbbell

collapse of a four-armed dumbbell. A residual ball separates off in the center and collapses smoothly through a spherical shape to a point.

Finally, a three-dimensional version of the spiral collapsing under mean curvature is computed. The three-dimensional spiral hypersurface shown in Figure 2.9 is actually hollow on the inside; the opening on the right end extends all the way through the object to the leftmost tip. The inner boundary of the spiral hypersurface is only a short thickness away from the outer boundary. As the hypersurface collapses under its mean curvature, the inner sleeve shrinks faster than the outer sleeve, and withdraws to the rightmost edge before the outer sleeve collapses around it.

2.5.1.2 Minimal Surfaces

The curvature flow algorithm can also be adapted to compute minimal surfaces. Consider a closed curve $\Gamma(s)$ in R^3; $\Gamma : [0,1] \rightarrow R^3$. The goal is to construct a membrane with boundary Γ and mean curvature zero. This can be accomplished by a type of relaxation method. Given a surface S spanning Γ, let S evolve by mean curvature flow until it reaches steady state. For a level set method implementation of this idea, the challenge is to ensure that

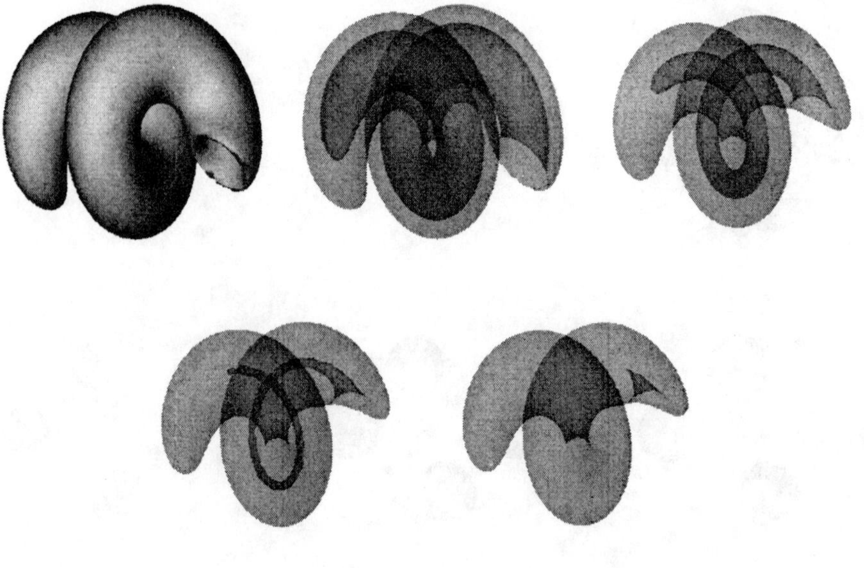

Figure 2.9: Collapse of a twisted testtube

the evolving zero level set always remains attached to the boundary Γ. This is accomplished by creating a set of intricate boundary conditions on those grid points closest to the wire frame linking together the neighboring values of ϕ to force $\phi = 0$ through Γ. The details of the construction of these boundary conditions are beyond the scope of this book. A complete description can be found in [4].

There is another issue that comes into play in the evolution of the level set function ϕ towards a minimal surface. By the above set of boundary conditions, only the zero level set $\phi = 0$ is constrained. This leads to stability problems at the boundary due to the development of a rapidly varying gradient near the boundary. Reinitialization is used restore a uniform $||\nabla\phi|| = 1$ everywhere.

As a test example, the minimal surface spanning two rings has an exact solution given by the catenoid

$$r(x) = a\cosh(x/a) \tag{2.61}$$

where $r(x)$ is the radius of the catenoid at a point x along the x axis, and a is the radius of the catenoid at the center point $x = 0$. Suppose that the boundary consists of two rings of radius R located at $\pm b$ on the x-axis. Then the parameter a is determined from the expression

$$R = a\cosh(b/a). \tag{2.62}$$

If there is no real value of a which solves this expression, then a catenoid solution between the rings does not exist.

In Figure 2.10, the minimal surface spanning two rings each of radius 0.5 and at positions $x = \pm.277259$ is computed. A cylinder spanning the two rings is taken as the initial level set $\phi = 0$. The final shape is shown from several different angles. Next, in Figure 2.11, this same problem is computed, but the rings are placed far enough apart so that a catenoid solution cannot exist. Starting with a cylinder as the initial surface, the evolution of this cylinder is computed as it collapses under mean curvature while remaining attached to the two wire frames. As the surface evolves, the middle pinches off and the surface splits into two surfaces, each of which quickly collapses into a disk. The final shape of a disk spanning each ring is indeed a minimal surface for this problem. This example illustrates one of the virtues of the level set method. No special cutting or *ad hoc* decisions are employed to decide when to break the surface. Instead the characterization of the zero level set as but one member of a family of flowing surfaces allows this smooth transition.

More examples of minimal surfaces are given in [4].

2.5.1.3 Extensions to Surfaces of Prescribed Curvature

The above technique can be extended to produce surfaces of prescribed mean curvature. To do so, the speed function used to produce minimal surfaces is replaced with the speed function $F = A(\mathbf{x}) - \kappa$. For this computation, the term $A(\mathbf{x})$ is taken as the advective component of the speed function, F_{adv} in Eqn. 2.32, while the parabolic term κ is the diffusive component, F_{diff}.

Using the two ring "catenoid" problem as a guide, in Figure 2.12 this technique is used to compute the surface of constant curvature spanning the two rings. In each case, the initial shape is the cylinder spanned by the rings. The final computed shapes for a variety of different mean curvatures are shown. In Figure 2.12a, a surface of mean curvature 2.50 spanning the rings is given: the rings are located a distance .61 apart and have diameter 1.0. The resulting surface bulges out to fit against the two rings. In Figure 2.12b, a surface of mean curvature 1.0 is found, which corresponds to the initial surface. In Figure 2.12c,

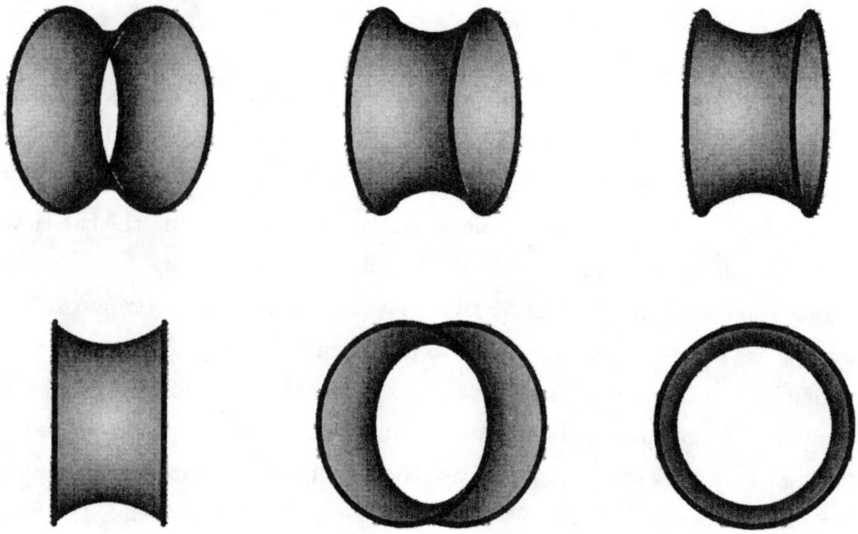

Figure 2.10: Euler's catenoid minimal surface

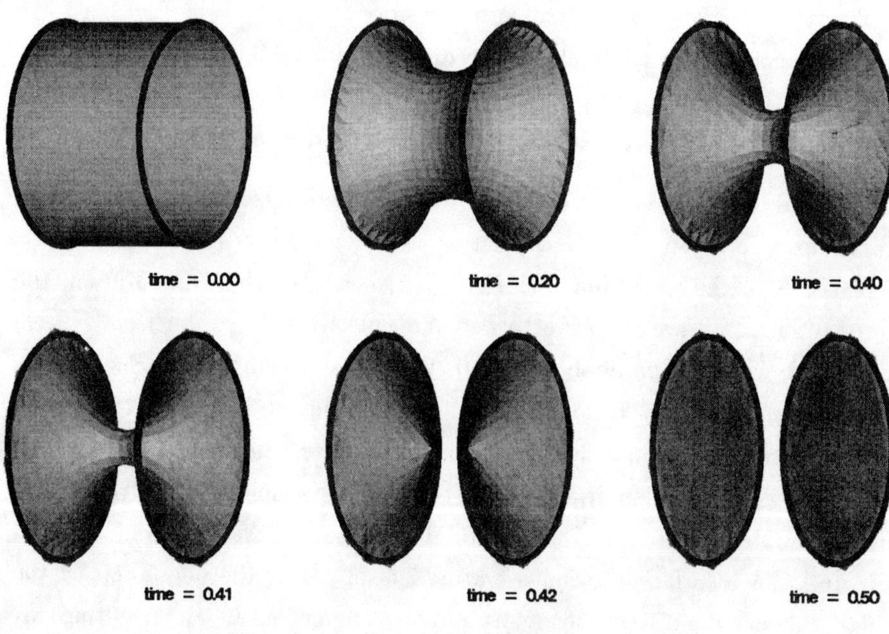

Figure 2.11: Splitting catenoid evolution

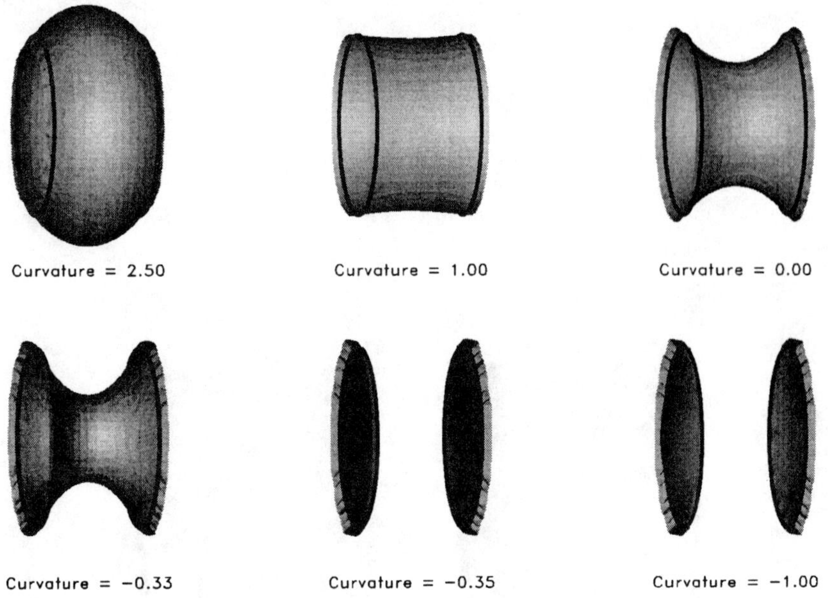

Figure 2.12: Constant mean curvature surfaces with fixed boundary

the catenoid surface of mean curvature 0 is given. The value of -0.33 is a value close to the breaking point as shown in Figure 2.12d. In Figure 2.12e, a mean curvature value of -0.35 is prescribed, causing the initial bounding cylinder to collapse onto the two rings and bulge out slightly. Finally, in Figure 2.12f, bowing out disks corresponding to surfaces of mean curvature -1 are shown.

For a non-constant, prescribed mean curvature surface, the surface spanning two rings with curvature at any point x along the x-axis given by $10\cos(10x)$ is constructed. The relaxation of the surface to the prescribed curvature is shown in Figure 2.13.

2.5.1.4 Self Similar Surfaces of Mean Curvature Flow

Without an analog of Grayson's theorem for higher dimensions, Self-similar solutions of motion by mean curvature are an important component in the current research of the singularities in that motion. There appears to be a link between singularities in motion by mean curvature and self-similar shapes. The best result showing the link between self-similarity and singularity is by Huisken [27] where he gives conditions when a surface evolving under mean curvature flow approaches a self-similar surface at a point of singularity.

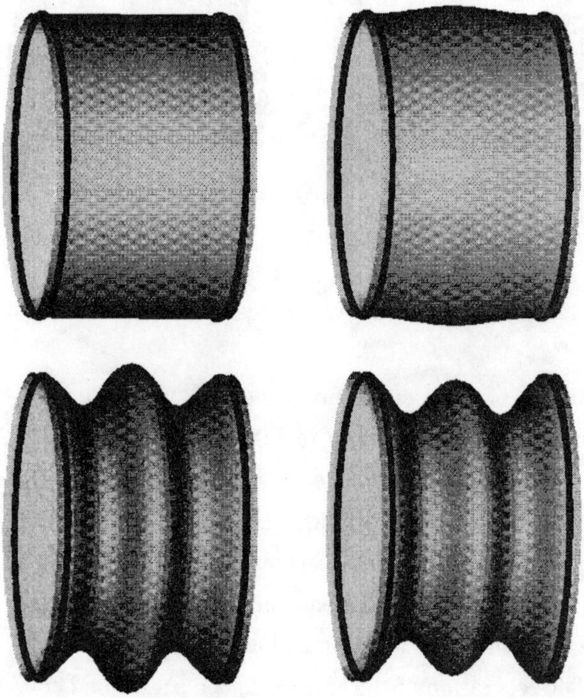

Figure 2.13: Non-constant prescribed curvature surface

At present, very few examples of two-dimensional embedded self-similar solutions for motion by mean curvature are proven to exist, all of them being surfaces of revolution. Here, the level set method is used to compute approximations of other self-similar solutions. The level set method is ideally suited for solving this problem because we can evolve a continuous family of surfaces simultaneously, each evolving by mean curvature flow. We then need a way to select the particular level set which is approaching a self-similar surface. The way this is accomplished is described through the example of finding a self-similar torus.

2.5.1.5 An Example: The Self-Similar Torus

We begin by building a parameterized family of nested torii. Let $C = \{\mathbf{x} = (x_1, x_2, x_3) \in R^3 : x_1^2 + x_2^2 = 1, x_3 = 0\}$ and define $S_\lambda(0) = \{\mathbf{x} \in R^3 : \text{dist}(\mathbf{x}, C) = \lambda\}$. Thus, $S_\lambda(0)$ is a one-dimensional family of torii parameterized by λ. Note that $\lambda = 0$ corresponds to a circle (a torus with outer radius 0), while for $\lambda > 1$, the center of the torus no longer exists, and the surface is topologically a ball. Let $S_\lambda(t)$ be the evolution of the initial surface $S_\lambda(0)$ by mean curvature flow at time t. Denote T_λ to be the time at which $S_\lambda(t)$ develops a singularity and is no longer a torus.

Next, define a ratio function $\rho : S_\lambda(t) \to R$, $\rho(S_\lambda(t)) = m_2/m_1$, where m_2 is the maximum height of the torus in the z direction and m_1 is the innermost radius of the torus as shown in Figure 2.14. A self-similar torus $S_{\lambda_0}(t)$ will be

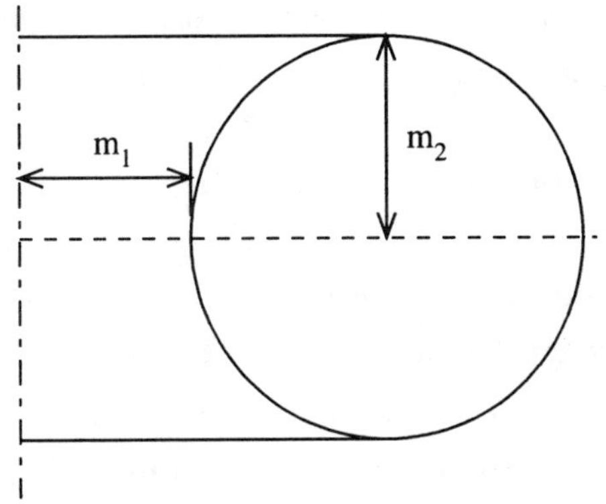

Figure 2.14: Measurements of a torus for computing ρ.

generated by the torus which has the property that $\frac{d}{dt}\rho(S_{\lambda_0}(t)) = 0$ as $t \to T_\lambda$.

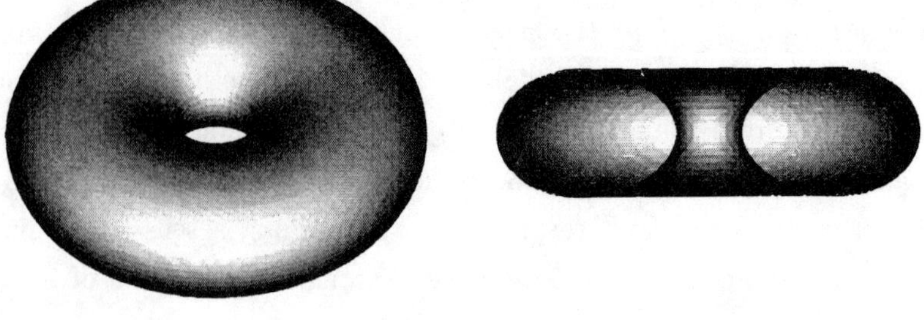

Figure 2.15: Pictures of the torus self-similar solution

Our goal then, is to locate the special trajectory $S_{\lambda_0}(t)$.

The level set method offers a unique way to solve this problem because we are simultaneously evolving the continuous family of surfaces for a range of λ, and the function ρ can be computed for any of the λ.

The self-similar torus will not take its final shape until it approaches singularity. Therefore, we must continually rescale so that the torus corresponding to λ_0 can be resolved. To accomplish this, the mean curvature flow evolution equation

$$\phi_t = \kappa \|\nabla \phi\| \tag{2.63}$$

is rewritten using a time-dependent spatial rescaling factor $\sigma(t)$ and an additional level set picking function $L(t)$. This is done by replacing ϕ with

$$\psi(x,t) = \phi(\sigma(t)x, t)/\sigma^2(t) - L(t). \tag{2.64}$$

The function $\sigma(t)$ is designed so that the zero level set of ψ remains a constant volume, and the function $L(t)$ uses ρ to give a best approximation for λ_0.

Applying this technique, a self-similar torus shape is generated, it is depicted in Figure 2.15. More shapes can be generated using this technique, the key is that enough symmetry be in the surfaces that a single function ρ can be used to parameterize the family of surfaces. More self-similar shapes are depicted in Figures 2.16, 2.17. Additional surfaces, and a complete description of the algorithm can be found in [5].

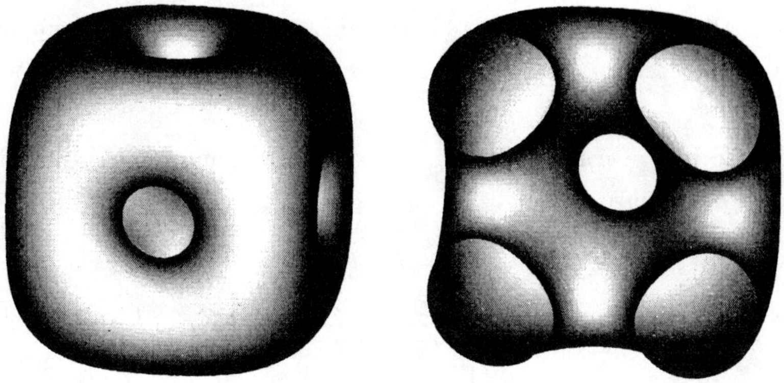

Figure 2.16: Pictures of the cube self-similar solution

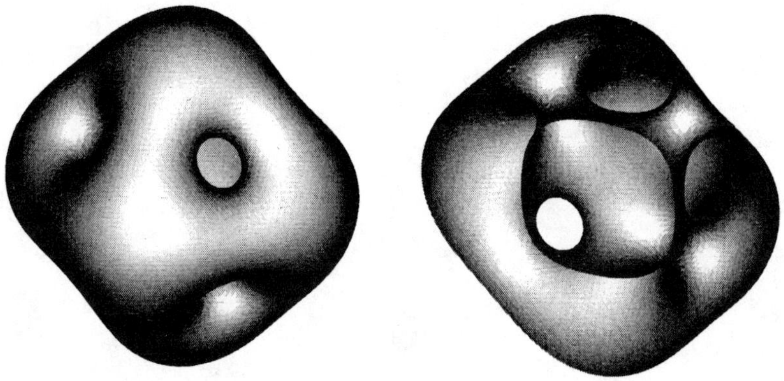

Figure 2.17: Self-similar octahedron surface

2.5.1.6 Laplacian of Curvature Flow

In addition to mean curvature flow, other curvature dependent flows can be modelled using the level set method. For example, in [10], the speed function $F = \kappa_{ss}$, the surface Laplacian of curvature is used. This flow is important in material science applications where it corresponds to surface diffusion of a solid.

Like the case of mean curvature flow, the speed function F can again be generated directly from the level set function ϕ. In this case,

$$F = -\kappa_{ss} = -\frac{\kappa_{xx}\phi_y^2 - 2\kappa_{xy}\phi_x\phi_y + \kappa_{yy}\phi_x^2}{\phi_x^2 + \phi_y^2} - \frac{(\kappa_x\phi_x + \kappa_y\phi_y)\kappa}{\sqrt{\phi_x^2 + \phi_y^2}} \tag{2.65}$$

One can see from this expression that κ_{ss} is a non-linear term involving up to four derivatives of the function ϕ. An example of this flow is depicted in Figures 2.18. In another example, Figure 2.19, it is shown how an initially con-

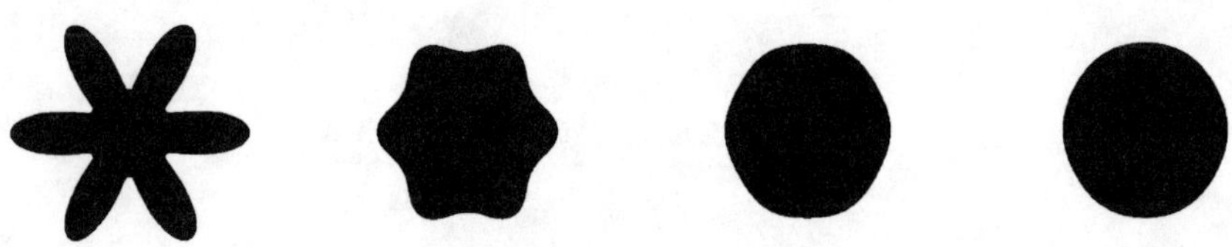

Figure 2.18: Evolution of star shape.

vex oval becomes non-convex before relaxing to a circle. Additional examples,

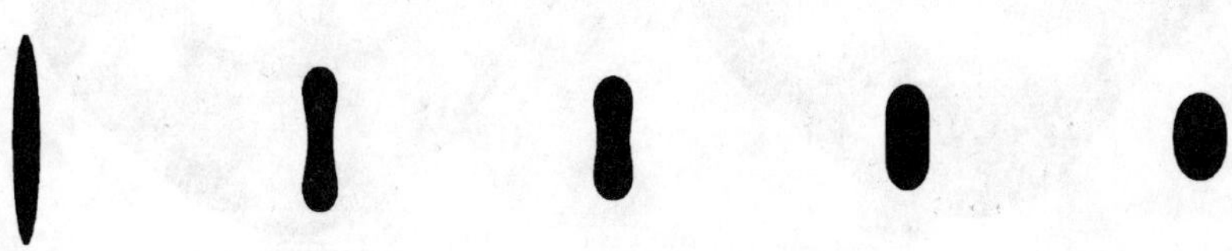

Figure 2.19: Evolution of oval shape.

including anisotropic surface diffusion, and the details of the implementation can be found in [10].

2.5.1.7 Linearized Laplacian of Curvature

Evolution by the surface Lapacian of curvature is important in many models of materials, but the resulting fourth-order partial differential equation can be exceedingly expensive to compute. In an effort to reduce the computational cost, while retaining the basic nature of the flow, a linearized version of the flow was developed in [12].

If the surface is near equilibrium, then the speed function in Equation (2.65) can be linearized resulting in the level set evolution equation

$$\phi_t = -\phi_{xxxx} - 2\phi_{xxyy} - \phi_{yyyy} + \frac{1}{R^3}. \tag{2.66}$$

where R is a constant given by the radius of the equilibrium shape. Since the flow is area preserving, R can be computed from the current interface location by computing the area A within the curve: $R = \sqrt{A/\pi}$. This equation can now be solved using a standard implicit time-stepping method. Figure 2.20 compares this linearized approach with the exact solution.

2.5.1.8 Gaussian Curvature Flow

For two-dimensional surfaces, there is an alternative measure of surface curvature called Gaussian curvature. While mean curvature is the average of the two principle curvatures, Gaussian curvature is the product of the two curvatures and is also an invariant of the manifold. The problem with Gaussian curvature is that the flow is unstable when the two principle curvatures have opposite sign, i.e. Gaussian curvature is negative. For this reason, this flow is only appropriate for convex bodies. For this flow, the speed function is given by

$$F = \kappa_{\text{Gauss}} = \frac{\begin{array}{l}\phi_x^2(\phi_{yy}\phi_{zz} - \phi_{yz}^2) + \phi_y^2(\phi_{xx}\phi_{zz} - \phi_{xz}^2) + \phi_z^2(\phi_{xx}\phi_{yy} - \phi_{xy}^2) \\ \quad + 2[\phi_x\phi_y(\phi_{xz}\phi_{yz} - \phi_{xy}\phi_{zz}) + \phi_y\phi_z(\phi_{xy}\phi_{xz} - \phi_{yz}\phi_{xx}) \\ \quad + \phi_x\phi_z(\phi_{xy}\phi_{yz} - \phi_{xz}\phi_{yy})]\end{array}}{(\phi_z^2 + \phi_y^2 + \phi_x^2)^2} \tag{2.67}$$

Another interesting observation about Gaussian curvature flow is that a non-concave surface with a region that is flat, i.e. both principle curvatures are zero, will remain flat for a finite amount of time [8]. This is different from mean curvature flow where the flat region becomes strictly convex instantly.

To illustrate the finite waiting time effects for Gauss curvature flows the level set numerical method was used to evolve two initial two-dimensional shapes

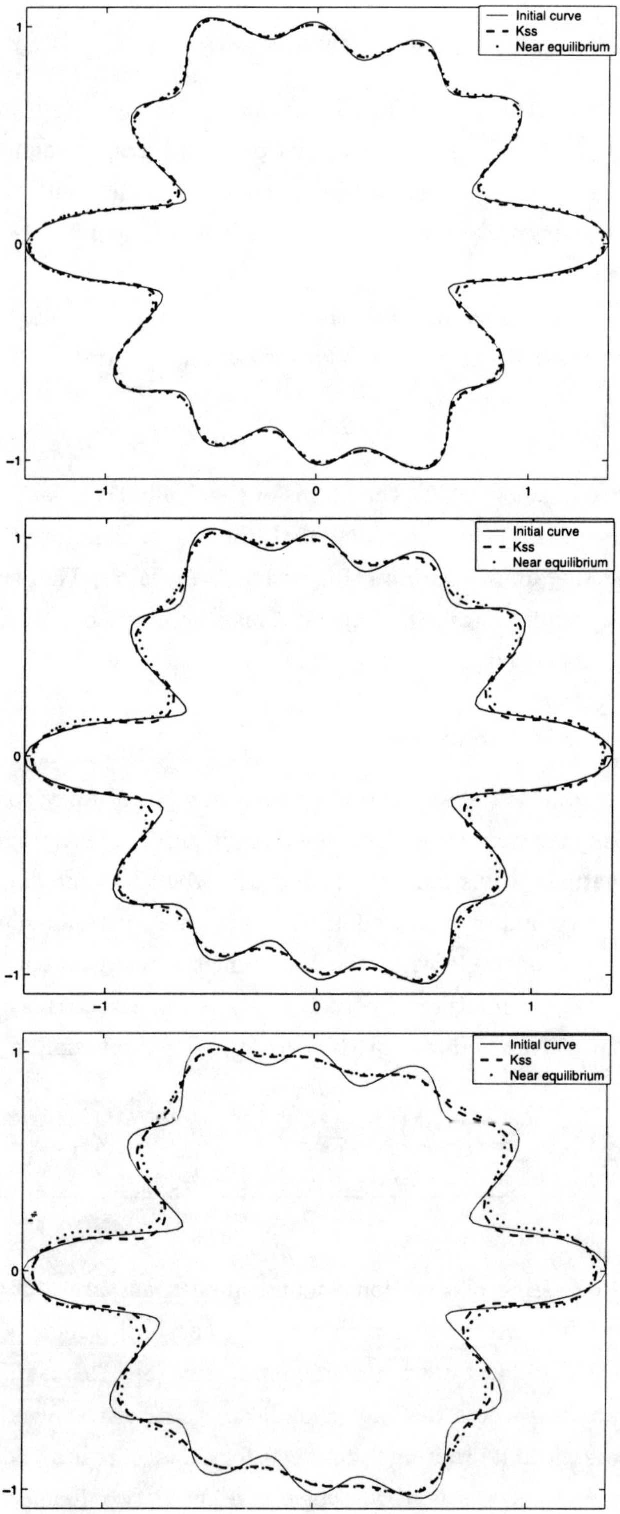

Figure 2.20: Comparison of a random small perturbation at different times

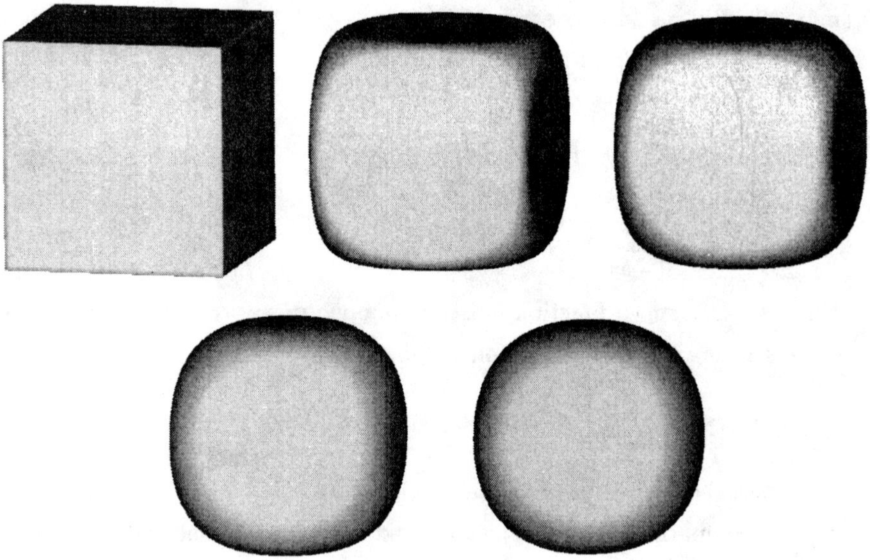

Figure 2.21: Collapse of a cube under Gauss curvature flow

with flat regions to illustrate how the flat regions remain flat for finite time. The first example is the evolution of a cube. In figure 2.21, the evolution of the cube surface shows the delayed rounding of the flat sides.

2.5.1.9 Geodesic Curvature Flow

The curvature flow algorithm can be generalized to more complicated two-dimensional spaces. For example, we may let the level set function ϕ be defined on a differentiable 2-manifold in R^3 with speed depending on geodesic curvature. By restricting the level set function ϕ to coordinate patches, it is possible to study single curves on non-simply connected manifolds, e.g. a torus. The fixed boundary condition techniques for minimal surfaces can also be applied here. In this case, a curve with fixed endpoints should flow towards a geodesic of the manifold, i.e. a curve with constant geodesic curvature zero.

First, assume the manifold M is given by $M = f^{-1}(0)$, where $f : R^3 \to R$. We break the manifold into a collection of coordinate maps, $\{(U_i, \pi_i)\}$ such that $M = \cup_i U_i$, each set U_i is simply connected, and $\pi_i : U_i \to V_i \subset R^2$ is a bijection. The computing is done on the collection of sets $V_i = \pi_i(U_i)$. We define the function $\Phi_i : V_i \to R$ by $\Phi_i(x,t) = \phi(\pi_i^{-1}(x), t)$, so that $\phi(x,t)|_{U_i} =$

$\Phi_i(\pi_i(x), t)$. Within this construction, the geodesic curvature of a level curve of ϕ defined on M is given by

$$\kappa_g = \frac{[N \times \tau] \cdot n}{1 - (n \cdot N)^2} \left\{ \tau \cdot \left[\left(\frac{n \cdot N}{\|\nabla f\|} \nabla^2 f - \frac{1}{\|\nabla \phi\|} \nabla^2 \phi \right) \cdot \tau \right] \right\} \tag{2.68}$$

where

$$n = \frac{\nabla \phi}{\|\nabla \phi\|}, \quad N = \frac{\nabla f}{\|\nabla f\|}, \text{ and } \quad \tau = \frac{\nabla f \times \nabla \phi}{\|\nabla f \times \nabla \phi\|}. \tag{2.69}$$

However, this speed function must be mapped down to each of the coordinate maps where the speed function becomes

$$\tilde{F}(\kappa_g) = F(\kappa_g) D\pi_i(v) \cdot \nabla \Phi_i / \|\nabla \Phi_i\|, \tag{2.70}$$

where $D\pi_i$ is the derivative of the projection map π_i.

Special compatibility conditions are used to make sure the overlap regions between the coordinate patches agree on the location of the interface. However, it is useful to note that the functions Φ_i do not need to agree on the sign of the function so long as the compatibility conditions adjust for the difference in sign. This allows for the evolution of a curve on a torus which wraps through the center of the torus. This would not be possible without breaking down the torus into coordinate patches which allow for an artificial change of sign in the overlap regions.

As an example of how this coordinate patch system works, Figure 2.22 shows a single curve flowing on a torus. This type of flow would not be possible without the coordinate patch system because there is no positive and negative side of the curve, i.e. the curve does not separate the torus into two distinct pieces.

By using the coordinate patches to essentially unhinge the sides of a cube, flows on a flat-sided cube can also be computed. To see that this is correct, the flow on a sharp-edged cube is compared with others with varying radii of curvature on each edge and corner to see that they agree in the motion of the curve (Figures 2.23–2.26).

Additional examples of surfaces and flows can be found in [9]

2.5.2 Multi-Phase Flow

An obvious application for use of the triple junction projection method described in Section 2.4.3 is to model multi-phase incompressible fluid flow [46,

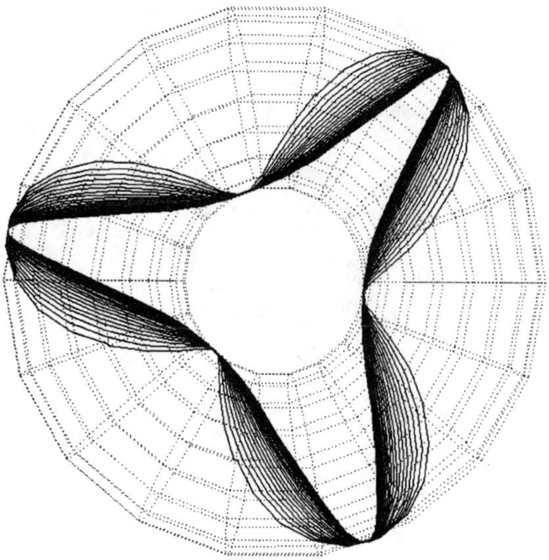

Figure 2.22: A single curve flowing on a torus

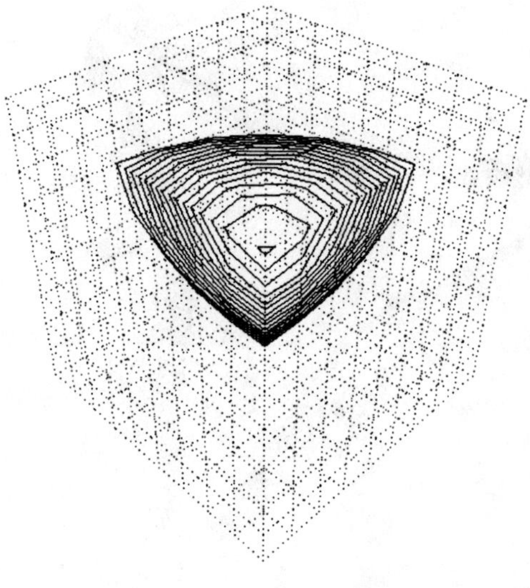

Figure 2.23: A single loop flowing on a cube with orthogonal edges

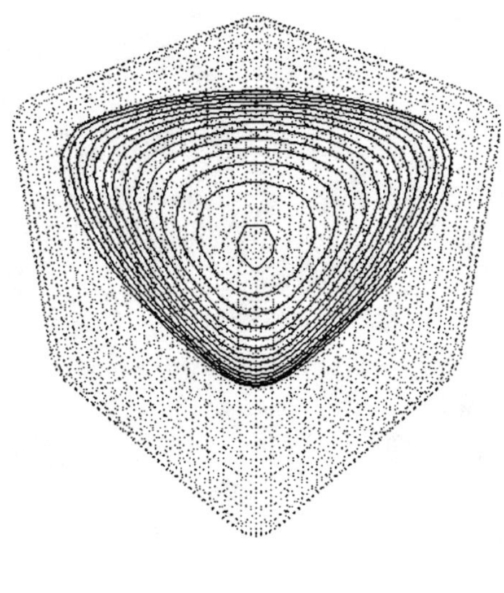

Figure 2.24: A single loop flowing on a cube with large rounded edges

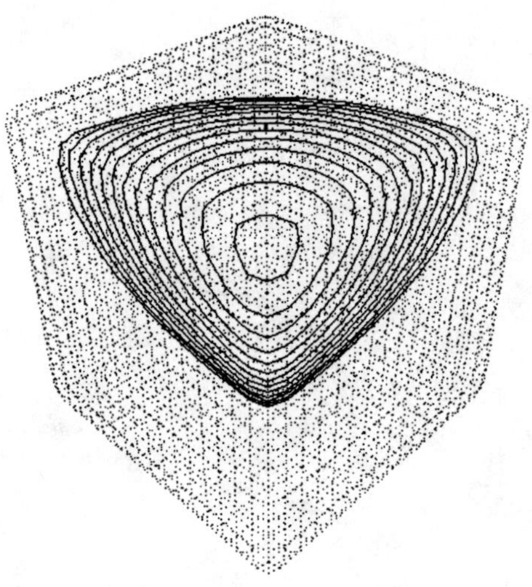

Figure 2.25: A single loop flowing on a cube with medium rounded edges

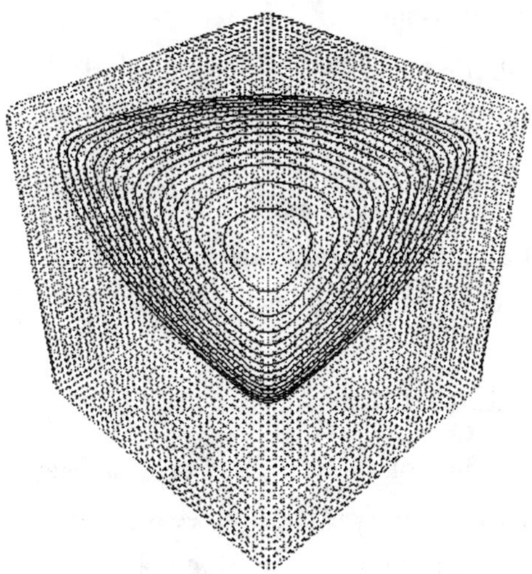

Figure 2.26: A single loop flowing on a cube with small rounded edges

45]. In this application, each fluid phase is represented by a level set function ϕ_i, and the speed function is derived from solving the incompressible Navier-Stokes equations with body forces derived from the inter-phase surface tension:

$$\frac{\partial \mathbf{u}}{\partial t} = -\nabla p - \mathbf{u} \cdot \nabla \mathbf{u} + \frac{1}{Re}\nabla^2 \mathbf{u} - \sum_{i=1}^{n} w_i \kappa(\phi_i) \nabla H(\phi_i) \tag{2.71}$$

$$\nabla \cdot \mathbf{u} = 0 \tag{2.72}$$

where Re is the Reynolds number, the w_i are such that the the Weber number for the i-j interface surface tension is given by $1/We_{ij} = w_i + w_j$, and H is the Heaviside function

Once the fluid velocity $\mathbf{u}$ is computed, a velocity extension is used so that the interface motion remains stable. The extended velocity is then used to advance the level set functions.

Figure 2.27 illustrates an example where a relatively high surface tension (between the middle drop and the bottom fluid) compared to the other surface tensions results in entrainment of the drop into the upper fluid where the surface tension is much lower. The method generalizes nicely to higher spatial dimensions without significant modification. In Figure 2.28, two drops in a shear flow are brought together and stick.

2.5.3 Ostwald Ripening

To model Ostwald ripening of a multi-tiered crystal facet, many level set functions are combined, each representing a layer of atoms on the crystal [6]. A diagram of the relationship between the single atomic layer surface structure and the level set functions are shown in Figure 2.29. The ith layer of the crystal surface is represented by a level set function ϕ_i, and the discrete height of the exposed surface corresponds to the highest index i such that $\phi_i \geq 0$. The collection of step edges are then given by the union of all the zero level sets.

On the open terraces, there is a density of adatoms, atoms which are freely diffusing on the crystal surface. The density ρ of the adatoms is computed via a system of ellpitic equations for each atomic layer given by

$$\Delta \rho(x) = 0, \; x \in \Phi \tag{2.73}$$

$$D\frac{\partial \rho}{\partial n} = -K(\rho_r^{\text{eq}} - \rho), \; x \in \Gamma^+ \tag{2.74}$$

$$D\frac{\partial \rho}{\partial n} = -\alpha \rho, \; x \in \Gamma^-. \tag{2.75}$$

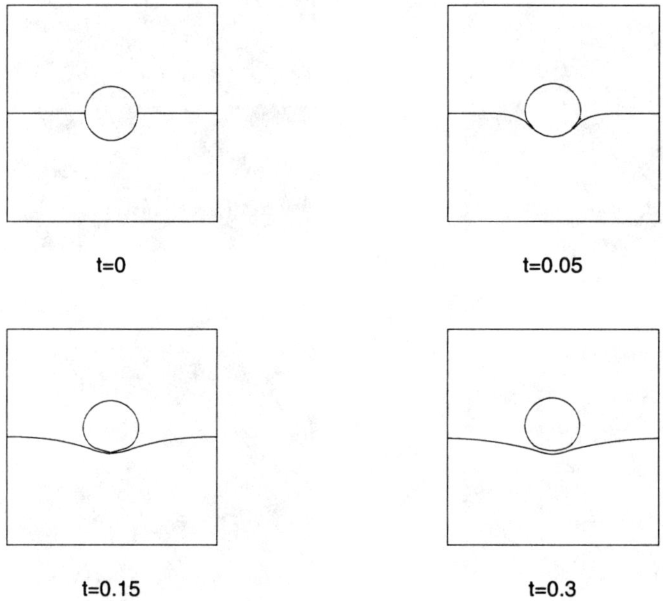

Figure 2.27: Time sequence of a droplet leaving an interface under surface tension forces. $w_{12} = w_{13} = 1, w_{23} = 10$

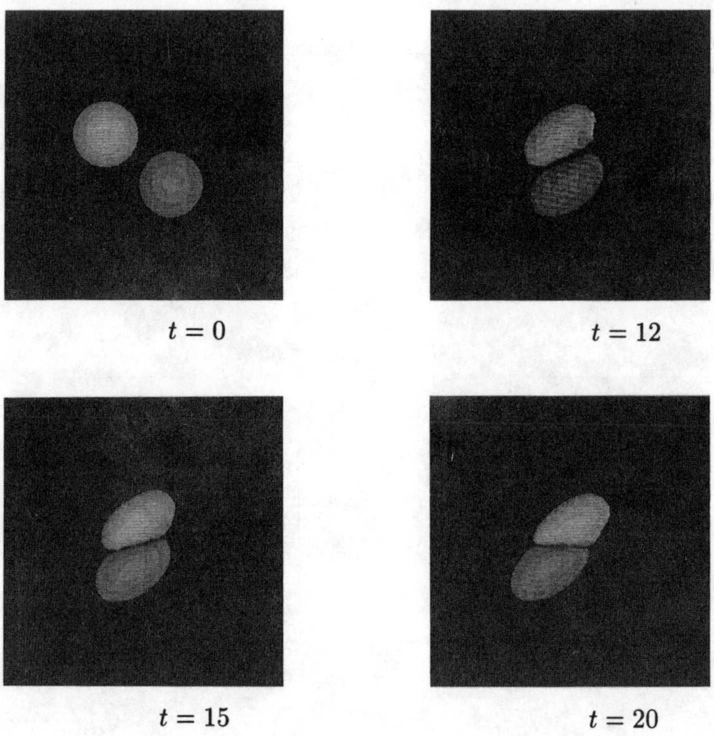

Figure 2.28: Time sequence of droplets colliding in 3D. $w_{12} = w_{13} = w_{23}$ where the droplets are phases 2 and 3 and the external fluid is phase 1.

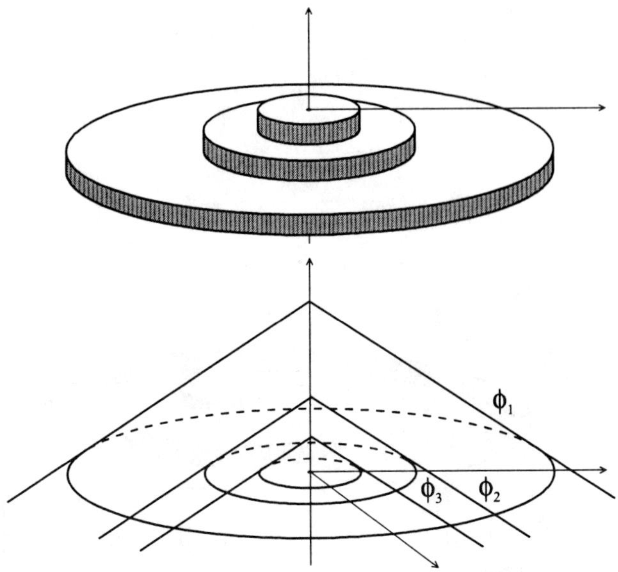

Figure 2.29: Level set representation of single atomic layer islands

where D is the surface diffusion rate, K is an attachment/detachment rate, ρ_r^{eq} is a curvature dependent equilibrium density constant, and α is the Ehrlich barrier step edge rate (the rate at which adatoms step down from one layer to the next lower). The two boundaries $\Gamma^{\pm}$ correspond to whether the open region is bounded by an up-step (+) or a down-step (−). An illustration of this structure is shown in Figure 2.30. Finally, the motion of the step edges (the zero level sets of the level set functions ϕ_i) is determined by the net flux. At a point x on the boundary, the net flux is given by the sum of the flux from below and above, thus

$$F(x) = -D\left(\frac{\partial \rho^-}{\partial n}(x) + \frac{\partial \rho^+}{\partial n}(x)\right) \tag{2.76}$$

$$= K(\rho_r^{\text{eq}}(x) - \rho^-(x)) + \alpha\rho^+(x) \tag{2.77}$$

where the + indicates the adatom density on the upper side of the step edge and the − indicates the adatom density of the lower side of the step edge. This is the front speed which is used to evolve the level set method.

It is worth noting that the solution of the elliptic equations (2.76) was done using a finite element boundary conforming method [6]. This predated the more recent development of the extended finite element method, but would

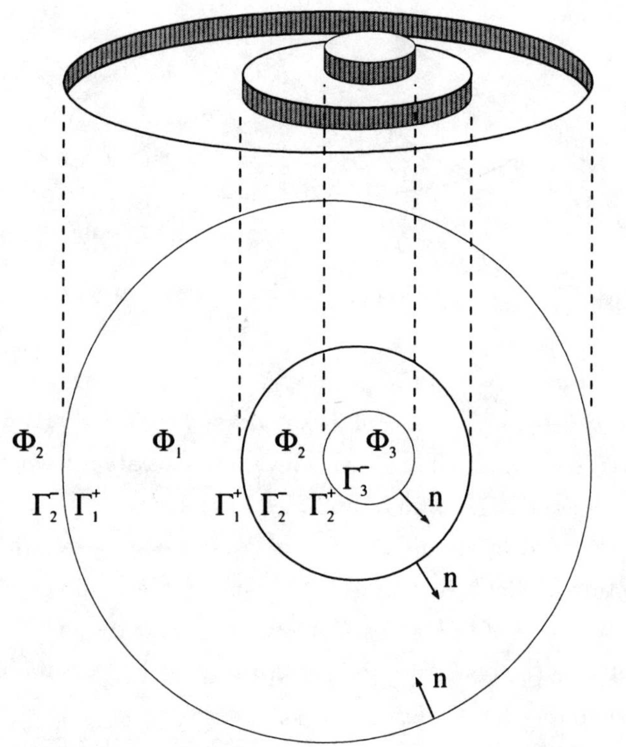

Figure 2.30: Illustration of the decomposition of the domain

be an ideal candidate for application of that technique. The first coupling of the level set method with the extended finite element method is described in Section 2.5.4.

For comparison purposes, the computed solution is compared with experimental data as shown in Figure 2.31. The experimental images are shown in the left column and our corresponding computed solution is in the right column. Note that our computed solution correctly predicts the expansion of a denuded zone around the larger islands. The fastest islands to decay are predicted to be the ones which are relatively small and begin near a much larger island. This leaves the larger islands gradually expanding a denuded zone around them as seen in the final image.

2.5.4 Crack Propagation

The coupling of the extended finite element method with the level set method is a recent development which has tremendous potential for many applications. More applications of this combination are certain to emerge as it gains prominence. The first application of this combination was used to solve problems in crack propagation. In this section, two such applications are presented.

2.5.4.1 One-Dimensional Cracks

For a one-dimensional crack, the crack is a segment embedded in a two-dimensional object as simple as a metal plate or as complicated as the surface of an airplane wing. The metal plate constitutes the domain Ω of the problem with boundary Γ. The boundary Γ is subdivided into four parts, Γ_u, Γ_t, and $\Gamma_c^{\pm}$. The displacement of the plate itself is prescribed on Γ_u, and the traction is prescribed on Γ_t. These are determined on the external boundary of the domain Ω. The crack surface is an additional internal boundary inside Ω. The crack surface is modelled as two coincident surfaces Γ_c^+, Γ_c^- and are assumed to be traction free. The domain Ω and its boundary Γ are illustrated in Figure (2.32).

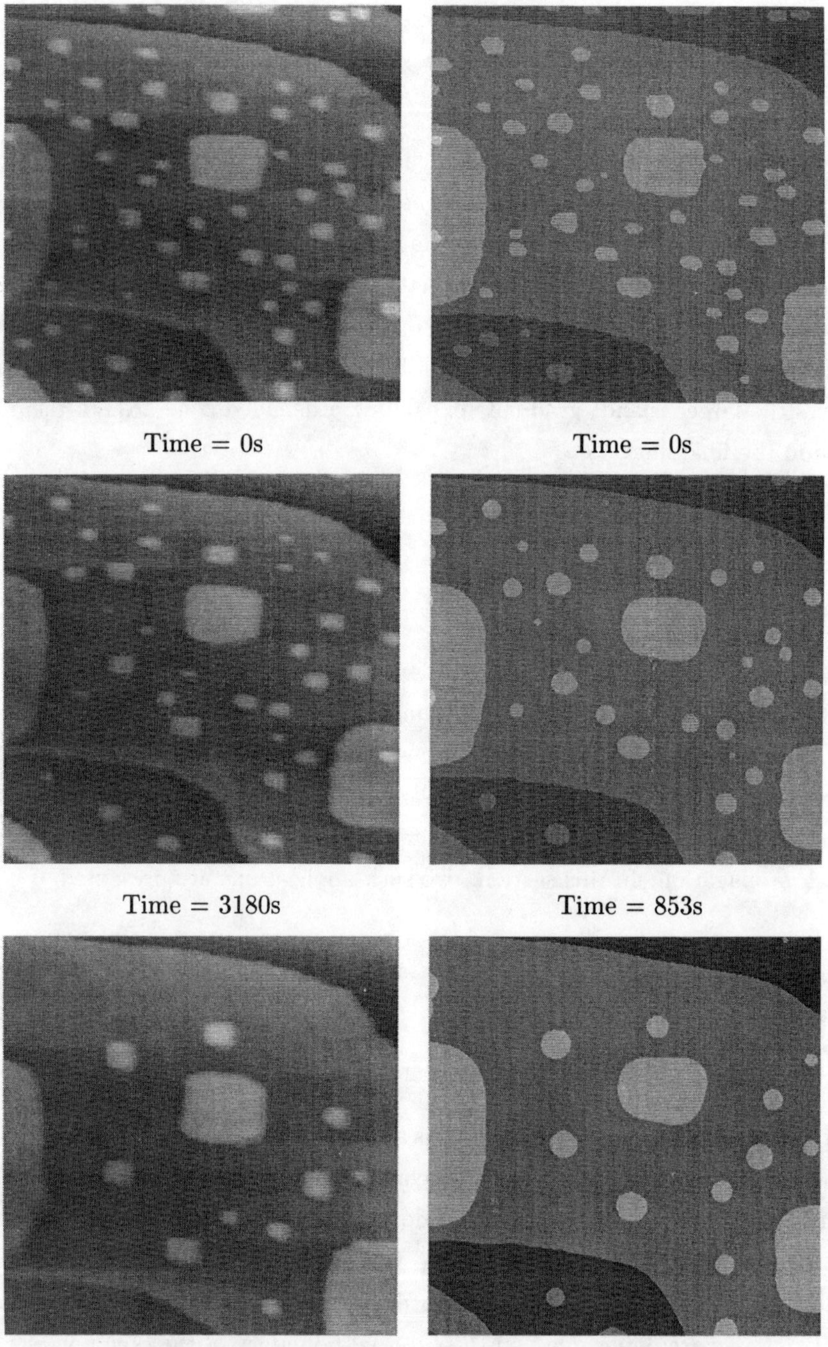

Figure 2.31: Time sequence of annealing TiN(002) at 800°C [30] compared with computed solution *(See color insert)*

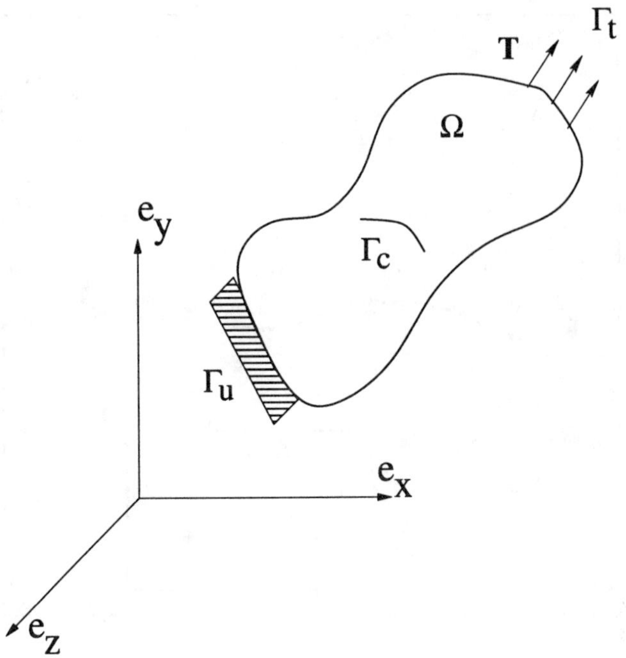

Figure 2.32: Domain Ω and its boundaries Γ.

The strong form of the equilibrium equations and boundary conditions is

$$\nabla \cdot \boldsymbol{\sigma} + \mathbf{b} = 0 \text{ in } \Omega \tag{2.78}$$

$$\boldsymbol{\sigma} \cdot \mathbf{n} = \mathbf{T} \text{ on } \Gamma_t \tag{2.79}$$

$$\boldsymbol{\sigma} \cdot \mathbf{n} = 0 \text{ on } \Gamma_{c+} \tag{2.80}$$

$$\boldsymbol{\sigma} \cdot \mathbf{n} = 0 \text{ on } \Gamma_{c-} \tag{2.81}$$

$$\mathbf{u} = \mathbf{U} \text{ on } \Gamma_u, \tag{2.82}$$

where $\boldsymbol{\sigma}$ is the Cauchy stress tensor, $\mathbf{u}$ is the displacement, $\mathbf{b}$ is the body force per unit volume, and $\mathbf{n}$ is the unit outward normal. The prescribed traction and displacement are respectively $\mathbf{T}$ and $\mathbf{U}$.

We consider small strains and displacements, so the strain-displacement relation is

$$\boldsymbol{\varepsilon} = \boldsymbol{\varepsilon}(\mathbf{u}) = \nabla_s \mathbf{u}. \tag{2.83}$$

In (2.83), ∇_s is the symmetric part of the gradient, and $\boldsymbol{\varepsilon}$ is the linear strain tensor. The constitutive relation is given by Hooke's Law,

$$\boldsymbol{\sigma} = \mathbf{C} : \boldsymbol{\varepsilon}, \tag{2.84}$$

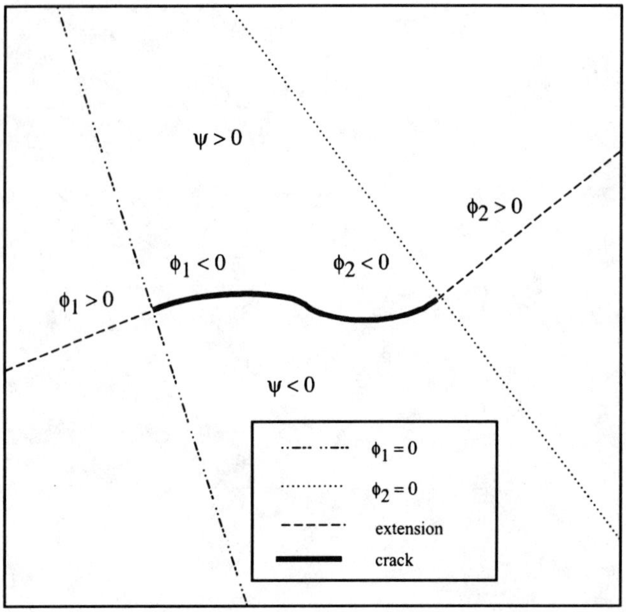

Figure 2.33: Construction of initial level set functions.

where **C** is the Hooke tensor.

For this application, the level set representation is used to model the location of the crack and the crack tips. Representing a line segment using a level set framework is a bit more challenging than might first appear because of the presence of the endpoints representing the crack tips. To handle this, one level set function ψ is used to represent the crack surface, and two additional level set functions ϕ_1, ϕ_2 are used to track the endpoints. An illustration of the relationship between these level set functions is depicted in Figure 2.33.

While this may appear to be a bit of overkill for modelling a simple segment, there are some definite advantages to this approach. The biggest advantage is in the evaluation of the enrichment functions from the extended finite element method. For this application, the enrichment functions consist of a jump discontinuity across the crack surface given by $H(y)$, and a branch function

$B_i(r, \theta)$ defined at each crack tip given by

$$H(y) = \begin{cases} 1 & \text{for } y > 0 \\ -1 & \text{for } y < 0. \end{cases} \tag{2.85}$$

$$B_l(r, \theta) = \left\{ \sqrt{r} \sin \frac{\theta}{2}, \sqrt{r} \cos \frac{\theta}{2}, \sqrt{r} \sin \frac{\theta}{2} \sin \theta, \sqrt{r} \cos \frac{\theta}{2} \sin \theta \right\}, \tag{2.86}$$

Here, the y value for the H function is the height above/below the crack surface and is therefore easily recovered from ψ. The r and θ values for the B function correspond to the distance and angle relative to the crack tip which is easily recovered by $\sqrt{\psi^2 + \phi_i^2}$ and $\arctan(\psi/\phi_i)$ respectively. Evaluating these functions without the level set framework requires more work, but using level sets, we get them essentially for free. It is this intimate coupling between the enrichment functions and the level set method that makes this combination method so intriguing.

The algorithm for advancing the crack tip now proceeds in a similar fashion as in Section 2.5.3. The elliptic system 2.82 is solved over the whole domain. The results are used to determine the crack tip direction and speed. The function ψ in the region where $\phi_i > 0$ is changed so that the zero contour of ψ coincides with the direction of the crack growth. The crack tip functions ϕ_i are then rotated and advanced according to the crack speed.

An example which shows the growth of a crack from a fillet in a structural member is shown in Figure 2.35. The configuration of the problem is taken from experimental work found in [55], the model was built in [18], and is shown in Figure 2.34. The computational domain is outlined by the dashed line. In this example, two different attachment schemes for the bottom of the fillet are compared. The upper path is for a rigid constraint of the fillet, while the lower path is for a flexible constraint. The crack tip and the associated level set functions ψ, ϕ_i are shown as cross-hairs on the end of the crack.

2.5.4.2 Two-Dimensional Planar Cracks

Two-dimensional planar cracks can also be modelled using the level set representation, but this time the crack front will be evolved using the fast marching method [13, 14]. The governing equations for the stress field are again given by the system (2.82), this time in three dimensions. Aside from the increased dimension and the different representation of the crack, the enrichment functions

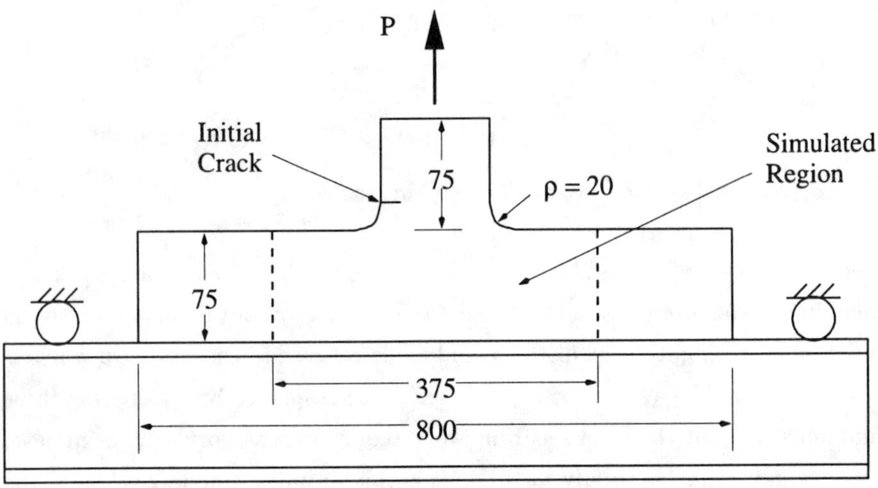

Figure 2.34: Experimental configuration of crack growth from a fillet taken from [55].

and the basic algorithm are essentially the same for two-dimensional cracks as for the one-dimensional cracks presented in the previous section.

The primary difference is the representation of the crack. In this example, the crack is confined to exist on a fixed plane, and hence the ψ component is fixed in space and can therefore be discarded. With this assumption, the crack tip can now be represented by a single level set function representing the one-dimensional crack tip on a two-dimensional plane contained in the three-dimensional domain. This time, only the crack speed is computed from the stress field since the direction is assumed to be confined to the plane. Separate meshes for the crack tip (two-dimensional) and the stress field (three-dimensional) are maintained.

Because the crack only expands, the speed function F is monotonic, $F > 0$, and hence the fast marching method can be used to determine the evolution of the crack tip. Using the fast marching method instead of the level set method offers a significant increase in speed because it computes the entire evolution of the crack tip for a single fixed speed function. This is a way in which the Courant-Friedrichs-Levy time-step restriction which affects the level set method can be side-stepped. Once the fast marching method is used to determine the evolution of the crack tip, the level set function is updated by simply subtracting the length of the time step from the fast marching solution.

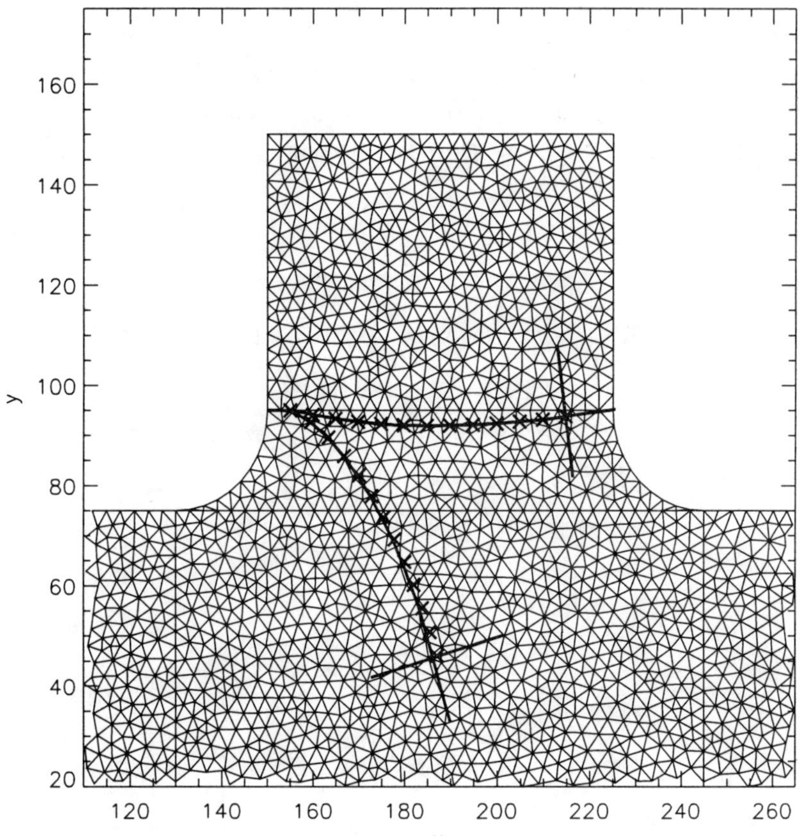

Figure 2.35: Crack paths for a rigid (upper crack) and flexible (lower crack) constraint. The path of the level set solution is shown as the solid line with the crack tip at the twelfth step shown as the intersection of the two zero level sets. The path of the explicit crack is shown by an X at the crack tip for each step.

This framework allows for the growth of multiple cracks which merge and continue to grow as illustrated in Figure 2.36.

2.6 Acknowledgements

I would like to acknowledge the very significant contributions from all the co-authors whose work has been presented in this chapter. In particular, I would like to mention the outstanding work of Magda Stolarska, Anthony Tongen, Natarajan Sukumar, Nic Moës, Kurt Smith, and Jamie Sethian.

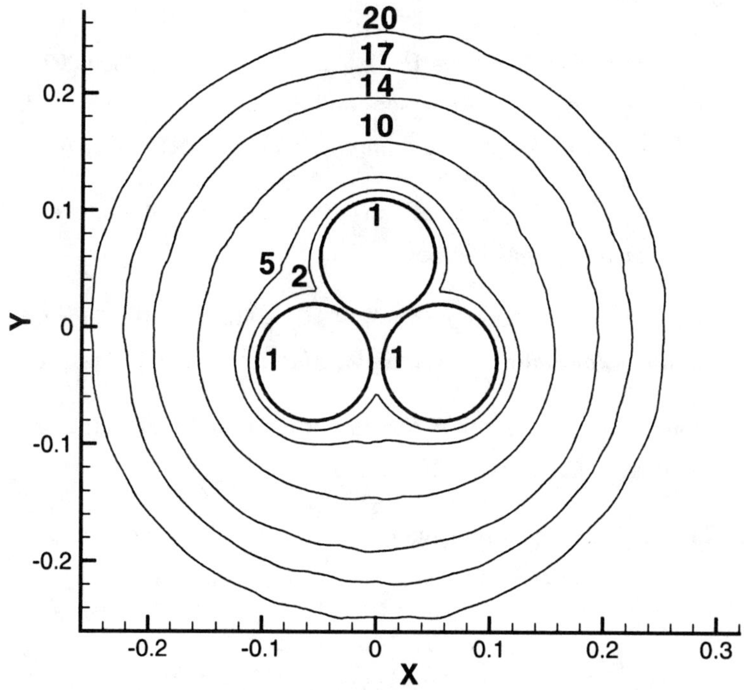

Figure 2.36: Fatigue crack growth simulation of three penny-shaped cracks. The step number is indicated in the plot.

Bibliography

[1] D. Adalsteinsson and J.A. Sethian. A fast level set method for propagating interfaces. *Journal of Computational Physics*, 118(2):269–277, 1995.

[2] D. Adalsteinsson and J.A. Sethian. The fast construction of extension velocities in level set methods. *Journal of Computational Physics*, 48(1):2–22, 1999.

[3] S. Chen, B. Merriman, M. Kang, R. E. Caflisch, C. Ratsch, L. T. Cheng, M. Gyure, R. P. Fedkiw, C. Anderson, and S. Osher. A level set method for thin film epitaxial growth. *J. Comput. Phys.*, 167:475–500, 2001.

[4] D. L. Chopp. Computing minimal surfaces via level set curvature flow. *Journal of Computational Physics*, 106(1):77–91, May 1993.

[5] D. L. Chopp. Numerical computation of self-similar solutions for mean curvature flow. *Journal of Experimental Mathematics*, 3(1):1–15, 1994.

[6] D. L. Chopp. A level-set method for simulating island coarsening. *Journal of Computational Physics*, 162:104–122, 2000.

[7] D. L. Chopp. Some improvements of the fast marching method. *SIAM J. Sci. Comp.*, 23(1):230–244, 2001.

[8] D. L. Chopp, L. C. Evans, and H. Ishii. Waiting time effects for Gauss curvature flows. *Indiana U. Math Journal*, 48(1):311–334, 1999.

[9] D. L. Chopp and J. A. Sethian. Flow under curvature: Singularity formation, minimal surfaces, and geodesics. *Journal of Experimental Mathematics*, 2(4):235–255, 1993.

[10] D. L. Chopp and J. A. Sethian. Motion by intrinsic Laplacian of curvature. *Interfaces and Free Boundaries*, 1:107–123, 1999.

[11] D. L. Chopp and N. Sukumar. Fatigue crack propagation of multiple coplanar cracks with the coupled extended finite element/fast marching method. *SIAM Journal of Scientific Computing*, 2001. submitted, preprint available at http://www.esam.northwestern.edu/chopp/pubs.html.

[12] D. L. Chopp, A. Tongen, and J. A. Sethian. Fast approximations of surface diffusion. preprint, 2000.

[13] D.L. Chopp. Computing minimal surfaces via level set curvature flow. *Journal of Computational Physics*, 106:77–91, 1993.

[14] M. H. Chung. A level set approach for computing solutions to inviscid compressible flow with moving solid boundary using fixed cartesian grids. *Int. J. Numer. Methods Fluids*, 36:373–389, 2001.

[15] C. Daux, N. Moës, J. Dolbow, N. Sukumar, and T. Belytschko. Arbitrary cracks and holes with the extended finite element method. *International Journal for Numerical Methods in Engineering*, 48(12):1741–1760, 2000.

[16] J. W. Deng and H. T. Tsui. A fast level set method for segmentation of low contrast noisy biomedical images. *Pattern Recognit. Lett.*, 23:161–169, 2002.

[17] T. Deschamps and L. D. Cohen. Fast extraction of minimal paths in 3d images and applications to virtual endoscopy. *Med. Image Anal.*, 5:281–299, 2001.

[18] J. Dolbow, N. Moës, and T. Belytschko. Discontinuous enrichment in finite elements with a partition of unity method. *Finite Elements in Analysis and Design*, 36:235–260, 2000.

[19] Q. Du, D. Z. Li, Y. Y. Li, R. Li, and P. W. Zhang. Simulating a double casting technique using level set method. *Comput. Mater. Sci.*, 22:200–212, 2001.

[20] T. Elperin and A. Vikhansky. Variational model of granular flow in a three-dimensional rotating container. *Physica A*, 303:48–56, 2002.

[21] M. Gage. An isoperimetric inequality with aplications to curve shortening. *Duke Math Journal*, 50(4):1225–1229, 1983.

[22] M. Gage. Curve shortening makes convex curves circular. *Inventiones Mathematica*, 76(2):357–364, 1984.

[23] M. Gage and R. S. Hamilton. The equation shrinking convex planes curves. *Journal of Differential Geometry*, 23:69–96, 1986.

[24] A. Gravouil, N. Moës, and T. Belytschko. Non-planar 3d crack growth by the extended finite element and the level sets. Part II: Level set update and discretization techniques. 2001. preprint.

[25] M. Grayson. The heat equation shrinks embedded plane curves to round points. *Journal of Differential Geometry*, 26(285):285–314, 1987.

[26] A. Harten, B. Engquist, S. Osher, and S. R. Chakravarthy. Uniformly high-order accurate essentially nonoscillatory schemes. *Journal of Computational Physics*, 71(2):231–303, 1987.

[27] G. Huisken. Asymptotic behavior for singularities of the mean curvature flow. *Journal of Differential Geometry*, 31:285–299, 1991.

[28] H. Ji, D. Chopp, and J. E. Dolbow. A hybrid extended finite element/level set method for modeling phase transformations. *International Journal of Numerical Methods for Engineering*, 2001. to appear.

[29] M. Khenner, A. Averbuch, M. Israeli, and M. Nathan. Numerical simulation of grain-boundary grooving by level set method. *J. Comput. Phys.*, 170:764–784, 2001.

[30] S. Kodambaka, V. Petrova, A. Vailionis, P. Desjardins, I. Petrov, and J. E. Greene. Time sequence images of annealing TiN(002) at 800°. Technical report, University of Illinois Urbana-Champaign, Dept. of Materials Science and Engineering and Matierals Research Laboratory, 1999. To be published.

[31] R. J. LeVeque. *Numerical Methods for Conservation Laws.* Birkhäuser Verlag, 1992.

[32] R. Malladi, J.A. Sethian, and B.C. Vemuri. Evolutionary fronts for topology-independent shape modeling and recovery. In *Proceedings of Third European Conference on Computer Vision, Stockholm, Sweden, Lecture Notes in Computer Science*, volume 800, pages 3–13, 1994.

[33] J. M. Melenk and I. Babuska. The partition of unity finite element method: Basic theory and applications. *Computer Methods in Applied Mechanics and Engineering*, 139:289–314, 1996.

[34] B. Merriman, J. Bence, and S.J. Osher. Motion of multiple junctions: A level set approach. *Journal of Computational Physics*, 112:334–363, 1994.

[35] N. Moës, J. Dolbow, and T. Belytschko. A finite element method for crack growth without remeshing. *International Journal for Numerical Methods in Engineering*, 46(1):131–150, 1999.

[36] N. Moës, A. Gravouil, and T. Belytschko. Non-planar 3d crack growth by the extended finite element and the level sets. Part I: Crack representation and stress intensity computation. 2001. preprint.

[37] S. Osher and J. A. Sethian. Fronts propagating with curvature-dependent speed: Algorithms based on Hamilton-Jacobi formulations. *Journal of Computational Physics*, 79(1):12–49, November 1988.

[38] S. J. Osher and F. Santosa. Level set methods for optimization problems involving geometry and constraints i. frequencies of a two-density inhomogeneous drum. *J. Comput. Phys.*, 171:272–288, 2001.

[39] S. B. Pillapakkam and P. Singh. A level-set method for computing solutions to viscoelastic twophase flow. *J. Comput. Phys.*, 174:552–578, 2001.

[40] J. A. Sethian. A review of recent numerical algorithms for hypersurfaces moving with curvature-dependent speed. *Journal of Differential Geometry*, 31:131–161, 1989.

[41] J. A. Sethian and J. Strain. Crystal growth and dendrite solidification. *Journal of Computational Physics*, 98(2):231–253, 1992.

[42] J.A. Sethian. *Level Set Methods: Evolving Interfaces in Geometry, Fluid Mechanics, Computer Vision and Material Science.* Cambridge University Press, 1996.

[43] J.A. Sethian. A marching level set method for monotonically advancing fronts. *Proceedings of the National Academy of Sciences*, 93(4):1591–1595, 1996.

[44] J.A. Sethian. Fast marching methods. *SIAM Review*, 41(2):199–235, 1999.

[45] K. A. Smith, F. J. Solis, and D. L. Chopp. A projection method for motion of triple junctions by level sets. *Interfaces and Free Boundaries*, 2001. to appear.

[46] K.A. Smith, F.J. Solis, L. Tao, K. Thornton, and M.O. de la Cruz. Domain growth in ternary fluids: A level set approach. *Phys. Rev. Lett.*, 84(1):91–94, 2000.

[47] G. H. Son. Numerical study on a sliding bubble during nucleate boiling. *KSME Int. J.*, 15:931–940, 2001.

[48] M. Stolarska, D. L. Chopp, N. Moës, and T. Belytschko. Modeling crack growth by level sets and the extended finite element method. *International Journal for Numerical Methods in Engineering*, 51(8):943–960, 2001.

[49] N. Sukumar, D. L. Chopp, N. Moes, and T. Belytschko. Modeling holes and inclusions by level sets in the extended finite-element method. *Comput. Meth. Appl. Mech. Eng.*, 190:6183–6200, 2001.

[50] N. Sukumar, D. L. Chopp, N. Moës, and T. Belytschko. Modeling holes and inclusions by level sets in the extended finite element method. *Computer Methods in Applied Mechanics and Engineering*, 190(46–47):6183–6200, 2001.

[51] N. Sukumar, D. L. Chopp, N. Moës, and T. Belytschko. Modeling holes and inclusions by level sets in the extended finite element method. *Computer Methods in Applied Mechanics and Engineering*, 190(46–47):6183–6200, 2001.

[52] N. Sukumar, D. L. Chopp, and B. Moran. Extended finite element method and fast marching method for three-dimensional fatigue crack propagation. 2001. submitted.

[53] N. Sukumar, D. L. Chopp, and B. Moran. Extended finite element method and fast marching method for three-dimensional fatigue crack propagation. *Engineering Fracture Mechanics*, 2001. to appear.

[54] N. Sukumar, N. Moës, B. Moran, and T. Belytschko. Extended finite element method for three-dimensional crack modeling. *International Journal for Numerical Methods in Engineering*, 48(11):1549–1570, 2000.

[55] Y. Sumi, C. Yang, and Z. Wang. Morphological aspects of fatigue crack propagation. part ii – effects of stress biaxiality and welding residual stresses. Technical report, Department of Naval Architecture and Ocean Engineering, Yokohama National University, Japan, 1995.

[56] M. Sussman, P. Smereka, and S.J. Osher. A level set method for computing solutions to incompressible two-phase flow. *Journal of Computational Physics*, 114:146–159, 1994.

[57] S. Y. Yeung, H. T. Tsui, and A. Yim. Global shape from shading for an endoscope image. *Lect Note Comput Sci*, 1679:318–327, 1999.

[58] K. Yokoi and F. Xiao. Mechanism of structure formation in circular hydraulic jumps: numerical studies of strongly deformed free-surface shallow flows. *Physica D*, 161:202–219, 2002.

[59] H.K. Zhao, T. Chan, B. Merriman, and S. Osher. A variational level set approach to multiphase motion. *Journal of Computational Physics*, 127:179–195, 1996.

[60] J. Zhu and J. A. Sethian. Projection methods coupled to level set interface techniques. *Journal of Computational Physics*, 102(1):128–138, 1992.

Chapter 3

Geometric Regularizers for Level Sets

Jasjit S. Suri[1], *Sameer Singh*[2] *and Swamy Laxminarayan*[3]

3.1 Introduction

The role of shape recovery has always been a critical component in 2-D[4] and 3-D[5] medical imagery since it assists largely in medical therapy (see the recent book by Suri *et al.* [1] and references therein). The applications of shape recovery have been increasing since scanning methods became faster, more accurate and less artifacted (see Chapter 4 by Suri *et al.* [1] and [2]). The recovery of shapes of the human body is more difficult compared to other imaging fields. This is primarily due to the large variability in shapes, complexity of medical structures, several kinds of artifacts and restrictive[6] body scanning methods. In spite of the above-mentioned complications, an exploration has begun into obtaining faster and more accurate software tools for shape recovery in 2-D and 3-D. This Chapter is an attempt to survey the latest techniques in 2-D and 3-D for fast shape recovery based on the class of deformable models, known as "level sets" or "geodesic active contours/surfaces."[7]

The application of the level sets in medical image segmentation became extremely popular because of its ability to capture the topology of shapes in medical imagery. Recently, Lachaud *et al.* (see [4], [5] and [6]) and Malgouyres

[1]Marconi Medical Systems, Inc., Cleveland, OH, USA
[2]University of Exeter, Exeter, UK
[3]New Jersey Institute of Technology, Newark, NJ, USA
[4]Two-dimensional
[5]Three-dimensional
[6]Scanning ability limited to acquiring in three orthogonal and oblique directions only.
[7]We will interchangeably use the phrase "level sets" and "geodesic active contour/surfaces".

PDE & Level Sets: Algorithmic Approaches to Static & Motion Imagery
Edited by Jasjit Suri and Swamy Laxminarayan, Kluwer Academic/Plenum Publishers, 2002

et al. [7] also recently published an excellent paper on topology preservation within digital surfaces. A detailed survey on digital topology in CVGIP[8] can be seen by Kong *et al.* [8] and also the related research work by Bertalmio *et al.* [9] and DeCarlo *et al.* [10]. The diversity of applications of level sets has reached into several fields. These applications and their relevent references are listed here: (**1**) *geometry:* (see Angenent *et al.* [11], Chopp [12], [13] and Sethian [14]); (**2**) *grid generation:* (see Sethian [15]); (**3**) *fluid mechanics:* (see Mulder *et al.* [16], Sethian [17] and Sussman *et al.* [18]); (**4**) *combustion:* (see Rhee *et al.* [19]); (**5**) *solidification:* (see Sethian *et al.* [20]); (**6**) *device fabrication:* (see Adalsteinsson *et al.* [21]); (**7**) *morphing:* (see Whitaker *et al.* [22], [23] and [24]); (**8**) *object tracking/image sequence analysis in images:* (see the recent work by Mansouri *et al.* [25], [26], [27] and Paragios *et al.* [28], [29] and Kornprobst *et al.* [30]); (**9**) *stereo vision:* (see the recent work by Faugeras and his coworkers at INRIA [31]); (**10**) *shape from shading:* (see Kimmel *et al.* [32], [33] and [34]); (**11**) *mathematical morphology:* (see Arehart *et al.* [35], Catte *et al.* [36], Sapiro [37] and Sochen *et al.* [38]); (**12**) *color image segmentation:* (see Sapiro *et al.* [39]); (**13**) *3-D reconstruction and modeling:* (see Caselles *et al.* [40] and [41]); (**14**) *surfaces and level sets:* (see Chopp [42] and Kimmel *et al.* [43]); (**15**) *topological evaluations:* (see DeCarlo *et al.* [10]); and (**16**) *2-D and 3-D medical image segmentation:* (see these works by Malladi *et al.* [44], [45], [46], [47], [48], [49] and [50], Yezzi *et al.* [51]); GM/WM[9] boundary estimation by Gomes *et al.* [52]; GM/WM boundary estimation with Fuzzy models by Suri [53]; GM/WM thickness estimation by Zeng *et al.* [54]; leaking prevention in fast level sets by Suri [55]; a recent survey article on brain segmentation by Suri *et al.* [57]; application of level sets for cortex unfolding by Faugeras and his coworkers from INRIA (see Hermosillo *et al.* [58]); application of the level set technique in cell segmentation (see Sarti and coworkers [59]); and Niessen *et al.* [60] for the application of geodesic active contours for cardiac image analysis. For a detailed review of some of these above applications, readers must see the works by Sethian [61], [62] published in 1989 and 1996, respectively and Kimmel *et al.* [63]. Though these survey publications cover a good collection of level set applications, with the advancement of image processing technology, these publications fall behind in: (**1**) the latest trends, the called design of the robust propagation forces, which is the crux of this Chapter; and (**2**) not having

[8]Computer Vision, Graphics and Image Processing

[9]GM-Gray Matter, WM-White Matter

a proper focus on the medical imaging area. Both these shortcomings will be removed in this Chapter. Having discussed the importance and application of level sets, the Chapter now presents the place of level sets in the segmentation tree and its taxonomy.

The taxonomy of level sets for segmentation of 2-D and 3-D medical imagery can be seen in Figure 3.1 (top). (For details on segmentation techniques, readers are referred to exhaustive reviews by Suri *et al.* [64] and [57].) Figure 3.1 (top) shows the classification of 2-D and 3-D segmentation techniques, divided into three core classes: (**1**) region-based; (**2**) boundary/surface-based; and (**3**) fusion of boundary/region-based. The second core class of segmentation is also known as "deformable models" and the third core class is also called the "fusion of regions with deformable models". The deformation process has played a critical role in shape representation. This Chapter uses "level sets" as its tool to capture deforming shapes in medical imagery. The research in deformation started in the late 1980's when the Chapter called "snakes" (the first class of deformable models) was published by Terzopoulous and coworkers (see Terzopoulous *et al.* [65] and Kass *et al.* [66]). Since then, there has been an extensive burst of publications in the area of parametric deformable models and their improvements, such as balloon force and template-based fitting (see all of these references in Chapter 3 and Chapter 4 by Suri *et al.* [1]). Discussions on these references are out of the scope of this Chapter. The second class of deformable models is level sets. These deformable models were started by Osher and Sethian [67], which started from Sethian's Ph.D. Thesis [68]. The fundamental difference between these two classes is: Parametric deformable curves (active contours) are local methods based on an energy-minimizing spline guided by external and image forces which pull or push the spline towards features such as lines and edges in the image. These classical active contour models solve the objective function to obtain the goal boundary, if the approximate or initial location of the contour is available. On the other hand, level set methods are active contour energy minimization techniques which solve computation of geodesics or minimal distance curves. Level set methods are governed by curvature dependent speeds of moving curves or fronts. Those familiar in the field of active-modeling will appreciate these major advantages and superiority of level sets compared to classical deformable models. These will be covered in this Chapter as well.

Geometric deformable models[10] or level set techniques are classified broadly into two classes (see Figure 3.1, top, shown in dotted line area): (**1**) without regularizers; and (**2**) with regularizers. The first class, level sets without regularizers, has techniques where the propagation force does not utilize the region-based strategy for its computation. These forces are constant and do not change. Sometimes they are also called "level sets stoppers". Earlier research called these "leakage prevention" techniques because they tried to prevent any bleeding of boundaries during propagation. These are further classified into five different kinds, depending upon the design of the stopping force: (**1**) gradient-based stopping force; (**2**) edge-based stopping force; (**3**) area-minimization-based stopping force; (**4**) curvature-based stopping force; and (**5**) application-driven level sets. The curvature-dependent class has four sub-classes: (**1**) plain curvature-based; (**2**) mean curvature flow based with directionality; (**3**) bubbles; and (**4**) morphing. Plain curvature based techniques are those which are driven solely by the curvature that is computed using differential geometry. Mean curvature flow with directionality-based techniques are those which use the combination of Euclidean curvature and direction together to achieve the deformation process. Such techniques are good for tiny, occluded and twisted objects like blood vessels. Bubbles are a set of seeds, or fourth order shocks, which grow, shrink, merge, split, disappear and deform under the influence of image information such as edges and gradients to segment objects in images and volumes. Morphing techniques are those which undergo shape deformation from one initial shape to the target shape driven by the combination of signed distance at coordinate transformation and the gradient of the signed distance transform functions. This transformation captures the similarity between user-defined shape and target shape.

The second core class of level sets uses regularizers or level sets that derive the propagation force using statistical means such as region-based strategy. This is further classified into four types depending upon the design of propagation force. They are: (**1**) clustering-based; (**2**) classification based on Bayesian statistics; (**3**) shape-based; and (**4**) constrained coupled level sets where the propagation force is derived from Bayesian strategies.

Having defined the taxonomy of level sets in medical image segmentation, the following goals of this Chapter are presented: (**1**) To present the tenta-

---

[10] We will interchangeably use the word "geometric deformable models" or "level sets" or "geodesic contours" during the course of this Chapter.

tive taxonomy of level sets and its place in 2-D and 3-D medical image segmentation; (**2**) To understand the curve/surface propagation of hypersurfaces based on differential geometry; (**3**) To present the mathematical foundations of different techniques as discussed in the level set taxonomy (see Figure 3.1 (top)). This also includes a discussion of the pros and cons of all techniques for curve/surface propagation; (**4**) To study different kinds of propagating forces[11] and their fusion in the level set formalism using PDE's[12] for curve/surface propagation and evolution; (**5**) To present the state-of-the-art 2-D and 3-D level set segmentation systems for medical imagery along with their merits and demerits; and finally, (**6**) To present the state-of-the-art ready references for readers interested in further exploring into the field of medical imaging segmentation using level sets. Note that the goal of this Chapter is not to discuss the PDE-based image processing approaches, even though it is closely related (for details on PDE-based applications to image processing, see the upcoming paper by Suri *et al.* [69] and their references therein).

The layout of the remainder of this Chapter is as follows: Section 3.2 presents the introduction to level sets and the derivation of the curve evolution equation. Section 3.3 presents the first core class of level sets, i.e., "level sets without regularizers" and their sub-classes. The second core class of level sets, i.e., "level sets fused with regularizers" for image segmentation, is discussed in section 3.4. This is the crux of the Chapter and discusses the state-of-the-art method for design of the "propagating force" used for the deformation/morphing process in 2-D/3-D medical imagery. Section 3.5 covers numerical methodologies of level sets using finite differences. Optimization techniques for segmentation in the level set framework and shape quantification techniques are discussed in section 3.6. Finally, merits, demerits, conclusions and the future on level sets are discussed in section 3.7.

3.2 Curve Evolution: Its Derivation, Analogies and the Solution

Since this Chapter is focused on level sets, this section first presents the derivation of the fundamental equation of level sets, known as "curve evolution". Let

[11] also called regularizers

[12] Partial Differential Equations

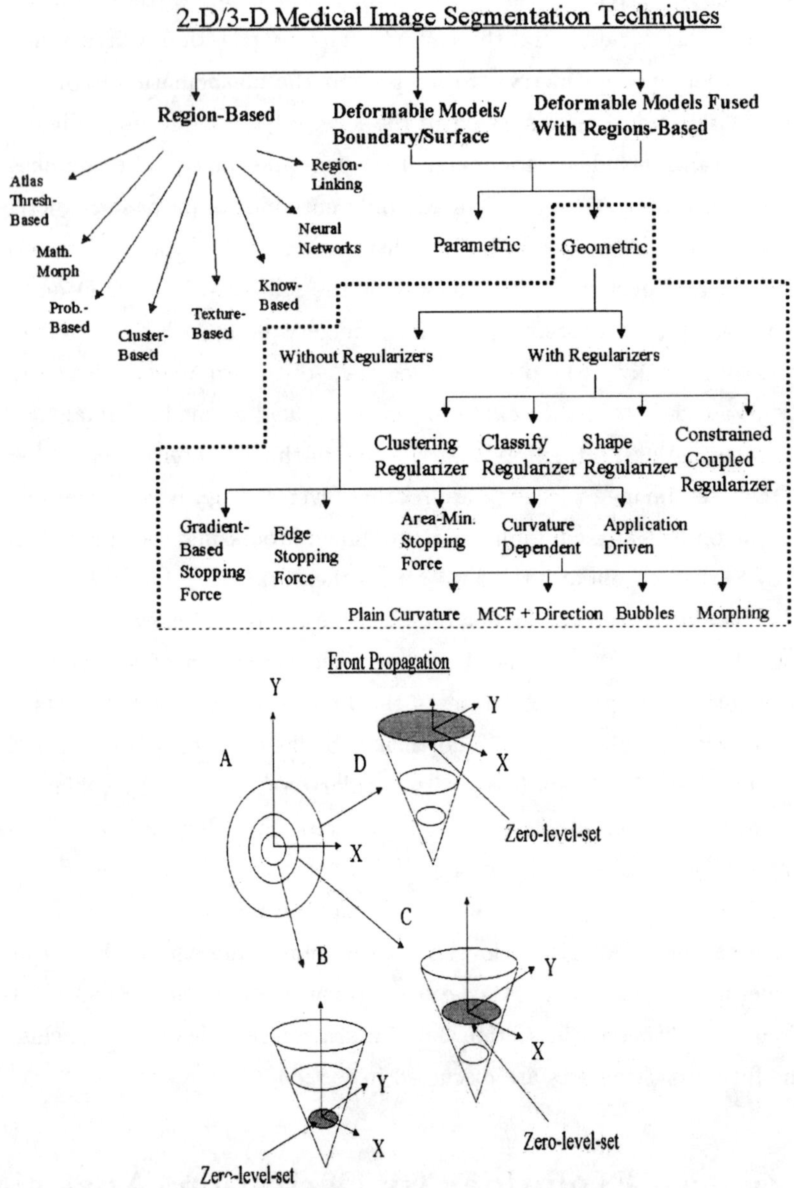

Figure 3.1: **Top**: The place of level sets in the medical segmentation tree. Note the classification sub-tree of geometric deformable models or level sets (shown in dotted line area). **Bottom**: Front propagation of the *zero level set.* Filled circles in figures (B), (C) and (D) show the position of the *zero level curve* as the front propagates. These three projected circles are seen in figure (A).

$\Gamma(t)$ be the closed interface or front propagating along its normal direction (see Figure 3.1, bottom). This closed interface $\Gamma(t)$: $[0, \infty) \rightarrow \Re^N$, can either be a curve in 2-D space or a surface in 3-D space. The main idea is to represent the front $\Gamma(t)$ as the *zero level set* of a higher dimensional function ϕ.

Let $\phi(x, t = 0)$, where $x \in \Re^N$ be defined by $\phi(x, t = 0) = d$, where d is the signed distance from position x to $\Gamma(0)$ and the plus (minus) sign is chosen if the point x is outside (inside) the initial front $\Gamma(0)$. Thus an initial function is: $\phi(x, t = 0) = \Re^N \rightarrow \Re$ with the property: $\Gamma(t = 0) = (x \mid \phi(x, t = 0) = 0)$. The goal now is to produce an equation for the evolving function $\phi(x, t)$ so that ϕ always remains zero on the propagating interface. Let $x(t)$, $t \in [0, \infty)$ be the path of a point on the propagation front (see Figure 3.1, bottom), i.e., $x(t = 0)$ is a point on the initial front $\Gamma(t = 0)$ and $x_t = V(x(t))$ with the vector x_t normal to the front at $x(t)$. Since the evolving function ϕ is always zero on the propagating front, thus $\phi(x(t), t) = 0$. By chain rule:

$$\phi_t + \sum_{i=1}^{N} \phi_{x_i} \, x_{i_t} = 0\,, \tag{3.1}$$

where x_i is the ith component of x. Since

$$\sum_{i=1}^{N} \phi_{x_i} \, x_{i_t} = (\phi_{x_1}, \phi_{x_2}, \phi_{x_3} ... \phi_{x_N}) \cdot (x_{1_t}, x_{2_t}, x_{3_t} ... x_{N_t}) = V(x(t)) \, |\nabla \phi|\,, \tag{3.2}$$

hence, using Equations 3.1 and 3.2, the final curve evolution equation is given as:

$$\frac{\partial \phi}{\partial t} = V(\kappa) \, | \, \nabla \phi \, |, \tag{3.3}$$

where ϕ is the level set function and $V(\kappa)$ is the speed with which the front (or *zero level curve*) propagates. This fundamental[13] equation describes the time evolution of the level set function (ϕ) in such a way that the *zero level curve* of this evolving function is always identified with the propagating interface. The term "level set function" will be interchangeably used with the term "flow

[13]Recently, Faugeras and his coworkers from INRIA (see Gomes *et al.* [52]) modified Eq. 3.3 into the "preserving distance function" as:

$$\frac{\partial \phi}{\partial t} = V(\mathbf{x}) \, (\mathbf{x} - \phi \nabla \phi), \tag{3.4}$$

where $\mathbf{x}$ was the vector of x and y coordinates, ϕ is the signed distance function. The main characteristic of this equation was that ϕ and V are orthogonal to each other (see details by Gomes *et al.* [52]).

field" or simply "field" during the course of this Chapter. The above equation is also called an Eulerian representation of evolution due to the work of Osher and Sethian [67]. Equation 3.3 for 2-D and 3-D cases can be generalized as: $\frac{\partial \phi}{\partial t} = V_{\kappa}(x,y)\,|\,\nabla\phi\,|$ and $\frac{\partial \phi}{\partial t} = V_{\kappa}(x,y,z)\,|\,\nabla\phi\,|$, respectively, where $V_{\kappa}(x,y)$ and $V_{\kappa}(x,y,z)$ are curvature dependent speed functions in 2-D and 3-D, respectively.

Three Analogies of the Curve Evolution Equation: (**1**) Note that these equations can be compared with the Euclidean geometric heat equation (see Grayson [70]), given as: $\frac{\partial \mathcal{C}}{\partial t} = \kappa \mathcal{N}$, where κ is the curvature and $\mathcal{N}$ is the inward unit normal and $\mathcal{C}$ is the curve coordinates. (**2**) Equation 3.3 is also called the curvature motion equation, since the rate of change of the length of the curve is a function of $\frac{\partial \mathcal{C}}{\partial t}$. (**3**) The above equations can be written in terms of differential geometry using divergence as: $\frac{\partial \phi}{\partial t} = \nabla \, . \, (\frac{\nabla\phi}{|\nabla\phi|})\,|\,\nabla\phi\,|$, where geometrical properties such as normal curvature ($\mathcal{N}$) and mean curvature ($\mathcal{H}$) are given as: $\mathcal{N} = \frac{\nabla\phi}{|\nabla\phi|}$ and $\mathcal{H} = \nabla \, . \, (\frac{\nabla\phi}{|\nabla\phi|})$.

3.2.1 The Eikonal Equation and its Mathematical Solution

In this sub-section, the mathematical solution is presented for solving the level set function with unity speed. Such a method is needed to compute the "signed distance transform" when the raw contour crosses the background grid. Consider a case of a "front" moving with a velocity $V = V(x,y)$, such that V is greater than zero. Using Osher-Sethian's [67] level set equation, consider a monotonically advancing front represented in the form: $\phi_t = V(x,y)\ ||\nabla\,\phi||$, where ϕ_t is the rate of change of the level set and $\nabla\,\phi$ is the gradient of the ϕ. Let $T(x,y)$ be the time at which the front crosses the grid point (x,y). In this time, the surface $T(x,y)$ satisfies the equation: $||\nabla T||\ .\ V = 1$. By approximation[14], the solution to the Eikonal Equation is:

$$\begin{aligned} &[\mathbf{max}\ (\ \mathbf{max}(D^{-x}\,T,0), -\mathbf{min}(D^{+x}\,T,0)\ )]^2 + \\ &[\mathbf{max}\ (\ \mathbf{max}(D^{-y}\,T,0), -\mathbf{min}(D^{+y}\,T,0)\ )]^2 = \frac{1}{{V^2}_{xy}}, \end{aligned} \tag{3.5}$$

[14]Numerical methodologies will be discussed in section 3.5.

where ${V^2}_{xy}$ is the square of the speed at location (x, y) and $D^{-x}T$, $D^{+x}T$, $D^{-y}T$, $D^{+y}T$ are the backward and forward differences in time, given as:

$$\begin{cases} D^{+x}T = \frac{T(x,y+1)-T(x,y)}{2} & \& \quad D^{-x}T = \frac{T(x,y)-T(x,y-1)}{2}, \\ D^{+y}T = \frac{T(x+1,y)-T(x,y)}{2} & \& \quad D^{-y}T = \frac{T(x,y)-T(x-1,y)}{2}. \end{cases} \tag{3.6}$$

There are efficient schemes for solving the Eikonal Equation 3.3. For details, see Sethian [71], Cao *et al.* [72] and Chen *et al.* [73]. Having discussed the taxonomy of level sets in medical imaging and the fundamental curve/surface evolution equation, the Chapter now presents the different types of level sets and their mathematical formalism along with their merits and demerits. Level sets without regularizers are discussed in section 3.3, and level sets fused with regularizers in the level set framework are discussed in section 3.4.

3.3 Level Sets without Regularizers for Segmentation

The main characteristic of the level set is its ability to pick up the desired topology of the shape being segmented. The accuracy of the segmentation process depends upon when and where the propagating hypersurface needs to stop. Consider the special case of a surface moving with a speed $V > 0$. Let T be the time at which the surface crosses a given point. The function T then satisfies $|\nabla T|\, V = 1$. This equation simply says that the gradient of the arrival time is inversely proportional to the speed of the surface. If the propagating surface needs to stop close to the vicinity of the segmenting topological shape, then the speed of the surface should approximate closely to zero near the final segmenting shape. This means that gradient values at the final shape boundary (in 2-D) or surface (in 3-D) should be very high (since the speed needed at the boundary is zero). Thus the accuracy of the segmentation process highly depends on how powerful the gradient values are at the final segmented shapes. This means the higher the gradient value, the faster the propagation of the curve/surface is, which results in a strong clamping force. As a result, one has robust and accurate segmentation. Thus the "stopping force" seen for the propagating surface is strongly dependent upon the gradient change of the final shape to be segmented. In the next few sub-sections, several kinds of stopping forces[15] will be discussed in the class of "level sets without regularizers" or "implicit deformable models".

The layout of this section is as follows: Sub-section 3.3.1 presents the stopping force due to the image gradient. Sub-section 3.3.2 presents the stopping force due to edge strength. Sub-section 3.3.3 presents the stopping force due to area minimization. Sub-section 3.3.4 presents the stopping force due to mean curvature flow (MCF). Finally, in curvature dependent level sets, we discuss the work on (i) plain curvature and (ii) mean curvature flow integrated with directionality.

3.3.1 Level Sets with Stopping Force Due to the Image Gradient (Caselles)

Using Osher and Sethian's [67] approach, Caselles *et al.* [75], Chopp *et al.* [42] and Rouy *et al.* [76] proposed the geometric active contours[16] followed by Malladi *et al.* [77]. The model proposed by Caselles and Malladi was based on the following equation: if $\phi(\mathbf{x}, t)$ was a 2-D scalar function that embedded the *zero level curve*, then the geometric active contour was given by solving:

$$\frac{\partial \phi}{\partial t} = \underbrace{c(\mathbf{x})}_{stopping-term-type-1} (\kappa + V_0) \mid \nabla \phi \mid, \tag{3.7}$$

where κ was the level set curvature, V_0 was the constant and $c(\mathbf{x})$ was the stopping term (type-1) based on the image gradient and was given as:

$$c(\mathbf{x}) = \frac{1}{1 + |\nabla [G_\sigma(\mathbf{x}) * I(\mathbf{x})]|}. \tag{3.8}$$

Note that Equation 3.7 is the same as Equation 5 from Malladi *et al.* [78]. Rewriting Equation 5 from Malladi *et al.* [78], the stopping force becomes:

$$c(\mathbf{x}) = e^{\alpha \, |\nabla [G_\sigma(\mathbf{x}) * I(\mathbf{x})]|}, \tag{3.9}$$

where α was the gradient constant and $|\nabla [G_\sigma(\mathbf{x}) * I(\mathbf{x})]|$ was the absolute of the gradient of the convoluted image. This convolved image was computed by convolving the original image by the Gaussian function with a known standard deviation σ. Taking the constant α as unity and using the exponential series, one can obtain Equation 3.8 from Equation 3.9.

---

[15] also called the data consistency term in the level set framework

[16] or the level set or curve evolution equation

Pros and Cons of Caselles ***et al.*** **'s Work:** Although Caselles and Malladi work is able to solve this problem, it has the following weaknesses: (**1**) The stopping term was not robust and hence could not stop the bleeding or leaking of the boundaries. (**2**) The pulling back feature was not strong. This meant that if the front propagated and crossed the goal boundary, then it could not come back.

3.3.2 Level Sets with Stopping Force Due to Edge Strength $(\nabla c.\nabla\,\phi)$ (Yezzi)

Kichenassamy *et al.* [74] and Yezzi *et al.* [51] tried to solve the above problems by introducing an extra stopping term (type-2), also called the pull back term. This was expressed mathematically as:

$$\frac{\partial \phi}{\partial t} = c(\mathbf{x})(\kappa + V_0)\,|\,\nabla\phi\,| \;\; + \;\; \underbrace{(\nabla c.\nabla\,\phi)}_{stopping-term-type-2} \tag{3.10}$$

Note that $(\nabla c.\nabla\,\phi)$ denoted the projection of an attractive force vector on the normal to the surface. This force was realized as the gradient of a potential field c. This potential field c for the 2-D and 3-D case was given as: $c(x,y) = -|\nabla G_\sigma * I(x,y)|$ and $c(x,y,z) = -|\nabla G_\sigma * I(x,y,z)|$, respectively. Note that Equation 3.10 is similar to Equation 7 given by Malladi *et al.* in [78]. Malladi *et al.* calls the equation as an additional constraint on the surface motion ϕ_t. Rewriting Equation 7 of Malladi *et al.* [78] becomes:

$$\phi_t + c(\mathbf{x})(\epsilon\,\kappa + V_0)\,|\,\nabla\phi\,| - \beta\,(\nabla c.\nabla\,\phi) = 0\,, \tag{3.11}$$

where β was the edge strength constant, V_0 was a constant (1 as used by Malladi *et al.*), κ was the curvature dependent speed, ϵ was the constant term controlling the curvature dependent speed and $(\nabla c.\nabla\,\phi)$ was the same as defined above.

Pros and Cons of Kichenassamy ***et al.*** **[74] and Yezzi** ***et al.*** **'s [51] Methods:** The weakness of the above technique include: (**1**) It still suffered from boundary leaking for complex structures, as pointed out by Siddiqi *et al.* [79].

3.3.3 Level Sets with Stopping Force Due to Area Minimization (Siddiqi)

Siddiqi *et al.* [79], [80] then changed Kichenassamy *et al.* [74] and Yezzi *et al.*'s [51] model by adding an extra term to it:

$$\frac{\partial \phi}{\partial t} = c(\mathbf{x})(\kappa + V_0) \,|\, \nabla \phi \,|\, + (\nabla c . \nabla \, \phi) \; + \underbrace{\frac{V_0}{2} \mathbf{x} \,.\, \nabla c \,|\nabla \phi|}_{stopping-term-type-3} \quad , \tag{3.12}$$

where $\frac{V_0}{2} \mathbf{x} \; (\nabla \, c) \, |\nabla \phi|$ was the area minimizing term and was mathematically equal to the product of the divergence of the stopping term times the gradient of the flow. This term provided an additional attraction force when the front was in the vicinity of an edge.

Pros and Cons of the Area Minimization Technique: The major advantage of this technique include: (**1**) It performed better compared to the first and second implicit models. The major weaknesses include: (**1**) The system was not very robust at handling the convolutedness of medical shapes. (**2**) The system did not take advantage of the regional neighbourhood for the propagation or evolution of level sets. To some extent, this weakness was temporarily removed using multiple level sets (see Niessen *et al.* [60]), however this was not a robust solution to the segmentation of complex shapes such as in brain cortical segmentation.

3.3.4 Level Sets with Curvature Dependent Stopping Forces

The layout of this sub-section is as follows: Plain curvature-driven techniques are presented in sub-section 3.3.4.1. Integrating the directionality into mean curvature flow is presented in sub-section 3.3.4.2. Note that the work on 3-D bubbles and free form deformations will not be discussed in this Chapter.

3.3.4.1 3-D Geometric Surface-Based Cortical Segmentation (Malladi)

The dominance of 3-D shape modeling using Geodesics active surfaces started with the UCLA group (see Osher and Sethian [67], Chopp *et al.* [3]) and then later used by the Berkeley Lab (see Malladi and Sethian, [78], [49]). Malladi's method was simply an extension from 2-D to 3-D of Equations 3.7 and 3.8 and an additional term, the called gradient of the potential field. Thus, if: $\frac{\partial \phi}{\partial t} = c(\mathbf{x})(\kappa + V_0) \mid \nabla \phi \mid$, where κ is the level set curvature, V_0 is the constant and $c(\mathbf{x})$ was the stopping term based on image gradient and given as: $c(\mathbf{x}) = \frac{1}{1+|\nabla[G_\sigma(\mathbf{x}) * I(\mathbf{x})]|}$. Then Malladi *et al.* 's final equation for cortical segmentation was:

$$\frac{\partial \phi}{\partial t} = \underbrace{c(\mathbf{x})(\epsilon\,\kappa + V_0) \mid \nabla \phi \mid}_{gradient+curvature+stopper} + \underbrace{\beta\, \nabla \mathbf{P}.\nabla \phi}_{attractive-force}\quad , \tag{3.13}$$

where $\mathbf{P}$ was the gradient of the potential field given as: $\mathbf{P}(x, y, z) = |(\nabla(G_{sigma} * I(x, y, z)))|$. Note that the term $\nabla \mathbf{P}.\nabla \phi$ denoted the projection of an attractive force on the surface normal. β controlled the strength of the attractive force. Also note that $V_0 = 1$ and κ was pre-multiplied by ϵ which controlled the mean curvature. The mean curvature κ in 3-D was: $\kappa = \frac{1}{(\phi_x^2+\phi_y^2+\phi_z^2)^{3/2}} \Big((\phi_{yy}+\phi_{zz})\, \phi_x^2 + (\phi_{xx}+\phi_{zz})\, \phi_y^2 + (\phi_{xx}+\phi_{yy})\, \phi_z^2 - 2(\phi_x\, \phi_y\, \phi_{xy} + \phi_x\, \phi_z\, \phi_{xz} + \phi_y\, \phi_z\, \phi_{yz}) \Big)$. So, the deformation was focused more on propagation based on curvature rather than on stopping force.

Pros and Cons of Malladi's Technique: The major advantages of this technique include: (**1**) This technique was one of the first in the application of level sets in the medical imaging world. (**2**) The recent work of Malladi *et al.* [78], [49] applied level sets for brain segmentation and showed the speed was N log (N), where N was the total number of points in the data set. The major disadvantages of this technique include: (**1**) It was not clear from this Chapter how the value of the arrival time T was selected to segment the cortex accurately, but their protocol followed a two-step process. He first reconstructed the arrival time function using the fast marching method (see Sethian [71], [114]). Then, he treated the final $T(x, y, z)$ function as an initial condition to their full model. This meant that they solved $\frac{\partial \phi}{\partial t} = c(\mathbf{x})(\epsilon\kappa + V_0) \mid \nabla \phi \mid$ in a few time steps using the finite difference with $\phi(x, y, z; t = 0) = T(x, y, z)$. (**2**) The system was not robust and did not take advantage of the region-based analysis. The modification of this technique will be seen in section 3.4, where four systems are presented with the design of propagation forces, a key to the success of robust segmentation.

3.3.4.2 Curvature Dependent Force Integrated with Directionality (Lorigo)

Recently, Lorigo *et al.* [81] presented an algorithm for brain vessel reconstruction based on curve evolution in 3-D, also know as "co-dimension two" in geodesic active contours. This method used two components: (i) mean curvature flow (MCF) and (ii) the directionality of vessels. The mean curvature flow component was used to derive the Eulerian representation of the level set equation. If ϕ was the Signed Distance Transform (SDT) and $\lambda(\nabla\,\phi(\mathbf{x},t), \nabla^2\phi(\mathbf{x},t))$ are the eigen values of the projection operator: $\mathcal{P}_{\nabla\,\phi}\,\nabla^2\,\phi\,P_{\nabla\phi}$, where $\mathcal{P} = I - \frac{qq^T}{|q|^2}$ and q was a non-zero vector, then using these eigen values, the Eulerian representation of the curve evolution was given by Lorigo as: $\frac{\partial\phi}{\partial t} = \lambda(\nabla\,\phi(\mathbf{x},t), \nabla^2\phi(\mathbf{x},t))$. The second component was the normal of these vessels projected onto the plane and was given as the product of $\nabla\phi$ with the projection vector d. This projection vector was computed using the Hessian of the intensity image, I and was given as: $\frac{g'}{g}(H\frac{\nabla I}{|\nabla I|})$, where g was the edge detector operator. Adding these two components, the complete level set equation was:

$$\frac{\partial\phi}{\partial t} = \underbrace{\lambda(\nabla\,\phi(\mathbf{x},t), \nabla^2\phi(\mathbf{x},t))}_{mean-curvature-force} + \underbrace{D \times S \times \frac{g'}{g}(H\frac{\nabla I}{|\nabla I|})}_{Angular-Balloon-force}, \tag{3.14}$$

where D was the directionality term which was the dot product of $\nabla\phi$ and ∇I which was the angle between these two vectors. S was the scale term. Note that the second term was like an angular balloon force which navigated the deformation process.

Pros and Cons of Lorigo's Technique: The major advantages of this technique include: **(1)** The method successfully demonstrated the segmentation of these vessels of the brain. **(2)** The method used the directional component in the level set framework, which was necessary for segmenting twisted, convoluted and occluded vessels. **(3)** The technique was used to compute vessel radii, a clinically useful measurement. The weaknesses of Lorigo's work include: **(1)** Not much discussion was available on the computation of the scale factor S. **(2)** The method has yet to show the analytical model since the output of the system showed relatively thinner vessels compared to maximum intensity projection

(MIP)[17] and thresholding schemes. (**3**) There was no comparison made between segmented results and the ground truth hence, this was not validated. So, we saw that the class of "level set without regularizers" primarily focused on stopping the deformation process by using the data consistency term, $c(\mathbf{x})$, or propagating the deformation process totally based on curvature-dependent speed. None of the above methods took advantage of the region-based strategy of neighbourhoods, hence they were not successful in capturing complex shapes of medical objects/organs such as brain cortex. The next section is focused on demonstrating the design of the propagating force based on region-strategy which is fused into the level set fundamental model to improve the robustness of the segmentation for medical imagery.

3.4 Level Sets Fused with Regularizers for Segmentation

Fusing regional statistics into parametric or geometric boundary/surfaces has brought a major success in medical imaging (see the recent work by Yezzi *et al.* [88], Guo *et al.* [89], Leventon *et al.* [117], Lorigo *et al.* [82] and recently by Suri [55], [56]). The main reason for this was that the segmentation system took advantage of the local and global shape information for pulling and pushing boundaries/surfaces to capture the topology in the level set framework based on PDE. Incorporating such regional-statistics, also known as "level sets with regularizers", makes the overall segmentation system more robust and accurate.

This section presents four different medical segmentation systems where regularizers are fused with geometric contour or geodesic active contours in the level set framework. Sub-section 3.4.1 presents the derivation of geodesic active contours from parametric deformable models. The same sub-section shows the design of the propagation force using fuzzy clustering, which was later fused in geodesic active contours or level sets. Sub-section 3.4.2 presents 3-D constrained level sets where two propagating surfaces are coupled by a constraint. The methodology of computing the propagation force using Bayesian statistics is shown in sub-section 3.4.3. Sub-section 3.4.4 presents the fusion of the shape-

[17]The MIP algorithm is a very popular technique. An example can be seen by Suri *et al.* [83].

based information as a propagating force in the level set formalism. Finally, a comparison among the designs of different propagation forces and their uses in level sets will be discussed in section 3.4.5.

3.4.1 2-D Regional Geometric Contour: Design of Regional Propagation Force Based on Clustering and its Fusion with Geometric Contour (Suri/Marconi)

Recently, Suri [2], [55], [56] derived the curve evolution equation by embedding the region statistics into the parametric classical energy model. This method was in the spirit of Xu's [90] attempt. Part of that derivation[18] will be discussed here (for details see Suri *et al.* [1]). To start with, the standard dynamic classical energy model as given by Kass *et al.* [66] was:

$$\gamma \frac{\partial \mathbf{X}}{\partial t} = \underbrace{\frac{\partial}{\partial s}(\alpha \frac{\partial \mathbf{X}}{\partial s}) - \frac{\partial^2}{\partial s^2}(\beta \frac{\partial^2 \mathbf{X}}{\partial s^2})}_{internal-energy} + \underbrace{F_{ext}(\mathbf{X})}_{external-energy} \quad , \tag{3.15}$$

where $\mathbf{X}$ was the parametric contour and γ was the damping coefficient. As seen in Equation 3.15, the classical energy model constituted an energy-minimizing spline guided by external and image forces that pulled the spline towards features such as lines and edges in the image. The energy-minimizing spline was named "snakes" because the spline softly and quietly moved while minimizing the energy term. The internal energy was composed of two terms: the first term was the first order derivative of the parametric curve which acted like a

[18]Aubert *et al.* [91] recently tried to give some remarks between classical snakes (given first by Kass *et al.* [66]) and geodesic snakes (given first by Caselles *et al.* [87]). Aubert *et al.* showed that the above two models are only valid for curves with a fixed length using the definition that "classical snakes and geodesic snakes are equivalent, if they have same extremas". Aubert *et al.* also showed that Mauperthuis' principle is not enough to show the equivalence between classical snakes and geodesic snakes. Aubert *et al.* mathematically showed that the derivation of the gradient flow from the classical snake and the geodesic snake have different expressions if Caselles *et al.*'s definition was used for developing the equivalence. Aubert *et al.* did, however, show equivalence between these two energy models to be the same if the following definition was used for equivalence: "Two minimization problems are equivalent if the direction which locally most decreases a criterion is also a decreasing direction for the other criterion and vice versa". In the forthcoming derivation, Caselles *et al.*'s idea was used for establishing equivalence between parametric and geodesic models.

membrane and the second term was the second derivative of the parametric curve which acted as a thin plate (also called the pressure force). These terms were controlled by elastic constants α and β. The second part of the classical energy model constituted the external force given by $F_{ext}(\mathbf{X})$. This external energy term depended upon image forces which were a function of image gradient. Parametric snakes had flexibility to dynamically control movements, but there were inherent drawbacks when they were applied to highly convoluted structures, sharp bends and corners, or on images with a large amount of noise. Suri *et al.* [1], [2], [64] and [57] tried to preserve the classical properties of these parametric contours but also brought these geometric properties which could capture the topology of convoluted shapes (say, cortical WM and GM). Since the curve evolution when embedded with regional statistics was the fundamental equation in the design of a propagation force, thus, the derivation will be presented next.

Derivation of the Geometric Snake: Since the second derivative term in Eq. 3.15 did not significantly affect the performance[19] of active geometric snakes (see Caselles *et al.* [87]), Suri dropped that term and replaced it with a new pressure force which was given by: $F_p(\mathbf{X})$. This pressure force was an outward force which was a function of the unit normal, $\mathcal{N}$ of the deforming curve. Suri defined the pressure force as: $F_p(\mathbf{X}) = w_p(\mathbf{X})\mathcal{N}(\mathbf{X})$, thus the new parametric active contour could be re-written by replacing $\beta\frac{\partial^2\mathbf{X}}{\partial s^2}$ by $w_p(\mathbf{X})\mathcal{N}(\mathbf{X})$, resulting in:

$$\gamma\frac{\partial \mathbf{X}}{\partial t} = \underbrace{\frac{\partial}{\partial s}\left(\alpha\frac{\partial \mathbf{X}}{\partial s}\right)}_{smoothing-force} - \underbrace{w_p(\mathbf{X})\mathcal{N}(\mathbf{X})}_{pressure-force} + \underbrace{F_{ext}(\mathbf{X})}_{external-force} \tag{3.16}$$

By redefining $\frac{\partial}{\partial s}(\frac{\partial \mathbf{X}}{\partial s})$ to be the curvature κ, and readjusting the terms by defining the constants $\epsilon = \frac{\alpha}{\gamma}$, $V_p = \frac{w_p(X)}{\gamma}\mathcal{N}(\mathbf{X})$ and $V_{ext} = \frac{F_{ext}}{\gamma}$, thus Eq. 3.16 was rewritten as: $\frac{\partial \mathbf{X}}{\partial t} = (\epsilon\kappa + V_p + V_{ext} \, . \mathcal{N})\mathcal{N}$. The above Eq. was analogous to Osher and Sethian's [67] Eq. of curve evolution, given as: $\frac{\partial \phi}{\partial t} = V(\kappa)\mathcal{N}$, where $\mathcal{N} = -\frac{\nabla\phi}{|\nabla\phi|}$. Note, ϕ was the level set function and $V(\kappa)$ was the curvature dependent speed with which the front (or *zero level curve*) propagated. The expression $\frac{\partial \phi}{\partial t} = V(\kappa)\mathcal{N}$ described the time evolution of the level set function (ϕ) in such a way that the *zero level curve* of this evolving function was always identified with the propagating interface. Comparing $\frac{\partial \mathbf{X}}{\partial t}$ and $\frac{\partial \phi}{\partial t} = V(\kappa)\mathcal{N}$, and using the geometric property of the curve's normal $\mathcal{N}$ and considering only

[19] see the previous footnote

the normal components of internal and external forces, $\frac{\partial}{\partial s}(\alpha\frac{\partial \mathbf{X}}{\partial s}).\mathcal{N} = (\alpha\kappa)$, Suri obtained the level set function (ϕ) in the form of a partial differential equation (PDE) as:

$$\frac{\partial \phi}{\partial t} = (\epsilon\,\kappa + V_p)\,|\nabla\phi| - V_{ext}.\nabla\phi\,. \tag{3.17}$$

Note, V_p was considered as a regional force term and was mathematically expressed as a combination of the inside-outside regional area of the propagating curve. This was defined as $\frac{w_R}{\gamma\,R}$, where R was the region indicator term that fell between 0 and 1 (the design of this propagation force will be seen in the next sub-section). So, the above derivation showed that the regional information was one of the factors which controlled the speed of the geometric snake or propagating curve in the level set framework. A framework in which a snake propagated by capturing the topology of the WM/GM, navigated by the regional, curvature, edge and gradient forces, was called regional geometric snakes. Also note that Eq. 3.17 had three terms: the product of ϵ and κ, V_p and V_{ext}. These three terms were the speed functions which controlled the propagation of the curve. These three speed functions were known as curvature, regional and gradient speed functions, since they contributed towards the three kinds of forces responsible for curve deformation.

3.4.1.1 Design of the Propagation Force Based on Fuzzy Clustering

Having discussed the embedding of the regional-force function in the level set framework in the previous section, this sub-section now presents how this regional force V_p was computed that navigated the deformation process for the final segmentation of the convoluted topology. As defined previously, the regional propagation force was mathematically given as: $\frac{w_R}{\gamma\,R}$, where R was the region indicator term that fell between 0 and 1. An example of such a region indicator was from a membership function of the fuzzy classifier. Thus Suri expressed the region indicator term as: $R_{ind} = 1 - 2\;u(x,y)$, where $u(x,y)$ was the fuzzy membership function which had a value between 0 to 1. R_{ind} was the region indicator function and fell in the range between -1 to +1. This membership function $u(x,y)$ was computed based on the fuzzy principle (see Bezdek *et al.* [93]).

Figure 3.3 (left) shows the system used for GM boundary estimation, whose results can be seen in Figure 3.2. Note thàt the last stage was the isocontour extraction. This was accomplished using an isocontour algorithm at sub-pixel resolution (for details on these methods, see Berger *et al.* [95], Sethian *et al.* [96], Tababai *et al.* [97], Huertas *et al.* [98] and Gao *et al.* [99]).

Pros and Cons When Clustering was Used as a Regularizer: The major advantages of embedding the clustering technique as a regularizer in the level set framework include: (**1**) robust implementation; (**2**) accurate boundary estimation depending upon the class chosen; (**3**) ease of implementation. The major weaknesses of this method include: (**1**) The algorithm was not fast enough to be implemented for real-time applications. (**2**) The performance of the algorithm depended upon a few parameters, such as: the error threshold and the number of iterations. (**3**) The choice of the initial cluster was important and needed to be carefully selected. (**4**) The algorithm was not very robust to MR images which had spatial variations due to large RF inhomogeneities.

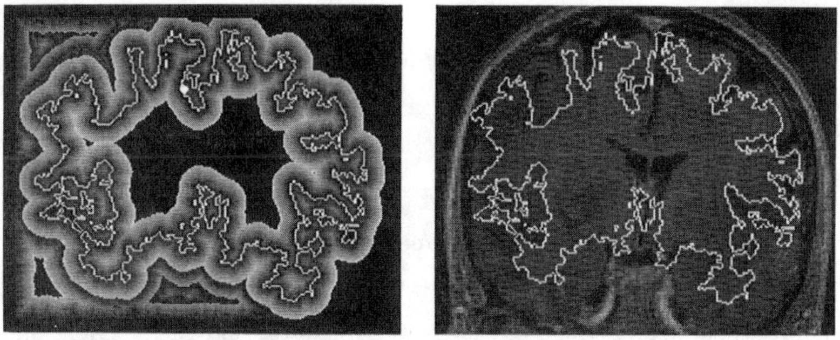

Figure 3.2: **Left**: Results of the superimposition of the ZLC and its level set function using the "fast marching method" in the narrow band (NB). Tube reconstruction. **Right**: Segmented GM boundary (results, courtesy of Jasjit Suri, Marconi Medical Systems, Inc. For details, see the articles by Suri [55], [56]).

3.4.2 3-D Constrained Level Sets: Fusion of Coupled Level Sets with Bayesian Classification as a Regularizer (Zeng/Yale)

Coupled constrained boundary estimation in medical imaging has been very successful when applying to shape analysis (see the derivation in the appendix

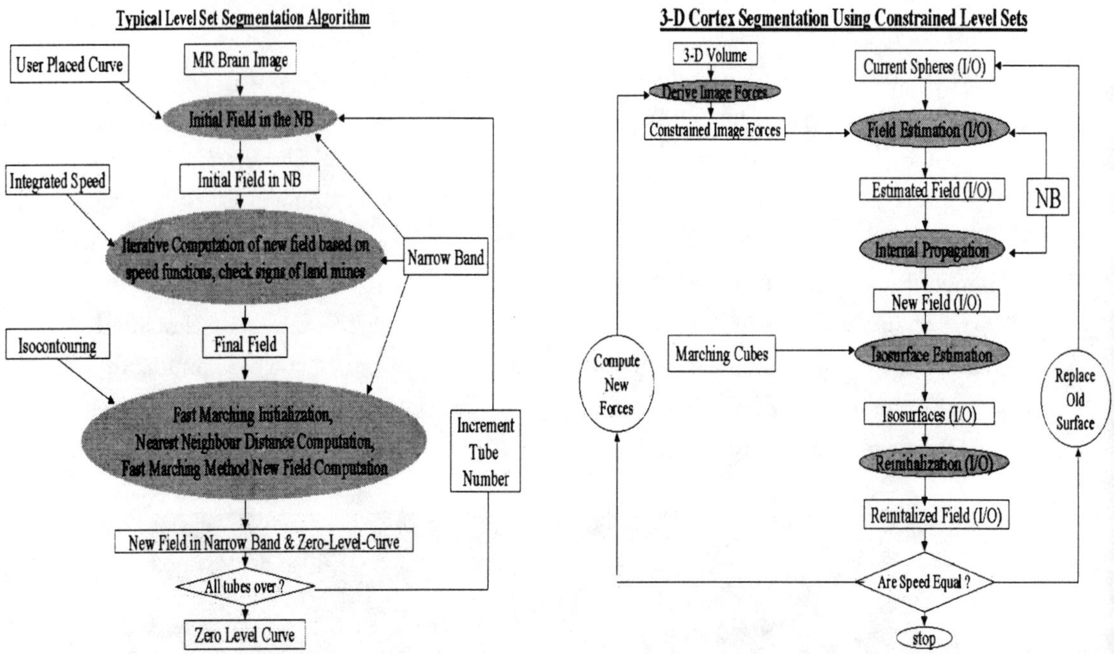

Figure 3.3: **Left**: Typical level set segmentation algorithm. This can be applied for brain segmentation. In such a case, the integrated speed will have regional, gradient and curvature speed terms. Note: the paradigm uses the fast marching method in the narrow band. **Right**: Constrained level set application: cortex segmentation algorithm. The user first specifies the initial spheres. Using the distance transform based on the shortest distance, the initial field is estimated in the narrow band. The surface is propagated in the narrow band and the new field distribution is estimated taking the propagation forces into account. These forces are computed using the likelihood measure. Using the marching cube algorithm, the *zero level surface* is computed, also known as isosurface extraction. The surfaces are reinitialized and the speeds of two new isosurfaces are compared. If they are equal to zero, the system stops the propagation, or else the next round is iterated. Before the new field is estimated in the next round, the constrained forces are derived again.

by Suri [64], where ED[20] and ES[21] shapes of the LV[22] were subjected to the "coupled constrained principle". These constraints were computed based on eigen values). In the level set framework, Zeng *et al.* [100], [54] recently had put the level set under constraints in neurological applications. For example, a volume has three tissue types, say T1, T2 and T3, and say tissue T2 was embedded in between tissues T1 and T3. Such an example is seen in the human brain where the GM is embedded between the WM and CSF. There is a coupling between WM-GM and GM-CSF volumes. Zeng *et al.*'s method had used constrained level sets in the application of human cortex segmentation from MR images. The proposed coupled level set formulation was motivated by the nearly constant thickness of the cortical mantle and took this tight coupling as an important constraint. The algorithm started with two embedded surfaces in the form of concentric sphere sets. The inner and outer surfaces were then evolved, driven by their own image-derived information, respectively, while maintaining the coupling in-between through a thickness constraint.

3.4.2.1 Overall Pipeline of Coupled Constrained Level Set Segmentation System

The cortical segmentation system based on level sets which was constrained by the coupling between the WM-GM and GM-CSF volumes can be seen in Figure 3.3 (right). This system will be briefly discussed next, since it has clinical value in neurological analysis. The input of the system was the 3-D gray scale volume and the initial spheres. From the gray scale volume, the propagating forces[23] were computed. This was called the likelihood function which drove the field distributions (to be discussed in sub-section 3.4.2.2). From the initial concentric spheres, the initial field was computed in the narrow band. Zeng *et al.* [54] then computed the new field driven by these propagating forces in this narrow band. This was where Zeng *et al.* ran the *coupled level set* equations (to be discussed in sub-section 3.4.2.3). From this new field the new surface was computed, known as the isosurface, which represented a unisurface value based on Marching Cubes (see Lorensen *et al.* [102]). The algorithm performed the re-initialization and was ready to repeat the above steps if the external

[20] end diastole
[21] end systole
[22] left ventricle
[23] also known as steering engines or image forces

and internal speeds of the spheres were not equal to zero. The algorithm used the fast marching method in the narrow band to optimize the performance. Thus a final representation of the cortical bounding surfaces and an automatic segmentation of the cortical volume was achieved. The intermediate and final results of the above coupled constrained level set algorithm can be seen in Figure 3.4. The following three sub-sections will discuss each of these components of this pipeline.

3.4.2.2 Design of the Propagation Force Based on the Bayesian Model

Capturing gray scale edges of the WM/GM interface and GM/CSF interface was a very critical component in the entire system. The image-derived information was obtained by using a local likelihood operator based on gray-level information rather than on image gradient alone, which gave the algorithm the ability in capturing the homogeneity of the tissue inside the volumetric layer. First, the 3-D field distribution[24] was estimated given the initial spheres[25]. From the initial field distribution, the normals and offsets at every voxel location were computed using the level set framework. These two offsets to a central voxel gave information on the neighbouring voxels. The first set of voxels belonged to the first distribution, while the second set of voxels belonged to the second distribution. Next, the likelihood values were computed using these two distributions. For the first distribution (here, WM), the WM likelihood probability was computed given a voxel and similarly, the GM likelihood was computed given the second distribution (here, GM). Assuming the distributions to be independent, the GM-WM likelihood computation was mathematically given as:

$$p_{GM-WM} = \prod_{g \in G} \frac{1}{\sqrt{2\pi\sigma_G}} e^{-\frac{(I_g-\mu_G)^2}{\sigma_G^2}} \prod_{w \in W} \frac{1}{\sqrt{2\pi\sigma_W}} e^{-\frac{(I_w-\mu_W)^2}{\sigma_W^2}}, \qquad (3.18)$$

where W and G were the WM and GM regions, μ_W and μ_G were mean values of the WM and GM regions. σ_W^2 and σ_G^2 were standard deviations of the WM and GM regions, I_w and I_g were the WM and GM pixel intensities. Note, the output of the GM-WM likelihood function was the image which had edge infor-

[24]Signed Distance Transform (SDT)

[25]inside and outside spheres

mation about the boundary of the GM-WM. Similarly, the WM-CSF likelihood function was an image which had the WM-CSF edge or gradient information.

3.4.2.3 Constrained Coupled Level Sets Fused with Bayesian Propagation Forces

The propagation of surfaces towards the final goal surface was performed in the level set framework. Instead of evolving two surface directly, two level functions whose *zero level set* corresponding to the cortical bounding surfaces were calculated. The equations of these evolving surfaces were:

$$\begin{cases} \psi_{in}(t) + F_{in}\,|\nabla\,\psi_{in}| &= 0\,, \\ \psi_{out}(t) + F_{out}\,|\nabla\,\psi_{out}| &= 0\,. \end{cases} \tag{3.19}$$

The coupling between these two surfaces was realized through propagation speed terms F_{out} and F_{in} which are dependent on the distance between the two surfaces and the propagation forces computed above. While the distance between the two surfaces was within the normal range, the inner and outer cortical surfaces propagated according to their own image features. When the distance started to fall out of the normal range, the propagation slowed down and finally stopped only when the distance was outside the normal range, or the image feature was strong enough. A coupled narrow band algorithm was customized for the coupled-surfaces propagation. The correspondence between points on the two bounding surfaces falls out automatically during the narrow band rebuilding, which was required for surface propagation at each iteration. This shortest distance-based correspondence was essential in imposing the coupling between two bounding surfaces through the thickness constraint. Once the new field was computed, the isosurface was extracted based on the marching cube technique (see Lorensen *et al.* [102]). Having discussed all the stages of the constrained coupled segmentation system, next will be presented the pros and cons.

Pros and Cons of Coupled Level Sets Fused with Bayesian Classification: The coupled-surfaces propagation with the level set implementation offered the following advantages: (**1**) easy initialization; (**2**) computational efficiency (one hour); (**3**) the ability to handle complex sulcal folds; (**4**) simultaneous "skull-stripping" (delineation of non-brain tissues) and GM/WM segmentation; (**5**) ready evaluation of several characteristics of the cortex, such

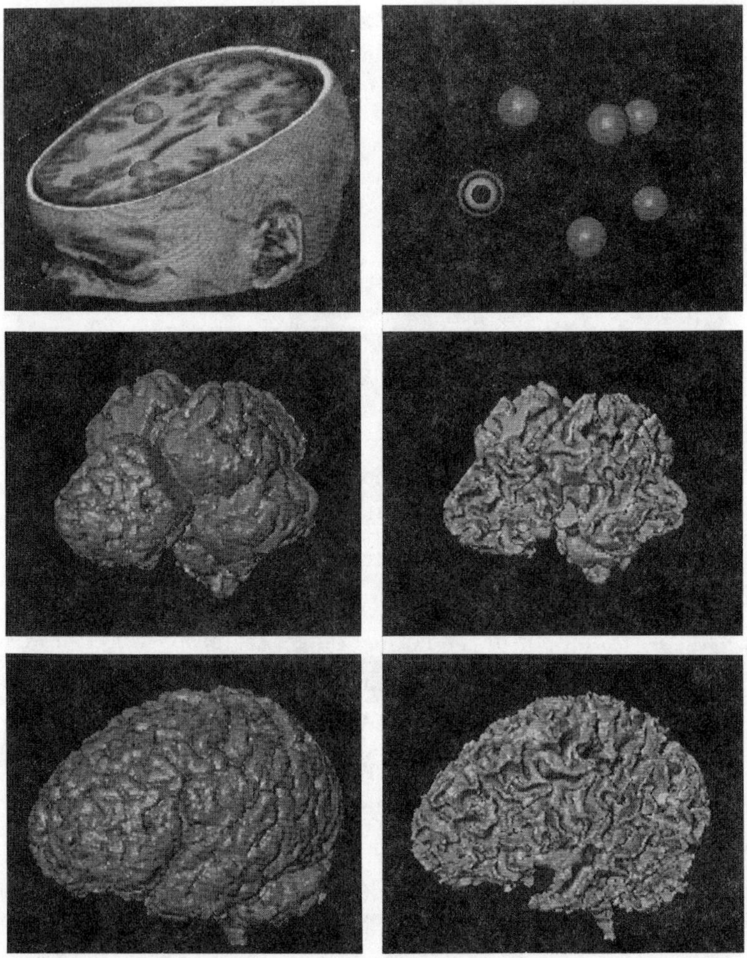

Figure 3.4: Propagation of the outer (pink) and inner (yellow) bounding surfaces. **Top Left**: embedded sphere sets as initializations shown in unedited 3-D MR brain volume. **Top Right**: outer (pink) and inner (yellow) bounding spheres. **Middle Left**: intermediate step in GM surface propagation. **Middle Right**: intermediate step in WM surface propagation. **Bottom Left**: final result of the segmented GM/CSF surface. **Bottom Right**: final result of the segmented WM/GM surface (Courtesy of Xiaolan Zeng, R2 Technology, Inc.). *(See color insert)*

as surface curvature and a cortical thickness map; (**6**) integration of efficiency and flexibility of level set methods with the power of shape constraint; (**7**) a promise towards the improved accuracy of brain segmentation through extensive experiments on both simulated brain images and real data. The major weaknesses include: (**1**) the method did not include a model that dealt with image inhomogeneity, unlike other research such as that of Wells *et al.* [101]; (**2**) the technique imposed no constraint to preserve the cortical surface topology, however it did take advantage of the topological flexibility of level set methods; (**3**) the resulting surface may not produce a two dimensional manifold. Other research work using coupled level sets was done by Gomes *et al.* [52].

3.4.3 3-D Regional Geometric Surface: Fusion of the Level Set with Bayesian-Based Pixel Classification Regularizer (Barillot/IRISA)

Baillot and his co-workers (see Baillard *et al.* [103], [104] and [105]) recently designed the brain segmentation system based on the fusion of region into boundary/surface estimation. This algorithm was quite similar in approach to Suri *et al.*'s method discussed previously in sub-section 3.4.1. This algorithm was another instance where the propagation force V_0 in the fundamental level set segmentation equation $\frac{\partial \phi}{\partial t} = c(\mathbf{x})(\kappa + V_0)\ |\nabla \phi|$ was changed into a regional force. There were in all three changes made to this equation by Barillot and co-workers. First was in the propagation force V_0, second was in the data consistency term or stopping term $c(\mathbf{x})$, and the third change was on the step size Δt. These equations and their interpretation will be briefly discussed next.

3.4.3.1 Design of the Propagation Force Based on Probability Distribution

The key idea was to utilize the probability density function inside and outside the structure to be segmented. The pixel/voxel in the neighbourhood of the segmenting structure was responsible for creating a pull/push force on the propagating front. This was expressed in the form of the probability density function to be estimated inside the structure, $p_i(u)$, the probability density function to be estimated outside the structure, $p_e(u)$ and the prior probability for a voxel to be inside the structure. Note here, u[26] was the intensity value of a voxel at location (x, y, z). Using the above concept, this bi-directional propagation force was estimated as:

$$V_0 = sgn\{\alpha_i\ p_i(u) - (1 - \alpha_i)\ p_e(u)\}, \tag{3.20}$$

where $sgn(x)$ was 1 if $x \geq 0$ and was -1 if $x < 0$. The second modification was to the data consistency term[27] that changed from the gradient term into the extended gradient term. This term was changed from $c(\mathbf{x}) = \frac{1}{1+|\nabla[G_\sigma(\mathbf{x})*I(\mathbf{x})]|}$ to a term which was based on the transitional probability of going from inside to outside the object to be segmented. This was mathematically given as: $c(\mathbf{x}) = g[p_T(x|I, C)]$, where $g[x]$ was $1 - 4x^3$ if $x < 0.5$ and was $4(1-x)^3$, if $x \geq 0.5$. The term p_T was computed based on these three parameters: α_i, $p_i(u)$ and $p_e(u)$, and mathematically estimated if the probability of a pixel/voxel class C belonged to a set inside and outside the object. If the class C was inside the region, then p_T was given as $\frac{(1-\alpha_i)\, p_e(I(x))}{\alpha_i\, p_i(I(x))+(1-\alpha_i)\, p_e(I(x))}$, while it was $\frac{(\alpha_i)\, p_i(I(x))}{\alpha_i\, p_i(I(x))+(1-\alpha_i)\, p_e(I(x))}$ if C was outside, derived from the simple Bayesian rule.

Pros and Cons of Baillard/Barillot's Technique: The major advantages of this technique were: (**1**) The Chapter was an excellent example of the fusion of region-based information into the boundary/surface. (**2**) The results were very impressive; however, it would have been valuable to see the enlarged version of the results. (**3**) The algorithm was adaptive since the data consistency term ($c(\mathbf{x})$) and the step size (Δt) were adaptively estimated in every iteration of the front propagation. This provided a good trade-off between convergence speed and stability. (**4**) This method used stocastic-EM (SEM) instead of expectation-minimization (EM), which was a more robust and accurate method for estimation of probability density function parameters. (**5**) The method had been applied to various brain structures and to various imaging modalities such as ultrasound. (**6**) The algorithm hardly needed any tuning parameters and thus it was very efficient. Both methods (Suri *et al.* 's and Baillard *et al.* 's) were designed to control the propagation force using region-based analysis. Suri's method used regional-force computed using pixel-classification based on clustering, while Baillard *et al.* 's method used pixel-classification

[26]Note, this symbol is not to be confused with the membership function used in sub-section 3.4.1.

[27]or stopping term

based on Bayesian-statistics.

3.4.4 2-D/3-D Regional Geometric Surface: Fusion of Level Set with Global Shape Regularizer (Leventon/MIT)

Another application of the fusion of Bayesian statistics into geometric boundary/surface to model the shape in the level set framework was done recently by Leventon *et al.* [117]. Though this technique did not show the segmentation of the cortex, rather it focused on the segmentation of the sub-cortical area such as the corpus callosum, and was a good example of the fusion of the boundary and region-based technique. Leventon *et al.* derived the shape information using *maximum a posterior probability* (MAP) and fused that with gradient and curvature driven boundary/surface in the level set framework. This MAP mode of shape used *priors* in the Bayesian framework from the training data set (analogous to Cootes *et al.*'s [118] technique). Using Eq. 3.10, the level set curve/surface evolution was given as:

$$\frac{\partial \phi}{\partial t} = c(\mathbf{x})(\kappa + V_0)\,|\,\nabla\phi\,| + \underbrace{(\nabla c.\nabla\,\phi)}_{extra-stopping-term} \tag{3.21}$$

Note that this equation was exactly the same as Eq. 8 used by Leventon *et al.* in [117], whose solution using finite difference was:

$$\phi(t+1) = \phi(t) + \lambda_1[\underbrace{c(\mathbf{x})(\kappa + V_0)\,|\,\nabla\phi\,|}_{Gradient+Curvature-Forces} + \underbrace{(\nabla c.\nabla\,\phi)}_{Image-Force}]. \tag{3.22}$$

If $[\phi^*(t) - \phi(t)]$ represented the optimized shape information at time t, then Leventon *et al.* added this term to the above equation to yield the final evolution equation in the level set framework as:

$$\phi(t+1) = \phi(t) + \lambda_1[\underbrace{c(\mathbf{x})(\kappa + V_0)\,|\,\nabla\phi\,|}_{Gradient+Curvature-Forces} + \underbrace{(\nabla c.\nabla\,\phi)}_{Image-Force}] + \underbrace{\lambda_2[\phi^*(t) - \phi(t)]}_{Global-Shape-Force} \tag{3.23}$$

3.4.4.1 Design of the External Propagation Force Based on Global Shape Information

The key to the above model was the extraction of the shape information from the training data (called "global shape" information) and fusing with the local information (gradient and curvature) in the level set framework based on partial differential equations. If α and β represented shape and pose parameters, then the optimized ϕ^*_{MAP} would be given as the *argmax* of $P(\phi^* | \phi, \nabla I)$. This model using Bayes' rule could be broken down as: $\frac{P(\phi|\alpha,\beta)\, P(\nabla I|\alpha,\beta,\phi)\, P(\alpha)\, P(\beta)}{P(\phi,\nabla I)}$, where $P(\alpha)$ and $P(\beta)$ were shape and pose priors. To understand the computation of $P(\alpha)$, Leventon took n-curves, each sampled N times and each surface was represented by ϕ_i. Then, the training set $\tau = \{\phi_i, ... \phi_n\}$. This mean shape could be computed as $\mu = \frac{1}{n}\Sigma\,\phi_i$ and the mean offset map was $\hat{\phi_i} = (\phi_i - \mu)$. Each of this map is a column vector of a matrix $(N \times n)$. If r, c represents the rows and columns of the matrix M, then $M = [\phi_{r,c}]$, where the limits r and c were: $1 \leq r \leq N$ and $1 \leq c \leq n$. Next, this matrix M undergoes SVD[28] to decompose to $U\,\Sigma\,V^T$. Taking k-principal components, that is k-rows and k-columns, gave the new matrix Σ_k. Thus the shape coefficients α were computed as: $\alpha = U_k^T(\phi - \mu)$. Using the Gaussian distribution, the priors shape model could be computed as:

$$P(\alpha) = \frac{1}{\sqrt{(2\pi)^k |\Sigma_k|}}\, exp(\frac{1}{2}\, \alpha^t\, \Sigma_k^{-1}\, \alpha)\,. \tag{3.24}$$

This equation was used in the computation of optimized ϕ^*. The pose prior was from the uniform distribution.

Pros and Cons of Shape Information Fused in Geometric Boundary/Surface: The major advantages of this system include: (**1**) Robustness and successful capture of topology based on the Bayesian shape information. (**2**) Shape and pose parameters converged on the shape to be segmented. The major disadvantages of such a system include: (**1**) The time taken for such a system was six minutes (for vertebral segmentation), which was relatively very long for spinal navigation real-time applications. (**2**) The system would need training data sets which had to be collected off-line. (**3**) This Chapter did not show results on cortical segmentation which had deep convolutions, large twists and bends. (**4**) The performance of systems which had coefficients estimated from training data off-line and application of these estimated coefficients on-line was dependent upon training data and test data sets. The above system was like a first layer of a neural network (see Suri *et al.* [119]) where the

---

[28]Singular Value Decomposition

performance was governed by shapes of training data and tuning parameters of the Gaussian model (see Lee [120]).

3.4.5 Comparison Between Different Kinds of Regularizers

Having discussed four different kinds of regularizers (or designs of propagating forces), this sub-section presents the comparison between them on the following points:

(**1**) *Internal Vs. External Propagating Force:* Primarily all of the regularizers design the propagating force and drive the speed term. Suri, Zeng and Barillot *et al.*'s technique designs the propagation force internal to the level set, while Leventon *et al.*'s technique designs the propagation force externally. The internal propagation force is accurate and robust since it directly acts on the speed function compared to the external propagation force. However, the internal propagation force is more sensitive to the overall system since these forces are computed directly based on region-based strategy and acted directly on speed functions.

(**2**) *Common to All Techniques:* Suri's method uses Fuzzy Clustering, Zeng *et al.*'s method uses the constrained Bayesian approach, Barillot *et al.*'s technique uses plain Bayesian classification, and Leventon *et al.*'s technique uses the global shape-based information using Eigen analysis based on SVD. All of these techniques had one objective in common, that is, they were after the extraction of the shape to be segmented by fusion of the region-based strategy in the level set framework.

(**3**) *Timings:* It is difficult to compare the speed since all of these four techniques do segmentation of different organs and volumes, and it also depended on the initial placement of the contour/surface. Individually, the claims of each of these techniques had the following timings: (i) Suri *et al.*'s 2-D GM/WM segmentation techniques took less than a minute per image. (ii) Zeng *et al.*'s 3-D technique took around one hour for cortical segmentation. (iii) Barillot *et al.*'s 3-D technique took around two hours for cortical segmentation. (iv) Leventon *et al.*'s 3-D technique took six minutes for the complete vertebrae.

(**4**) *User Interaction:* Suri's technique was automatic except for the placement of the initial contour. Zeng *et al.*'s method did initialization of sphere sets in white matter, which was at a minimum. Barillot's technique also involved minimal interaction. Leventon *et al.*'s technique used an off-line method for tracing the boundaries of shapes which was needed for training data sets. This was time consuming.

(**5**) *Number of Parameters and Adaptability Towards Step Size:* The number of parameters used in Suri's technique was at a minimum for a particular tissue type for the MR image (e.g., T_1, T_2 or PD). The fuzzy clustering had two parameters, the error threshold and the number of iterations. The technique was not self-adaptive as far as the step sizes went. It was kept constant at unity. Zeng *et al.*'s method used a minimum number of parameters and was also not adaptive; however, the constrained force generation was dynamic. Barillot's method had also a minimum number of parameters but was self-adaptive. Leventon *et al.*'s method was not self-adaptive and used a greater number of parameters compared to the other techniques.

(**6**) *Stability of the Method:* This factor depended upon a ratio, the Courant number[29]. No discussion was given about the CFL number by Suri, Zeng or Leventon. Barillot did discuss stability issues in which they talked about the dynamic nature of the CFL number that automatically changed to adjust for any instabilities.

3.5 Numerical Methodologies for Solving Level Set Functions

The relationship between conservation laws and the evolution of curves was introduced in the classic paper by Osher and Sethian [67]. This paper presented a new formulation for curve evolution by considering the evolution of a higher dimensional function in which the curve was embedded as a "level set". This was a stable and efficient numerical scheme (for the non-convex Hamiltonian numerical scheme, readers are referred to Osher and Shu [106]).

This section has three parts: (**1**) Part one (sub-section 3.5.1) is the derivation of the finite difference equation in terms of level sets using the Hamilton-Jacobi (HJ) and hyperbolic conservation law; (**2**) Part two (sub-section 3.5.2) is on the ratio $\frac{\Delta t}{\Delta x}$, called CFL number[30]; and (**3**) Part three (sub-section 3.5.3) consists of the application of the numerical scheme using finite difference for

[29] see sub-section 3.5.2

[30] Courant number, named after the author Courant *et al.* [107]

cortical segmentation.

3.5.1 Hamilton-Jacobi Equation and Hyperbolic Conservation Law

Here, the numerical approximation of the Hamilton-Jacobi formulation of the level set function will be briefly derived. To start with, the hyperbolic conservation law stated that "the rate of change of the total amount of substance contained in a fixed domain G is equal to the flux of that substance across the boundary of G". If v was the density of the substance and f the flux, then the conservation law was mathematically given as: $\frac{d}{dt}\int_G v\, dx = -\int_{\partial G} < f, n > dS$, where n was the outward normal to G, dS is the surface element of ∂G. Using vector calculus, the differential conservation law was: $v_t + \nabla . f = 0$. The HJ equation in $\mathcal{R}^d$ had the form: $\phi_t + H(\phi_{x1} ... \phi_{xd})$ and in 1-D, the HJ equation became the conservation law, and as a result, the methodologies used for solving the conservation law were used for solving the HJ equation. A finite difference method was in the conservation form if it could be written as:

$$\frac{v_j^{n+1} - v_j^n}{\Delta t} = -(\frac{c_{j+1/2}^n - c_{j-1/2}^n}{\Delta x}), \tag{3.25}$$

where c was the potential field or the numerical flux, which was Lipschitz and consistent[31]. Thus using the relationship between the level set function, the HJ equation and the conservation law, we have: $\phi(x,t) = \int_{\infty}^{x} v(\hat{x}, t) d\hat{x}$. By integration over the monotone numerical scheme and shifting from $j + 1/2$ to j, the HJ formulation was given as: $\phi_j^{n+1} = \phi_j^n - \Delta t\; c(D_-\phi_j^n, D_+\phi_j^n)$, where $c(D_-\phi_j^n, D_+\phi_j^n) = h[(\mathbf{min}(v_j^n, 0))^2 + (\mathbf{max}(v_j^n, 0))^2]$ [32]. This equation will be used in the segmentation example in sub-section 3.5.3, but first, the ratio $\frac{\Delta t}{\Delta x}$, the called CFL number, will be discussed.

3.5.2 CFL Number

For the stability of the numerical scheme, it was observed by Courant *et al.* [107] that a necessary stability condition for any numerical scheme was that the *domain of dependence* (DoD) of each point in the *domain of numerical scheme* should include the DoD of the partial differential equation itself. This condition

---

[31] numerical flux becomes continuous flux, i.e., c(v,....v)=H(v)

[32] Note, D_- and D_+ are the backward and forward difference operator.

was necessary for the stability of the numerical scheme. The ratio $\frac{\triangle t}{\triangle x}$ under the limit $\Delta x \rightarrow 0$ and $\Delta t \rightarrow 0$ is the CFL number, or called the Courant number. This CFL number was determined by the maximal possible flow of information. This flow of lines of information depended upon the type of the data and was thus called as "characteristics of the PDE". If these "characteristics" collide, then "shocks" occur. Interested readers can see the work by Kimia *et al.* [84] on shocks. Recently, Goldenberg *et al.* [108] fused the AOS[33] scheme in level sets for numerical stability. The original AOS model was presented by Perona-Malik [109] for non-linear diffusion in image processing. Interested readers can explore the AOS model and its fusion in level sets by Goldenberg.

3.5.3 A Segmentation Example Using a Finite Difference Method

Here, speed control functions and their integration in terms of the level set function ϕ to estimate the ϕ over time are presented. The time step restrictions for solving the partial differential equation will not be discussed here (the reader can refer to the work by Osher and Sethian *et al.* [67] and the recent work by Barillot and his co-workers [103]). Using the finite difference method (see also Sethian [71] and Rouy *et al.* [76]), the level set Eq. 3.17 was given in terms of time n as (for details, see Suri [55] and [56]):

$$\phi_{x,y}^{n+1} = \phi_{x,y}^{n} - \Delta t \; \{ \; V_{reg}(x,y) + V_{grad}(x,y) - V_{cur}(x,y) \; \}, \tag{3.26}$$

where $\phi_{x,y}^{n}$ and $\phi_{x,y}^{n+1}$ were level set functions at pixel location (x, y) at times n and $n+1$, Δt was the time difference, and $V_{reg}(x,y)$, $V_{grad}(x,y)$ and $V_{cur}(x,y)$ were the regional, gradient and curvature speed terms, respectively. Now, these terms are presented as under: **(1)** The regional speed term expressed in terms of the level set function (ϕ) was given as: $V_{reg}(x,y) = \mathbf{max}(V_p(x,y),0)\ \nabla^{+} + \mathbf{min}(V_p(x,y),0)\ \nabla^{-}$, where terms $V_p(x,y)$, ∇^{+} and ∇^{-} were given as: $V_p(x,y) = \frac{w_R}{\gamma\, R_{ind}(x,y)}$, $R_{ind} = 1 - 2\,u(x,y)$, $\nabla^{-} = [\nabla_x^{-} + \nabla_y^{-}]^{\frac{1}{2}}$ and $\nabla^{+} = [\nabla_x^{+} + \nabla_y^{+}]^{\frac{1}{2}}$.

$$\left\{ \begin{array}{lcl} \nabla_x^{+} & = & [\mathbf{max}(D^{-x}(x,y),0))^2 + \mathbf{min}(D^{+x}(x,y),0))^2] \\ \nabla_y^{-} & = & [\mathbf{max}(D^{-y}(x,y),0))^2 + \mathbf{min}(D^{+y}(x,y),0))^2], \end{array} \right. \tag{3.27}$$

where $u(x,y)$ took a value between 0 and 1. This could be coming from, say, a fuzzy membership function or any other clustering technique. R_{ind} was the

[33]additive operator splitting

region indicator function that was in the range between -1 to +1. (**2**) The gradient speed term, called the edge strength of the object boundaries, was expressed in terms of the level set function (ϕ) as the x and y components of the gradient speed as: $V_{grad}(x,y) = V_{gradx}(x,y) + V_{grady}(x,y)$, where:

$$\begin{cases} V_{gradx}(x,y) &= \mathbf{max}(p^n(x,y),0)\ D^{-x}(x,y) + \mathbf{min}(q^n(x,y),0)\ D^{+x}(x,y) \\ V_{grady}(x,y) &= \mathbf{max}(q^n(x,y),0)\ D^{-y}(x,y) + \mathbf{min}(q^n(x,y),0)\ D^{+y}(x,y) \\ p^n(x,y) &= \nabla_x(w_e\ \nabla(G_\sigma * I))\ \&\ q^n(x,y) = \nabla_y(w_e\ \nabla(G_\sigma * I)), \end{cases} \tag{3.28}$$

where w_e was the weight of the edge and was also a fixed constant. $p^n(x,y)$ and $q^n(x,y)$ were defined as the x and y components of the gradient strength at a pixel location (x,y). Note that the regional and edge speed terms depended upon the forward and backward difference operator which was defined in terms of the level set function ϕ defined as:

$$\begin{cases} D^{-x}(x,y) = \frac{(\phi(x,y)-\phi(x-1,y))}{\Delta x} & \&\ \ D^{+x}(x,y) = \frac{(\phi(x+1,y)-\phi(x,y))}{\Delta x} \\ D^{-y}(x,y) = \frac{(\phi(x,y)-\phi(x,y-1))}{\Delta y} & \&\ \ D^{+y}(x,y) = \frac{(\phi(x,y+1)-\phi(x,y))}{\Delta y}, \end{cases} \tag{3.29}$$

where $\phi(x,y)$, $\phi(x-1,y)$, $\phi(x+1,y)$, $\phi(x,y-1)$, $\phi(x,y+1)$ were the level set functions at pixel locations (x,y), $(x-1,y)$, $(x+1,y)$, $(x,y-1)$, $(x,y+1)$, being the four neighbours of (x,y). (**3**) The curvature speed term expressed in terms of the level set function (ϕ) was given as: $V_{cur}(x,y) = \epsilon\,\kappa^n(x,y)\,[\,(D^{0x}(x,y))^2 + ((\,D^{0y}(x,y))^2\,]^{\frac{1}{2}}$, where ϵ was a fixed constant, $\kappa^n(x,y)$ was the curvature at a pixel location (x,y) at n^{th} iteration as: $\kappa^n(x,y) = \frac{\phi_{xx}^2\,\phi_y^2 - \phi_x^2\,\phi_y^2\,\phi_{xy}^2 + \phi_{yy}^2\,\phi_x^2}{(\phi_x^2+\phi_y^2)^{\frac{3}{2}}}$ and $D^{0x}(x,y)$ and $D^{0y}(x,y)$ were defined as:

$$D^{0x}(x,y) = \frac{(\phi(x+1,y) - \phi(x-1,y))}{2\,\Delta x}\ \ \&\ \ D^{0y}(x,y) = \frac{(\phi(x,y+1) - \phi(x,y-1))}{2\,\Delta y}. \tag{3.30}$$

Thus, to numerically solve Eq. 3.26, all that was needed was: (i) the gradient speed values (p,q), (ii) the curvature speed κ at pixel location (x,y), and (iii) the membership function $u(x,y)$ for a particular class K. In the next section, how these speeds control mathematical functions will be discussed and how they are used to compute the field flow (level set function, ϕ) in the "narrow band" using the "fast marching method", also called the "optimization technique".

3.6 Optimization and Quantification Techniques Used in Conjunction with Level Sets: Fast Marching, Narrow Band, Adaptive Algorithms and Geometric Shape Quantification

The level set method could be computatively very expensive as the dimensionality of the surface increases. If d is the dimension of the surface, and $n = \frac{1}{\delta}$ where δ is the length scale of the computational resolution, then the cost of tracking the surface can be reasonably expected to be of the order $O(n^{\delta})$ per time step. There are two ways by which the speed can be improved. One way is by running the level set implementation in the narrow band (see Malladi *et al.* [77]) and the second is by using the adaptive mesh technique (see Milne [116]). These will be discussed in this section. The algorithms in 2-D will be discussed, but it is straightforward to convert it into 3-D.

3.6.1 Fast Marching Method

The fast marching method (FMM) was used to solve the Eikonal Equation (see Adalsteinsson *et al.* [110], [111] and [112]), or a level set evolution with speed where the sign did not change. Its main usage was to compute the signed distance transform from a given curve (say, one with speed = 1). This signed distance function was the level set function that was used in the narrow band algorithm. The FMM can also be used for a simple active contour model if the contour only moved either inward (pressure force in terms of parametric snakes) or outward (balloon force in terms of parametric snakes). The FMM algorithm consisted of three major stages: (**1**) initialization stage; (**2**) tagging stage; and (**3**) marching stage. A discussion on these follows next.

1. *Initialization Stage:* If the curve cuts the grid points exactly, this means that the curve passed through the intersection of the horizontal and vertical grid lines. If the curve did not pass through the grid points, then it was necessary to find where the curve intersected the grid lines using the simple method recently developed by Adalsteinsson *et al.* [111]. The method consisted of checking the neighbors (E, W, N, S) of a given cen-

tral pixel and finding 16 different combinations where the given contour could intersect the grid. Since the central pixel could be inside or outside, there were 16 positive combinations and 16 negative combinations. At the end of this process, the distances of all the grid points were noted which were closest to the given curve.

2. *Tagging Stage:* Here, three sets of grid points were created: *Accepted set*, *Trial set* and *Far set*. The *Accepted set* were those points which fell on the given curve. All these points obviously had a distance of zero. Those points were tagged as ACCEPTED. If the curve did not pass through the grid points, then those points were points of the initialization stage and were tagged as ACCEPTED. The *Trial set* included all points that were nearest neighbors to the point in the *Accepted set*. Those were tagged as TRIAL. Then their distance values were computed by solving the Eikonal Eq. 3.5. Those points and their distances were put on the heap. The *Far set* were grid points which were neither tagged as ACCEPTED nor TRIAL. Those were tagged as FAR. They did not affect the distance computation of trial grid points. These grid points were not put onto the heap.

3. *Marching Stage:*

   (a) Here, the grid point (say, P) was popped from the top of the heap. It should have the smallest distance value among all grid points in the heap. This point was tagged as ACCEPTED so that its value would not change anymore. Heap sort methodology was used for bubbling the least distance value on the heap.

   (b) Four nearest neighbors of the popped point P were found. If its tag was ACCEPTED, nothing was done; otherwise, the distance was re-computed by solving the Eikonal Eq. 3.5. If it was FAR, it was relabled as TRIAL and was put on the heap. If it is already labeled as TRIAL, its value was updated in the heap. This prevented the same point from appearing twice in the heap.

   (c) Go back to step (a) until there were no more points in the heap, i.e., all points had been tagged as ACCEPTED.

Note that the above method was an exhaustive search like the greedy algorithm discussed by Suri *et al.* [92]. The superiority of this method was evidenced by the fact that every visited grid point was visited no more than four times. The crux of the speed was due to the sorting algorithm. Suri *et al.* used the back pointer method at the grid or pixel location (x, y), similar to the approach taken by Sethian [113], [114].

3.6.2 A Note on the Heap Sorting Algorithm

Heap sorting based on the back pointer method was first applied by Sethian/Malladi in their work (see Malladi *et al.* [49]). Since then, almost all researchers have used this technique in their implementations. The heap sorting algorithm was basically used to select the smallest value (see Sedgewick [115]). Briefly, a heap can be viewed as a tree or a corresponding ordered array. A binary heap had the property that the value at a given "child" position int(i) was always larger than or equal to the value at its "parent" position (int (i/2)). The minimum travel time in the heap was stored at the top of the heap. Arranging the tentative travel time array onto a heap effectively identified and selected the minimum travel time in the array. The minimum travel time on the heap identified a corresponding minimum travel time grid point. Values could be added or removed from the heap. Adding or removing a value to/from the heap included re-arranging the array so that it satisfied the heap condition ("heapifying the array"). Heapifying an array was achieved by recursively exchanging the positions of any parent-child pair violating the heap property until the heap property was satisfied across the heap. Adding or removing a value from a heap generally has a computational cost of order $\mathcal{O}(log\ N)$, where N was the number of heap elements.

3.6.3 Narrow Band Method

Malladi *et al.* [77] were one of the beginners who first applied the narrow banding scheme for medical image segmentation. Almost all the recent applications using level sets have used narrow banding in their implementations. Below are the steps that were followed for optimization of the level set function ϕ using narrow banding. The level set function computation was implemented in the narrow band, given the speed functions.

1. *Narrow Band and Land Mine Construction*

   Here, a narrow band was constructed around the given curve where the absolute distance value was less than half the width of the narrow band. These grid points were put onto the list. Now some points in the narrow band were tagged as land mines. They were the grid points whose absolute distance value was less than $\frac{W}{2}$ and greater than $(\frac{W}{2} - \Delta_l)$, where W was the band-width and Δ_l was the width of the land mine points. Note that the formation of the narrow band was equivalent to saying that the first external iteration or a new tube had been formed.

2. *Internal Iteration for Computing the Field Flow (ϕ)*
   This step evolved the active contour inside the narrow band until the land mine sign changed. For all the iterations, the level set function was updated by solving the level set Eq. 3.26. Now the land mine sign of its ϕ was checked. If the sign was changed, the system was re-initialized, otherwise the loop was continued.

3. *Re-Initialization (zero level curve (ZLC) and signed distance transform computation)*
   This step consisted of two parts: (i) Determination of the *zero level curve* given the field flow ϕ. (ii) Given the *zero level curve*, estimation was done of the signed distance transform (SDT). Part (i) is also called isocontour extraction since the front in the field flow is estimated which had a value of zero. The modified version of the Adalsteinsson *et al.* [111] algorithm was used for estimating the ZLC, however the signs of the field flow were needed. In part (ii), the fast marching method was run to estimate the signed distance transform. The signed-distance-function was computed for all the points in the computational domain. At the end of step 3, the algorithm moved to step 1 and the next external iteration was started.

At the end of the process, a new *zero level curve* was estimated which represented the final object boundary. Note, this technique was used for all the global information integrated into the system.

3.6.4 A Note on Adaptive Level Sets Vs. Narrow Banding

Adaptive level sets were attempted by Milne [116] while working towards his Ph.D. In this method, the resolution of the grid was changed during the marching stage. Figure 3.5 shows an example where the mesh resolution changed for the high curvature zones. This scheme had three major benefits: (**1**) The algorithm does not need to be re-initialized. (**2**) The computational domain was extended beyond the surface of interest without the incurrence of a performance penalty. Thus the boundary conditions were not a serious threat to the stable solution. (**3**) Adaptive level sets allowed for a non-uniform resolution of the surface itself. This meant one can selectively redistribute the density of information across the surface. As a result, one could match itself to the small scale features of the surface. Thus adaptive level sets are more powerful than plain narrow band level set methods. Even though adaptive level sets had done well compared to narrow band methods, the application of adaptive level sets in high curvature areas is not very stable. If the interface changed from coarse to fine, then stability issues of the propagating fronts are in question (see Berger *et al.* [94], [95]).

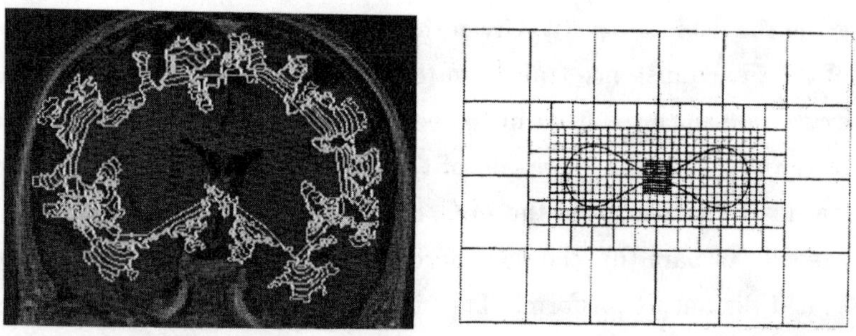

Figure 3.5: **Left**: Ripples formed during the growth evolution of *zero level curves*. Also seen is the large capture range of the segmentation scheme along with the shape change as per the topology. This figure shows superimposition of 6 *zero level set* curves (MR Data Set: Courtesy of Marconi Medical Systems, Inc.). **Right**: Adaptive mesh refinement. Reprinted with permission of R.B. Milne, Lawrence Berkeley National Laboratory, Berkeley, CA, LBNL-39216, pg. 33, 1995.

3.7 Merits, Demerits, Conclusions and the Future of 2-D and 3-D Level Sets in Medical Imagery

3.7.1 Advantages of Level Sets

Level set formulation offers a large number of advantages that are as follows: (**1**) *Capture Range*: The greatest advantage of this technique is that this algorithm increases the capture range of the field flow and thereby increases the robustness of the initial contour placement. (**2**) *Effect of Local Noise*: When the regional information is integrated into the system, then the local noise or edge will not distract the growth process. This technique is non-local and thus the local noise cannot distract the final placement of the contour or the diffusion growth process. (**3**) *No Need of Elasticity Coefficients*: The technique is not controlled by elasticity coefficients, unlike parametric contour methods. There is no need to fit tangents to the curves and compute normals at each vertex. In this system, the normals are embedded in the system using the divergence of the field flow. This technique has an ability to model incremental deformations in shape. (**4**) *Suitability for Medical Image Segmentation*: This technique is very suitable for medical organ segmentation since it can handle any of the cavities, concavities, convolutedness, splitting or merging. (**5**) *Finding the Global Minima*: There is no problem finding the local minima or global minima, unlike optimization techniques of parametric snakes. (**6**) *Normal Computation*: This technique is less prone to the normal computational error which is very easily incorporated in classical balloon force snakes for segmentation. (**7**) *Automaticity*: It is very easy to extend this model from semi-automatic to completely automatic because the region is determined on the basis of prior information. (**8**) *Integration of Regional Statistics*: This technique is based on the propagation of curves (just like the propagation of ripples in the tank or propagation of the fire flames) utilizing the region statistics. (**9**) *Flexible Topology*: This method adjusts to the topological changes of the given shape. Diffusion propagation methods handle a very natural framework for handling the topological changes (joining and breaking of the curves). (**10**) *Wide Applications*: This technique can be applied to unimodal, bimodal, and multi-modal imagery, which means it can have multiple gray level values in it. These methods have a wide range of applications in 3-D surface modeling. (**11**) *Speed of the System*: This technique implements the fast marching method in the narrow band for solving the Eikonal Equation for computing signed distances. (**12**) *Extension*: The technique is an easy extension from 2-D to 3-D. (**13**) *Incorporation of Regularizing Terms*: This can easily incorporate other features for controlling the speed of the curve. This is done by adding an extra term to the region, gradient and curvature speed terms. (**14**) *Handling Corners*: The system takes care of the corners easily unlike parametric curves, where it needs special handling at corners of the boundary. (**15**) *Resolution Changes*: The technique is extendable to multi-scale resolutions, which means that at lower resolutions, one can compute regional segmentations. These segmented results can then be used for higher resolutions. (**16**) *Multi-phase Processing*: This technique is extendable to multi-phase, which means that if there are multiple level set functions, then they automatically merge and split during the course of the segmentation process. (**17**) *Surface Tracking*: Tracking surfaces are implemented using level sets very smoothly. (**18**) *Quantification of 3-D Structures*: Computation of geometrical computations is done in a natural way, for example, one can compute the curvature of 3-D surfaces directly while performing normal computations. (**19**) *Integration of Regularization Terms*: Allows easy integration of vision models for shape recovery such as in fuzzy clustering, Gibbs model, Markov Random Fields and Bayesian models (see Paragios *et al.* [29]). This makes the system very powerful, robust and accurate for medical shape recovery. (**20**) *Concise Descriptions*: One can give concise descriptions of differential structures using level set methods. This is because of background mesh resolution controls. (**21**) *Hierarchical Representations*: Level set offers a natural scale space for hierarchical representations. (**22**) *Reparameterization*: There is no need for reparameterization for curve/surface estimation during the propagation, unlike in the classical snakes model.

3.7.2 Disadvantages of Level Sets

Even though level sets have dominated several fields of imaging science, these front propagation algorithms have certain drawbacks. They are as follows: (**1**) *Initial placement of the contour:* One of the major drawbacks of parametric active contours was its initial placement. It does not have either enough capture range or enough power to grab the topology of shapes. Both of these drawbacks were removed by level sets provided the initial contour was placed *symmetrically* with respect to the boundaries of interest. This ensures that level sets reached object boundaries almost at the same time. On the contrary, if the initial contour is much closer to the first portion of the object boundary compared to the second portion, then the evolving contour crosses over the first portion of the object boundary. This is because the stop does not turn out to be zero. One of the controlling factors for the stop function is the gradient of the image. The relationship of the stop function to the gradient is its inverse, and also depends upon the index power m in the ratio $\frac{1}{1+|\nabla G_\sigma * I(x,y)|^m}$. For stopping the propagation, the denominator should be large, which means image forces due to the gradient should be high. This means index m should be high. In other words, if m is high, then the gradient is high, which means weak boundaries are not detected well and will be easily crossed over by the evolving curve. If m is low (low threshold), then the level set will stop at noisy or at isolated edges. (**2**) *Embedding of the object:* If some objects (say, inner objects) are embedded in another object (the outer object), then the level set will not capture all objects of interest. This is especially true if embedded objects are asymmetrically situated. Under such conditions, one needs multiple initializations of active contours. This means only one active contour can be used per object. (**3**) *Gaps in boundaries:* This is one of the serious drawbacks of the level set method and has been pointed out by Siddiqi and Kimia. Due to gaps in the object, the evolving contour simply leaks through gaps. As a result, objects represented by incomplete contours are not captured correctly and fully. This is especially prominent in realistic images, such as in ultrasound and multi-class MR and CT images. (**4**) *Problems due to shocks:* Shocks are the most common problem in level sets. Kimia and co-workers (see Kimia *et al.* [84], Siddiqi *et al.* [85] and Stoll *et al.* [86]) developed such a framework by representing shape as the set of singularities (called shocks) that arise in a rich space of shape deformations as classified into four types: (i) first-order shocks are orientation discontinuities (corners) and arise from protrusions and indentations; (ii) second-order shocks are formed when a shape breaks into two parts during a deformation; (iii) third-order shocks represent bends; and (iv) fourth-order shocks are seeds for each component of a shape. These shocks arise in level sets and can cause sometimes serious problems.

3.7.3 Conclusions and the Future on Level Sets

The class of differential geometry, also called level sets, has been shown to dominate medical imaging in a major way. There is still a need to understand how regularization terms can be integrated into level sets to improve medical segmentation schemes. Even though the application of level sets has gone well in fields of medical imaging, biomedicine, fluid mechanics, combustion, solidification, CAD/CAM, object tracking/image sequence analysis, and device fabrication, this is still far away from achieving stable 3-D and a standard segmentation technique in real-time. By standard, this means that which can segment the 3-D volume with a wide variation of pulse sequence parameters. In the near future will be seen the modelling of front propagation that takes into account physical constraints of the problem, for example, minimization of variation geodesic distances, rather than simple distance transforms. Also will be seen more incorporation of likelihood functions and adaptive fuzzy models to prevent leaking of curves/surfaces. A good example of the integration of low level processes into the evolution process would be given as: $\frac{\partial \phi}{\partial t} = L(x,y)\,(\beta_0 - \beta_1 \kappa)\,|\nabla \phi|$, where $L(x,y) = 1 - max(S_1, S_2, S_3, ..., S_n)$, where S_i is the low level process from edge detection, optical flow, stereo disparity, texture, etc. The better the $S(x,y)$, the more robust would be the level set segmentation process. It is also hoped that more papers in level sets will be seen where the segmentation step does require a reinitialization stage (see Zhao *et al.* [121] and Evans *et al.* [122]). It would also, however, be helpful if a faster triangulation algorithm can be incorporated for isosurface extraction in 3-D segmentation methods.

A massive effort has been seen by the computer vision community to integrate regularization terms to improve robustness and accuracy of 3-D segmentation techniques. How curve/surface propagation hypersurfaces based on differential geometry are used was shown for the segmentation of medical objects in 2-D and 3-D. Also shown in this Chapter is the relationship between parametric deformable models and curve evolution framework; incorporation of clamping/stopping forces to improve the robustness of these topologically independent curves/surfaces; and finally, state-of-the-art 2-D and 3-D level set segmentation systems was presented for medical imagery. With time, more adaptive schemes will be seen buffered with knowledge-based methods to yield more efficient techniques for 2-D and 3-D segmentation.

3.7.4 Acknowledgements

Special thanks go to John Patrick and Elaine Keeler, both with Marconi Medical Systems, Inc., for their encouragements. Special thanks go also to Marconi Medical Systems, Inc., for their MR data sets. Thanks go also to the anonymous reviewers for their valuable suggestions.

Bibliography

[1] Suri, J. S., Setarehdan, S. K. and Singh, S., Advanced Algorithmic Approaches to Medical Image Segmentation: State-of-the-Art Applications in Cardiology, Neurology, Mammography and Pathology, ISBN 1-85233-389-8, First Eds. In Press, 2001.

[2] Suri, J. S., Two Dimensional Fast MR Brain Segmentation Using a Region-Based Level Set Approach, Accepted for Publication in Int. Journal of Engineering in Medicine and Biology, 2001.

[3] Chopp, D. L., Computing Minimal Surfaces via Level Set Curvature Flow, Journal of Comput. Physics, Vol. 106, No. 1, pp. 77-91, 1993.

[4] Lachaud, J. O. and Montanvert, A., Deformable Meshes with Automated Topology Changes for Coarse-to-Fine 3D Surface Extraction, Medical Image Analysis, Vol. 3, No. 2, pp. 187-207, 1999.

[5] Lachaud, J. O. and Bainville, E., A discrete adaptative model following topological modifications of volumes, In Proc. of the 4th Discrete Geometry for Computer Imagery (DGCI), Grenoble, France, pp. 183-194, 1994.

[6] Lachaud, J. O. and Montanvert, A., Continuous analogs of digital boundaries: A topological approach to iso-surfaces, Graphical Models and Image Processing (GMIP), Vol. 62, No. 3, pp. 129-164, 2000.

[7] Malgouyres, R. and Lenoir, A., Topology Preservation within Digital Surfaces, Graphical Models, Vol. 62, No. 2, pp. 71-84, 2000.

[8] Kong, T. Y. and Rosenfeld, A., Digital Topology: Introduction and Survey, Computer Vision, Graphics and Image Processing, Vol. 48, No. 3, pp. 357-393, 1989.

[9] Bertalmio, M., Sapiro, G. and Randall, G., Region tracking on level-sets methods, IEEE Trans. on Med. Imaging, Vol. 18, No. 5, pp. 448-51, May 1999.

[10] DeCarlo, D. and Gallier, J., Topological Evolution of Surfaces, Graphics Interface, pp. 194-203, 1996.

[11] Angenent, S., Chopp, D. and Ilmanen, T., On the singularities of cones evolving by mean curvature, Communications in Partial Differential Equations (CPDE), Vol. 20, No. 11/12, pp. 1937-1958, 1995.

[12] Chopp, D. L., Flow under curvature: Singularity formation, minimal surfaces and geodesics, Experimental Mathematics, Vol. 2, No. 4, pp. 235-255, 1993.

[13] Chopp, D. L., Numerical computation of self-similar solutions for mean curvature flow, Experimental Mathematics, Vol. 3, No. 1, pp. 1-15, 1993.

[14] Sethian, J. A., Numerical algorithms for propagating interfaces: Hamilton-Jacobi equations and conservation laws, J. of Differential Geometry, Vol. 31, No. 1, pp. 131-161, 1990.

[15] Sethian, J. A., Curvature flow and entropy conditions applied to grid generation, J. Computational Physics, Vol. 115, No. 1, pp. 440-454, 1994.

[16] Mulder, W., Osher, S. J. and Sethian, J. A., Computing interface motion in compressible gas dynamics, J. Computational Physics, Vol. 100, No. 1, pp. 209-228, 1992.

[17] Sethian, J. A., Algorithms for tracking interfaces in CFD and material science, Annual Review of Computational Fluid Mechanics, 1995.

[18] Sussman, M., Smereka, P. and Osher, S. J., A level set method for computing solutions to incompressible two-phase flow, J. Computational Physics, Vol. 114, No. 1, pp. 146-159, 1994.

[19] Rhee, C., Talbot, L. and Sethian, J. A., Dynamical study of a premixed V-flame, J. of Fluid Mechanics, Vol. 300, pp. 87-115, 1995.

[20] Sethian, J. A. and Strain, J. D., Crystal growth and dentritic solidification, J. Computational Physics, Vol. 98, No. 2, pp. 231-253, 1992.

[21] Adalsteinsson, D. and Sethian, J. A., A unified level set approach to etching, deposition and lithography I: Algorithms and two-dimensional simulations, J. Computational Physics, Vol. 120, No. 1, pp. 128-144, 1995.

[22] Whitaker, R. T., Algorithms for Implicit Deformable Models, International Conference on Computer Vision (ICCV), pp. 822-827, June 1995.

[23] Whitaker, Ross, T., A Level-Set Approach to 3D Reconstruction From Range Data, International J. of Computer Vision (IJCV), Vol. 29, No. 3, pp. 203-231, October 1998.

[24] Whitaker, R. T. and Breen, D. E., Level-Set Models for the Deformation of Solid Objects, Proceedings of Implicit Surfaces, Eurographics/Siggraph, pp. 19-35, June 1998.

[25] Mansouri, A. R. and Konrad, J., Motion segmentation with level sets, In Proc. IEEE Int. Conf. Image Processing (ICIP), Vol. II, pp. 126-130, Oct. 1999.

[26] Mansouri, A. R., Sirivong, B. and Konrad, J., Multiple motion segmentation with level sets, Image and Video Communications and Processing, Bhaskaran, V. T., Russell, H., Tescher, A. G. and Stevenson, R. L., Eds., Proc. SPIE, Vol. 3974, pp. 584-595, April 2000.

[27] Mansouri, A.-R. and Konrad, J., Minimum description length region tracking with level sets, in Proc. SPIE Image and Video Communications and Process., Vol. 3974, pp. 515-525, Jan. 2000.

[28] Paragios, N. and Deriche, R., Geodesic Active Contours and Level Sets for the Detection and Tracking of Moving Objects, IEEE Transactions on Pattern Analysis and Machine Intelligence, Vol. 22, No. 3, pp. 266-280, March 2000.

[29] Paragios, N. and Deriche, R., Coupled Geodesic Active Regions for Image Segmentation: a level set approach, In the Sixth European Conference on Computer Vision (ECCV), Trinity College, Dublin, Ireland, Vol. II, pp. 224-240, 26th June - 1st July, 2000.

[30] Kornprobst P., Deriche R. and Aubert, G., Image Sequence Analysis via Partial Differential Equations, J. of Mathematical Imaging and Vision, Vol. 11, No. 1, pp. 5-26, 1999.

[31] Faugeras, O. and Keriven, R., Variational principles, surface evolution, PDE's level set methods and the stereo problem, IEEE Trans. on Image Proc., Vol. 7, No. 3, pp. 336-344, May 1998.

[32] Kimmel, R., Siddiqi, K. and Kimia, B., Shape from Shading: Level Set Propagation and Viscosity Solutions, International Journal of Computer Vision, Vol. 16, No. 2, pp. 107-133, 1995.

[33] Kimmel, R., Tracking Level Sets by Level Sets: A Method for Solving the Shape from Shading Problem, Computer Vision and Image Understanding, Vol. 62, No. 2, pp. 47-58, 1995.

[34] Kimmel, R. and Bruckstein, A. M., Global Shape from Shading, Computer Vision and Image Understanding, Vol. 62, No. 3, pp. 360-369, 1995.

[35] Arehart, A., Vincent, L. and Kimia, B. B., Mathematical Morphology: The Hamilton-Jacobi Connection, In Int. Conference in Computer Vision (ICCV), pp. 215-219, 1993.

[36] Catte, F., Dibos, F. and Koepfler, G., A morphological scheme for mean curvature motion and applications to anisotropic diffusion and motion of level sets, in SIAM Jour. of Numerical Analysis, Vol. 32, No. 6, pp. 1895-1909, 1995.

[37] Sapiro, G., Kimmel, R., Shaked, D., Kimia, B. B. and Bruckstein, A. M., Implementing continuous-scale morphology via curve evolution, Pattern Recognition, Vol. 26, No. 9, pp. 1363-1372, 1997.

[38] Sochen, N., Kimmel, R. and Malladi, R., A Geometrical Framework for Low Level Vision, IEEE Trans. on Image Processing, Vol. 7, No. 3, pp. 310-318, 1998.

[39] Sapiro, G., Color Snakes, Computer Vision and Image Understanding (CVIU), Vol. 68, No. 2, pp. 247-253, 1997.

[40] Caselles, V., Kimmel, R., Sapiro, G. and Sbert, C., Three Dimensional Object Modeling via Minimal Surfaces, Proc. of the European Conf. Computer Vision (ECCV), pp. 97-106, 1996.

[41] Caselles, V., Kimmel, R., Sapiro, G. and Sbert, C., Minimal surfaces: A geometric three dimensional segmentation approach, Numerische Mathematik, Vol. 77, No. 4, pp. 423-451, 1997.

[42] Chopp, D. L., Computing Minimal Surfaces via Level Set Curvature Flow, J. Computational Physics, Vol. 106, No. 1, pp. 77-91, 1993.

[43] Kimmel, R., Amir, A. and Bruckstein, A. M., Finding Shortest Paths on Surfaces Using Level Sets Propagation, IEEE Trans. on Pattern Analysis and Machine Intelligence, Vol. 17, No. 6, pp. 635-640, June 1995.

[44] Malladi, R., Kimmel, R., Adalsteinsson, D., Sapiro, G., Caselles, V. and Sethian, J. A., A Geometric Approach to Segmentation and Analysis of 3-D Medical Images, Proc. of IEEE/SIAM Workshop on Mathematical Morphology and Biomedical Image Analysis (MMBIA), San Francisco, CA, pp. 244-252, June 1996.

[45] Malladi, R. and Sethian, J. A., Image Processing via Level Set Curvature Flow, Proc. Natl. Acad. Sci. (PNAS), Vol. 92, No. 15, pp. 7046-7050, 1995.

[46] Malladi, R. and Sethian, J. A., Image processing: flows under min/max curvature and mean curvature, Graphics Models Image Processing (GMIP), Vol. 58, No. 2, pp. 127-141, 1996.

[47] Malladi, R., Sethian, J. A., A Unified Approach to Noise Removal, Image-Enhancement and Shape Recovery, IEEE Trans. in Image Processing, Vol. 5, No. 11, pp. 1554-1568, Nov. 1996.

[48] Malladi, R., Sethian, J.A. and Vemuri, B. A., A fast level set based algorithm for topology independent shape modeling, Journal of Mathematical Imaging and Vision, Special Issue on Topology and Geometry in Computer Vision, Ed., Rosenfeld, A. and Kong, Y., Vol. 6, Nos. 2 and 3, pp. 269-290, April 1996.

[49] Malladi, R. and Sethian, J. A., A real-time algorithm for medical shape recovery, Int. Conference on Computer Vision, Mumbai, India, pp. 304-310, Jan. 1998.

[50] Malladi, R., Sethian, J. A. and Vemuri, B. C., Evolutionary fronts for topology-independent shape modeling and recovery, Proc. of the 3rd European Conf. Computer Vision, Stockholm, Sweden, By Lect. Notes Comput. Sci., Vol. 800, pp. 3-13, 1994.

[51] Yezzi, A., Kichenassamy, S., Kumar, A., Olver, P. and Tannenbaum, A., A geometric snake model for segmentation of medical imagery, IEEE Trans. on Med. Imag., Vol. 16, No. 2, pp. 199-209, 1997.

[52] Gomes, J. and Faugeras, O., Level sets and distance functions, In Proc. of the 6th European Conference on Computer Vision (ECCV), pp. 588-602, 2000.

[53] Suri, J. S., Fast WM/GM Boundary Segmentation From MR Images Using the Relationship Between Parametric and Geometric Deformable Models, Chapter 8, in the book edited by Suri, Setarehdan and Singh, titled Advanced Algorithmic Approaches to Medical Image Segmentation: State-of-the-Art Applications in Cardiology, Neurology, Mammography and Pathology, In Press, First Eds., to be published in 2001.

[54] Zeng, X., Staib, L. H., Schultz, R. T. and Duncan, J. S., Segmentation and measurement of the cortex from 3-D MR images using coupled-surfaces propagation, IEEE Trans. on Med. Imag., Vol. 18, No. 10, pp. 927-37, Sept. 1999.

[55] Suri, J. S., Leaking Prevention in Fast Level Sets Using Fuzzy Models: An Application in MR Brain, Inter. Conference in Information Technology in Biomedicine (ITAB-ITIS), pp. 220-226, Nov. 2000.

[56] Suri, J. S., White Matter/Gray Matter Boundary Segmentation Using Geometric Snakes: A Fuzzy Deformable Model, Proc. International Conference on Advances in Pattern Recognition, Lecture Notes in Computer Science (LNCS) No. 2013, Singh, S., Murshed, N. and Kropatsch, W. (Eds.), Springer-Verlag, Rio, De Janerio, Brazil (11-14 March), pp. 331-338, 2001.

[57] Suri, J. S., Singh, S. and Reden, L., Computer Vision and Pattern Recognition Techniques for 2-D and 3-D MR Cerebral Cortical Segmentation: A State-of-the-Art Review, To Appear in Journal of Pattern Analysis and Applications, Vol. 4, No. 3, Sept. 2001.

[58] Hermosillo, G., Faugeras, O. and Gomes, J., Unfolding the Cerebral Cortex Using Level Set Methods, Proceedings of the Second International Conference on Scale-Space Theories in Computer (SSTC), Lecture Notes in Computer Sci., Vol. 1682, pg. 58, 1999.

[59] Sarti, A., Ortiz, C., Lockett, S. and Malladi, R., A Unified Geometric Model for 3-D Confocal Image Analysis in Cytology, Int. Symposium on Computer Graphics, Image Processing and Vision, (SIBGRAPI), Rio de Janeiro, Brazil, pp. 69-76, Oct. 20-23, 1998.

[60] Niessen, W. J., ter Haar Romeny, B. M. and Viergever, M. A., Geodesic deformable models for medical image analysis, IEEE Trans. Med. Imag., Vol. 17, No. 4, pp. 634-641, Aug. 1998.

[61] Sethian, J. A., A review of recent numerical algorithms for hypersurfaces moving with curvature dependent flows, J. Differential Geometry, Vol. 31, pp. 131-161, 1989.

[62] Sethian, J. A., Theory, algorithms and applications of level set methods for propagating interfaces, Acta Numerica, Vol. 5, pp. 309-395, 1996.

[63] Kimmel, R., Kiryati N. and Bruckstein, A. M., Analyzing and Synthesizing Images by Evolving Curves with the Osher-Sethian Method, International Journal of Computer Vision, Vol. 24, No. 1, pp. 37-55, 1997.

[64] Suri, J. S., Computer Vision, Pattern Recognition, and Image Processing in Left Ventricle Segmentation: Last 50 Years, Journal of Pattern Analysis and Applications, Vol. 3, No. 3, pp. 209-242, 2000.

[65] Terzopoulous, D. and Fleischer, K., Deformable Models, The Visual Computer, Vol. 4, No. 6, pp. 306-331, Dec. 1988.

[66] Kass, W. and Terzopolulous, D., Snakes: Active Contour Models, Int. Jour. of Computer Vision, Vol. 1, No. 4, pp. 321-331, 1988.

[67] Osher, S. and Sethian, J., Fronts propagating with curvature-dependent speed: algorithms based on Hamiltons-Jacobi formulations, J. Comput. Physics, Vol. 79, No. 1, pp. 12-49, 1988.

[68] Sethian, J. A., An Analysis of Flame Propagation, Ph.D. Thesis, Department of Mathematics, University of California, Berkeley, CA, 1982.

[69] Suri, J. S. *et al.*, Modeling Segmentation Issues via Partial Differential Equations, Level Sets, and Geometric Deformable Models: A Revisit, To be submitted to International Journal, 2001.

[70] Grayson, M., The heat equation shrinks embedded plane curves to round points, J. of Differential Geometry, Vol. 26, pp. 285-314, 1987.

[71] Sethian, J. A., Level Set Methods and Fast Marching Methods: Evolving interfaces in computational geometry, fluid mechanics, Computer Vision and Material Science, Cambridge University Press, Cambridge, UK, 2nd Edition, ISBN: 0-521-64204-3, 1999.

[72] Cao, S. and Greenhalgh, S., Finite-difference solution of the Eikonal equation using an efficient, First-arrival, wavefront tracking scheme, Geophysics, Vol. 59, No. 4, pp. 632-643, April 1994.

[73] Chen, S., Merriman, B., Osher, S. and Smereka, P., A Simple Level Set Method for Solving Stefan Problems, Journal of Comput. Physics, Vol. 135, No. 1, pp. 8-29, 1997.

[74] Kichenassamy, S., Kumar, A., Olver, P., Tannenbaum, A. and Yezzi, A., Conformal curvatures flows: from phase transitions to active vision, Arch. Rational Mech. Anal., Vol. 134, No. 3, pp. 275-301, 1996.

[75] Caselles, V., Catte, F., Coll, T. and Dibos, F., A geometric model for active contours, Numerische Mathematik, Vol. 66, No. 1, pp. 1-31, 1993.

[76] Rouy, E. and Tourin, A., A viscosity solutions approach to shape-from-shading, SIAM J. of Numerical Analysis, Vol. 23, No. 3, pp. 867-884, 1992.

[77] Malladi, R., Sethian, J. A. and Vemuri, B. C., Shape modeling with Front Propagation, IEEE Trans. on Pattern Analysis and Machine Intelligence, Vol. 17, No. 2, pp. 158-175, Feb. 1995.

[78] Malladi, R. and Sethian, J. A., An O(N log N) algorithm for shape modeling, Applied Mathematics, Proc. Natl. Acad. Sci. (PNAS), Vol. 93, No. 18, pp. 9389-9392, Sept. 1996.

[79] Siddiqi, K., Lauriere, Y. B., Tannenbaum, A. and Zucker, S. W., Area and Length Minimizing Flows for Shape Segmentation, IEEE Trans. on Img. Proc., Vol. 7, No. 3, pp. 433-443, 1998.

[80] Siddiqi, K., Tannenbaum, A. and Zucker, S. W., Hyperbolic Smoothing of Shapes, Sixth International Conference on Computer Vision (ICCV), Mumbai, India, Vol. 1, pp. 215-221, 1998.

[81] Lorigo, L. M., Faugeras, O., Grimson, W. E. L., Keriven, R., Kikinis and R., Westin, Carl-Fredrik, Co-Dimension 2 Geodesic Active Contours for MRA Segmentation, In Proceedings of 16th International Conference of Information Processing in Medical Imaging, Visegrad, Hungary, Lecture Notes in Computer Science, Vol. 1613, pp. 126-139, June/July 1999.

[82] Lorigo, L. M., Grimson, W. Eric L., Faugeras, O., Keriven, R., Kikinis, R., Nabavi, A. and Westin, Carl-Fredrick, Two Geodesic Active Contours for the Segmentation of Tubular Structures, In Proc. of the Computer Vision and Pattern Recognition (CVPR), pp. 444-451, June 2000.

[83] Suri, J. S. and Bernstien, R., 2-D and 3-D Display of Aneurysms from Magnetic Resonance Angiographic Data, 6th International Conference in Computer Assisted Radiology, pp. 666-672, 1992.

[84] Kimia, B. B., Tannenbaum, A. R. and Zucker, S. W., Shapes, shocks and deformations, I: The components of shape and the reaction-diffusion space, Int. Journal of Computer Vision (IJCV), Vol. 15, No. 3, pp. 189-224, 1995.

[85] Siddiqi, K., Tresness, K. J. and Kimia, B. B., Parts of visual form: Ecological and psychophysical aspects, Perception, Vol. 25, No. 4, pp. 399-424, 1996.

[86] Stoll, P., Tek, H. and Kimia, B. B., Shocks from images: Propagation of orientation elements, In Proceedings of Computer Vision and Pattern

Recognition, Puerto Rico, IEEE Computer Society Press, pp. 839-845, June 15-16, 1997.

[87] Caselles, V., Kimmel, R. and Shapiro, G., Geodesic Active Contours, Int. J. of Computer Vision (IJCV), Vol. 22, No. 1, pp. 61-79, 1997.

[88] Yezzi, A., Tsai, A. and Willsky, A., A statistical approach to snakes for bimodal and trimodal imagery, In Proc. of Int'l Conf. Comp. Vision (ICCV), pp. 898-903, 1999.

[89] Guo, Y. and Vemuri, B., Hybrid geometric active models for shape recovery in medical images, In Proc. of Int'l Conf. Inf. Proc. in Med. Imaging (IPMI), Springer-Verlag, pp. 112-125, 1999.

[90] Xu, C., On the relationship between the parametric and geometric active contours, Internal Technical Report, Department of Electrical and Computer Engineering, Johns Hopkins University, Baltimore, MD, 1999.

[91] Aubert, G. and Blanch-Féraud, L., Some Remarks on the Equivalence Between 2D and 3D Classical Snakes and Geodesic Active Contours, Int. Journal of Computer Vision, Vol. 34, No. 1, pp. 19-28, 1999.

[92] Suri, J. S., Haralick, R. M. and Sheehan, F. H., Greedy Algorithm for Error Correction in Automatically Produced Boundaries from Low Contrast Ventriculograms, Int. Journal of Pattern Applications and Analysis, Vol. 1, No. 1, pp. 39-60, Jan. 2000.

[93] Bezdek, J. C. and Hall, L. O., Review of MR image segmentation techniques using pattern recognition, Medical Physics, Vol. 20, No. 4, pp. 1033-1048, March 1993.

[94] Berger, M. and Colella, P., Local adaptive mesh refinement for shock hydrodynamics, Mathematics of Computation, Vol. 45, No. 142, pp. 301-318, Oct. 1985.

[95] Berger, M. J., Local Adaptive Mesh Refinement, J. Computational Physics, Vol. 82, No. 1, pp. 64-84, 1989.

[96] Sethian, J. A., Curvature Flow and Entropy Conditions Applied to Grid Generation, J. Computational Physics, Vol. 115, No. 2, pp. 440-454, 1994.

[97] Tababai, A. J. and Mitchell, O. R., Edge location to subpixel values in digital imagery, IEEE Transactions on Pattern Analysis and Machine Intelligence (PAMI), Vol. 6, No. 2, pp. 188-201, March 1984.

[98] Huertas, A. and Medioni, G., Detection of intensity changes with subpixel accuracy using Laplacian-Gaussian masks, IEEE Trans. on Pattern Analysis and Machine Intelligence (PAMI), Vol. 8, No. 5, pp. 651-664, Sept. 1986.

[99] Gao, J., Kosaka, A. and Kak, A. C., A deformable model for human organ extraction, Proceedings IEEE Int. Conference on Image Processing (ICIP), Chicago, Vol. 3, pp. 323-327, Oct. 1998.

[100] Zeng, X., Staib, L. H., Schultz, R. T. and Duncan, J. S., Segmentation and measurement of the cortex from 3-D MR images, Medical Image Computing and Computer-Assisted Intervention, pp. 519-530, 1998.

[101] Wells III, W. M., Grimson, W. E. L., Kikinis, R. and Jolesz, F. A., Adaptive Segmentation of MRI Data, IEEE Trans. on Med. Imag., Vol. 15, No. 4, pp. 429-442, Aug. 1992.

[102] Lorenson, W. E. and Cline, H., Marching Cubes: A high resolution 3-D surface construction algorithm, ACM Computer Graphics, Proceedings of Siggraph, Vol. 21, No. 4, pp. 163-169, July 1987.

[103] Baillard, C., Hellier, P. and Barillot, C., Segmentation of 3-D Brain Structures Using Level Sets, Research Report 1291, IRISA, Rennes Cedex, France, 16 pages, Jan. 2000.

[104] Baillard, C., Barillot, C. and Bouthemy, P., Robust Adaptive Segmentation of 3-D Medical Images with Level Sets, Research Report 1369, IRISA, Rennes Cedex, France, 26 pages, Nov. 2000.

[105] Baillard, C., Hellier, P. and Barillot, C., Cooperation between level set techniques and dense 3d registration for the segmentation of brain structures, In Int. Conference on Pattern Recognition, Vol. 1, pp. 991-994, Sept. 2000.

[106] Osher, S. and Shu, C. W., Higher-order essentially non-oscillatory schemes for Hamilton-Jacobi Equations, SIAM J. Numer. Anal., Vol. 28, No. 4, pp. 907-922, 1991.

[107] Courant, R., Friedrichs, K. O. and Lewy, H., On the partial difference equations of mathematical physics, IBM Journal, Vol. 11, pp. 215-235, 1967.

[108] Goldenberg, R., Kimmel, R., Rivlin, E. and Rudzsky, M., Fast Geodesic Contours, In Proc. of Scale-Space Theories in Computer Vision (SSTCV), pp. 34-45, 1999.

[109] Perona, P. and Malik, J., Scale space and edge detection using anisotropic diffusion, IEEE Trans. on Pattern Analysis and Machine Intelligence, Vol. 12, No. 7, pp. 629-639, Apr. 1993.

[110] Adalsteinsson, D. and Sethian, J. A., A fast level set method for propagating interfaces, J. Computational Physics, Vol. 118, No. 2, pp. 269-277, May 1995.

[111] Adalsteinsson, D. and Sethian, J. A., The fast construction of extension velocities in level set methods, J. Computational Physics, Vol. 148, No. 1, pp. 2-22, 1999.

[112] Adalsteinsson, D., Kimmel, R., Malladi, R. and Sethian, J. A., Fast Marching Methods for Computing the Solutions to Static Hamilton-Jacobi Equations, CPAM Report 667, Univ. of California, Berkeley, CA, also submitted for publication, SIAM J. Numerical Analysis, Feb. 1996.

[113] Sethian, J. A., A fast marching level set method for monotonically advancing fronts, Proceedings Natl. Acad. Sci., Applied Mathematics, Vol. 93, No. 4, pp. 1591-1595, Feb. 1996.

[114] Sethian, J. A., Three-dimensional seismic imaging of complex velocity structures, US Patent #: 6,018,499, Jan. 25, 2000.

[115] Sedgewick, R., Algorithms in C, Fundamentals, data structures, sorting, searching, Addison-Wesley, ISBN: 0201314525, Vol. 1, 1998.

[116] Milne, R. B., An Adaptive Level Set Method, Ph.D. Thesis, Report Number LBNL-39216, Department of Mathematics, Lawrence Berkeley National Laboratory, Berkeley, CA, Dec. 1995.

[117] Leventon, M. E., Grimson, W. Eric L. and Faugeras, O., Statistical Shape Influence in Geodesic Active Contours, Proceedings of the Computer Vision and Pattern Recognition (CVPR), Vol. 1, pp. 316-323, June 2000.

[118] Cootes, T. F., Taylor, C. J., Cooper, D. H. and Graham, J., Active Shape Models: Their Training and Applications, Computer Vision and Image Understanding, Vol. 61, No. 1, pp. 38-59, Jan. 1995.

[119] Suri, J. S., Haralick, R. M. and Sheehan, F. H., Automatic Quadratic Calibration for Correction of Pixel Classifier Boundaries to an Accuracy of 2.5 mm: An Application in X-ray Heart Imaging, International Conference in Pattern Recognition, (ICPR) Brisbane, Australia, pp. 30-33, Aug 17-20, 1998.

[120] Lee, C. K., Automated Boundary Tracing Using Temporal Information, Ph.D. Thesis, Department of Electrical Engineering, University of Washington, Seattle, WA, 1994.

[121] Zhao, H. K., Chan, T., Merriman, B. and Osher, S., A variational level set approach to multiphase motion, J. Computational Physics, Vol. 127, No. 1, pp. 179-195, 1996.

[122] Evans, L. C. and Spruck, J., Motion of level sets by mean curvature: Part I, J. of Differential Geometry, Vol. 33, No. 3, pp. 635-681, 1991.

Chapter 4

Image Segmentation Via PDEs

Jasjit S. Suri[1], *S. Laxminarayan*[2], *Jianbo Gao*[3] *and Laura Reden*[4]

4.1 Introduction

Partial Differential Equations (PDEs)[5] have recently dominated the fields of computer vision, image processing and applied mathematics due to the following reasons: their ability to transform a segmentation modeling problem into a PDE framework; their ability to embed and integrate regularizers into these models; their ability to solve PDEs using finite difference methods (FDM); their ability to link between PDEs and the level set framework for implementing finite difference methods; their ability to extend the PDE framework from 2-D to 3-D or even higher dimensions; their ability to control the degree of PDE in the image processing domain; their ability to provide solutions in a fast, stable and closed form; and lastly, their ability to interactively handle image segmentation in the PDE framework.

Application of PDE has recently become more prominent in the biomedical and non-biomedical imaging fields (see Suri *et al.* [1], [2], [3], [4], [5], [6], Haker [7], Chambolle [8] and Morel *et al.* [9]) for shape recovery and the recently published book by Sapiro [10]. This is because the role of shape recovery has always been a critical component in 2-D and 3-D medical and non-medical imagery. This assists largely in medical therapy and object detection/tracking in industrial applications, respectively (see the recent book by Suri *et al.* [4]

[1]Marconi Medical Systems, Inc., Cleveland, OH, USA
[2]New Jersey Institute of Technology, Newark, NJ, USA
[3]KLA-Tencor, Milpitas, CA, USA
[4]Marconi Medical Systems, Inc., Cleveland, OH, USA
[5]Whenever PDE is seen in this Chapter, it means that it is a PDE-based method.

PDE & Level Sets: Algorithmic Approaches to Static & Motion Imagery
Edited by Jasjit Suri and Swamy Laxminarayan, Kluwer Academic/Plenum Publishers, 2002

and the references therein and also see Weickert *et al.* [11], [12] and the references therein). Shape recovery of medical organs in medical images is more difficult compared to other imaging fields. This is primarily due to the large shape variability, structure complexity, different kinds of artifacts and restrictive body scanning methods. With PDE-based segmentation techniques, it has been possible to integrate low level vision techniques to make the segmentation system robust, reliable, fast, closed-form and accurate. This Chapter revisits the application of PDE in the field of computer vision and image processing and demonstrates the ability to model segmentation in PDE and the level set framework. Before discussing PDE techniques in detail, we will first discuss the different kinds of PDE applications.

Figure 4.1 shows the classification tree of non-coupled and coupled PDE applications. Even though the applications are very large in number, we have narrowed them down to discuss the CVGIP (Computer Vision, Graphics and Image Processing) domain only. Although the tree shows applications such as image smoothing/filtering, image segmentation, optic flow, mathematical morphology, image matching and coupled PDEs, the main focus of this Chapter is on modeling segmentation using non-coupled and coupled PDEs in the level set framework by fusing geometric regularizers (also known as geometric deformable models). Thus under the class of geometric segmentation techniques, PDEs have become almost an integral part of deformable modeling (see the segmentation classification paper by Suri *et al.* [5] and all the references therein. In [5], the three major techniques of segmentation were discussed: region-based, boundary-based and the fusion of region and boundary-based. Boundary-based were further classified into parametric and geometric. Similarly, the fusion of region and boundary-based techniques were also further classified into parametric and geometric). The deformation class of segmentation is so naturally handled in the level set framework that PDE and the level set framework go side-by-side in achieving the objectives of segmentation. PDE-based techniques have recently replaced finite element models (FEM) and finite difference methods (FDM), only because FEM and FDM are expensive in time and tedious to use in the design phases. PDE-based techniques are also less sensitive to complex structures and are extremely accurate. Having discussed the advantages of PDE in segmentation modeling and the broad classification tree for PDE applications, we will now classify the geometric deformable models and see their relationship to PDEs and level sets along with conclusions and a discussion on where this may lead to in the future.

Referring back to Figure 4.1, geometric deformable models (GDM's) are classified broadly into two classes: first, GDM without regularizers and second, GDM with regularizers. The *first core class* of segmentation based on the PDE/level set framework is GDM without regularizers. These are techniques where the propagation force, i.e., the force which navigates the propagation front inwards and outwards, does not utilize the region-based strategy for its computation. These forces are constant and do not change. Sometimes they are also called "level set stoppers". Earlier research called these "leakage prevention" techniques because they tried to prevent any bleeding of boundaries during propagation. These are further classified into five different kinds, depending upon the design of the stopping force: (**1**) gradient-based stopping force; (**2**) edge-based stopping force; (**3**) area-minimization-based stopping force; (**4**) curvature-dependent stopping force; and (**5**) application-driven level sets. The curvature-dependent class has four sub-classes: (**1**) plain curvature-based; (**2**) mean curvature flow (MCF) with directionality-based; (**3**) bubbles; and (**4**) morphing. Plain curvature based techniques are those which are driven solely by the curvature that is computed using differential geometry. Mean curvature flow with directionality-based techniques are those which use the combination of Euclidean curvature and direction together to achieve the deformation process. Such techniques are good for tiny, occluded and twisted objects like blood vessels. Bubbles are a set of seeds, or fourth order shocks, which grow, shrink, merge, split, disappear and deform under the influence of image information such as edges and gradients to segment objects in images and volumes. Morphing techniques are those which undergo shape deformation from one initial shape to the target shape, driven by the combination of signed distance at coordinate transformation and the gradient of the signed distance transform functions. This transformation captures the similarity between user-defined shape and target shape.

The *second core class* of PDE-based segmentation techniques uses regularizers or level sets that derive the propagation force using statistical means such as region-based strategy. This is further classified into four types, depending upon the design of propagation force. They are: (**1**) fuzzy clustering-based; (**2**) classification based on Bayesian statistics; (**3**) shape-based; and (**4**) constrained coupled level sets where the propagation force is derived from Bayesian strategies.

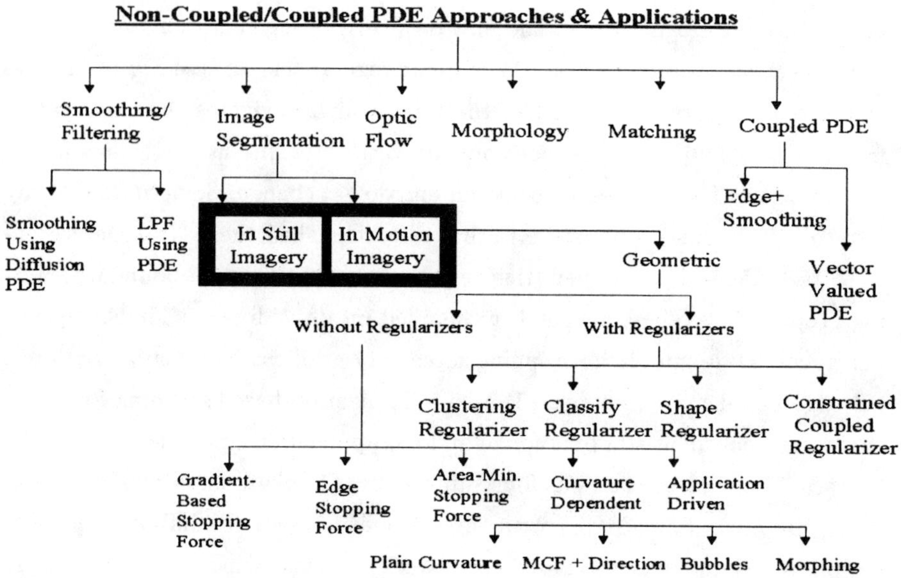

Figure 4.1: Classification of PDE tree of non-coupled and coupled PDE applications applied to Computer Vision, Image Processing and Computer Graphics.

This Chapter will survey and discuss the role of regularizers in PDEs and the level set framework. We will take a few sample representation techniques from Suri *et al.* [6] where regularizers are designed and used in the PDE and the level set framework, but details on GDM with/without regularizers can be seen explictly in the paper by Suri *et al.* [6]. Thus, the fundamental differences between this Chapter and [6] are: (**1**) this Chapter focuses on PDEs and level sets for segmentation modeling, while [6] focused on different kinds of level set methods. (**2**) This Chapter shows applications of PDE in the area of CVGIP for *still* and *motion* imagery, while [6] showed applications of level sets for static 2-D and 3-D medical imagery only. (**3**) This Chapter covers a wide variety of PDE applications such as image smoothing, coupled PDE, low pass filtering and miscellaneous applications such as mathematical morphology, missing shape recovery from partial information. On the contrary, [6] focused on the "optimization techniques" based on the fast marching method, narrow banding and adaptive level sets. In other words, [6] was a detailed version on the growth of level sets and was a good tutorial for researchers who wished to design medical image segmentation techniques in 2-D and 3-D based just on level sets. Having discussed the previous work in the area of PDE and level sets, we will next discuss the goals of this Chapter.

The goals of this Chapter are the following: (**1**) to understand the role of PDE in different image processing applications, particularly in segmentation for *still* and *motion* imagery. (**2**) To understand the relationship between PDE, level sets and regularizers. (**3**) To understand how one can derive the image segmentation process by fusing the regional-based PDE information with boundary-based PDE models, which is the crux of this Chapter. (**4**) To discuss the state-of-the-art research published in the area of PDE applications in relation to image processing, computer graphics and numerical algorithms. (**5**) To present state-of-the-art ready references for readers interested in further exploring into the field of image segmentation using PDE and summarizing the state-of-the-art work done by major research groups such as: Osher and Sethian (UCLA, University of California, Los Angeles, CA, USA), Faugeras and Deriche (INRIA, Institut National de Recherche en Informatique et Automatique, Sophia-Antipolis, France), Kimmel (Technion, Israel Institute of Technology, Haifa, Israel), Sapiro and Tannenbaum (UM, University of Minnesota, Minneapolis, MN, USA), Malladi (LBL, Lawrence Berkeley Labs., Berkeley, CA, USA), Paragios (Siemens, Siemens Corporate Research, Siemens Medical Systems, Inc., Iselin, NJ, USA), Suri (Marconi, Marconi Medical Systems, Inc., Cleveland, OH, USA), Vemuri (UF, University of Florida, Gainesville, FL, USA) and Zhang (UW, University of Wisconsin, Milwaukee, WI, USA). Also note that this Chapter does not discuss: (**1**) PDE-based approaches to vector-valued, i.e., color images or hyper-stack images or multi-band images; (**2**) coupled PDE approaches to image processing. These topics are out of the scope of this Chapter.

The remaining sections of this Chapter are as follows: Section 4.2 presents the fundamentals on level sets, curve evolution and the Eikonal Equation. Image smoothing and the anisotropic diffusion method based on PDE are covered in section 4.3. Segmentation in *still* imagery via PDE in the level set framework is covered in section 4.4. Segmentation in *motion* imagery using PDE and the level set framework is discussed in section 4.5. Miscellaneous applications of PDEs in mathematical morphology, surface smoothing and missing shape recovery are covered in section 4.6. Finally, this Chapter concludes in section 4.7 by discussing the advantages and the disadvantages of segmentation modeling via geometric deformable models (GDM), PDE and level sets along with conclusions and the future.

4.2 Level Set Concepts: Curve Evolution and Eikonal Equation

The level set framework has provided one of the beds which implements the PDE. The concept of level sets was introduced by Osher and Sethian [47], which bubbled out from the Ph.D. Thesis of Sethian [48]. The diversity of applications of level sets has reached into several fields of engineering. Although this Chapter will not go in depth on level sets, it will cover the fundamental equation of the level sets. Before discussing the level set equation, we present a list of authors who have covered the level sets in the following fields: (**1**) *geometry*: (see Angenent *et al.* [49], Chopp [50], [51] and Sethian [52]), (**2**) *grid generation*: (see Sethian [53]), (**3**) *fluid mechanics* (see Mulder *et al.* [54], Sethian [80], Sussman *et al.* [55]), (**4**) *combustion*: (see Rhee *et al.* [56]), (**5**) *solidification*: (see Sethian *et al.* [81]), (**6**) *device fabrication*: (see Adalsteinsson *et al.* [57]), (**7**) *deformation modeling*: (see Whitaker *et al.* [58], [59] and [60]), (**8**) *object tracking/image sequence analysis in images*: (see the recent work by Paragios *et al.* [61], [62] and Kornprobst *et al.* [63]), (**9**) *stereo vision*: (see the recent work by Faugeras and his coworkers at INRIA [64]), (**10**) *mathematical morphology*: (see Sapiro *et al.* [65], Arehart *et al.* [66], Catte *et al.* [67] and Sochen *et al.* [68]), (**11**) *color image segmentation*: (see Sapiro [82]) and (**12**) *2-D and 3-D medical image processing*: (see the works by Malladi *et al.* [69], [70], [71], [72] and [73], Gray-Matter/White-Matter (GM/WM) boundary estimation by Gomes *et al.* [78], GM/WM boundary estimation with fuzzy models by Suri [1], [83], GM/WM thickness estimation by Zeng *et al.* [84], leakage prevention in fast level sets using fuzzy models by Suri [2], also a survey article on brain segmentation by Suri *et al.* [5] and a recent article for cell segmentation by Sarti *et al.* [85]). For a detailed review of some of the above mentioned applications, the reader must see Sethian [86] and [87]. Although both of these publications cover a good collection of the level set applications, with the advancement of image processing technology, these publications are behind the latest trends. Recently, Suri *et al.* [6] wrote another extensive survey on level sets and their applications. Having stated the applications of level sets, next will be covered the fundamental equation of curve evolution.

4.2.1 Fundamental Equation of Curve Evolution

Since this Chapter uses level sets as the framework, this sub-section first presents the derivation of the fundamental equation of level sets, known as "curve evolution". Let $\Gamma(t)$ be the closed interface or front propagating along its normal direction (see Figure 4.2). This closed interface $\Gamma(t)$: $[0,\infty) \to \mathcal{R}^N$, is either be a curve in 2-D space or a surface in 3-D space. The main idea is to represent the front $\Gamma(t)$ as the *zero level set* of a higher dimensional function ϕ.

Let $\phi(x, t = 0)$, where $x \in \mathcal{R}^N$ is defined by $\phi(x, t = 0) = d$, where d is the signed distance from position x to $\Gamma(0)$ and the plus (minus) sign is chosen if the point x is outside (inside) the initial front $\Gamma(0)$. Thus, an initial function is: $\phi(x, t = 0) = \mathcal{R}^N \to \mathcal{R}$ with the property: $\Gamma(t = 0) = (x \mid \phi(x, t = 0) = 0)$. The goal now is to produce an equation for the evolving function $\phi(x, t)$ so that ϕ always remains zero on the propagating interface. Let $x(t)$, $t \in [0, \infty)$ be the path of a point on the propagation front (see Figure 4.2), i.e., $x(t = 0)$ is a point on the initial front $\Gamma(t = 0)$ and $x_t = V(x(t))$ with the vector x_t normal to the front at $x(t)$. Since the evolving function ϕ is always zero on the propagating front, thus $\phi(x(t), t) = 0$. By chain rule:

$$\phi_t + \sum_{i=1}^{N} \phi_{x_i} x_{i_t} = 0\,, \tag{4.1}$$

where x_i is the ith component of x. Since

$$\sum_{i=1}^{N} \phi_{x_i} x_{i_t} = (\phi_{x_1}, \phi_{x_2}, \phi_{x_3} ... \phi_{x_N}) \cdot (x_{1_t}, x_{2_t}, x_{3_t} ... x_{N_t}) = V(x(t))\,|\nabla\phi|\,, \tag{4.2}$$

thus, using Equations (4.1) and (4.2), the final curve evolution equation is given as:

$$\frac{\partial \phi}{\partial t} = V(\kappa) \mid \nabla\phi \mid, \tag{4.3}$$

where ϕ is the level set function and $V(\kappa)$ is the speed with which the front (or *zero level curve*) propagates. This fundamental equation describes the time evolution of the level set function (ϕ) in such a way that the *zero level curve* of this evolving function is always identified with the propagating interface. The term "level set function" will be interchangeably used with the term "flow field" or simply "field" during the course of this Chapter. The above equation is also called an Eulerian representation of evolution due to the work of Osher and Sethian [47]. Equation (4.3) for the 2-D and 3-D cases is generalized as: $\frac{\partial \phi}{\partial t} = V_\kappa(x,y)\,|\,\nabla\phi\,|$ and $\frac{\partial \phi}{\partial t} = V_\kappa(x,y,z)\,|\,\nabla\phi\,|$, respectively, where $V_\kappa(x,y)$ and $V_\kappa(x,y,z)$ are curvature dependent speed functions in 2-D and 3-D, respectively.

Three Analogies of the Curve Evolution Equation: First, the above mentioned equations can be compared with the Euclidean geometric heat equation (see Grayson [79]), given as: $\frac{\partial \mathcal{C}}{\partial t} = \kappa \mathcal{N}$, where κ is the curvature and $\mathcal{N}$ is the inward unit normal and $\mathcal{C}$ is the curve coordinates. Second, equation (4.3) is also called the curvature motion equation, since the rate of change of the length of the curve is a function of $\frac{\partial \mathcal{C}}{\partial t}$. Third, the above equations can be written in terms of differential geometry using divergence as: $\frac{\partial \phi}{\partial t} = \nabla\,.\,(\frac{\nabla\phi}{|\nabla\phi|})\,|\,\nabla\phi\,|$, where geometrical properties such as normal curvature ($\mathcal{N}$) and mean curvature ($\mathcal{H}$) are given as: $\mathcal{N} = \frac{\nabla\phi}{|\nabla\phi|}$ and $\mathcal{H} = \nabla\,.\,(\frac{\nabla\phi}{|\nabla\phi|})$. Note that the above equation remains the fundamental form but recently, Faugeras and his coworker from INRIA (see Gomes *et al.* [78]) modified Eq. (4.3) into the "preserving distance function" as:

$$\frac{\partial \phi}{\partial t} = V(\mathbf{x})\,(\mathbf{x} - \phi\nabla\phi), \tag{4.4}$$

where $\mathbf{x}$ is the vector of x and y coordinates, ϕ is the signed distance function. The main characteristic of this equation is that ϕ and V are orthogonal to each other (see details by Gomes *et al.* [78]).

4.2.1.1 The Eikonal Equation and its Mathematical Solution

In this sub-section, we present the mathematical solution for solving the level set function with unity speed. Such a method is needed to compute the "signed distance transform" when the raw contour crossed the background grid. Consider a case of a "front" moving with a velocity $V = V(x,y)$, such that V is greater than zero. Using Osher-Sethian's [47] level set equation, consider a monotonically advancing front which represents in the form: $\phi_t = V(x,y)\;||\nabla\,\phi||$, where ϕ_t is the rate of change of the level set and $\nabla\,\phi$ is the gradient of the ϕ. Let $T(x,y)$ be the time at which the front crosses

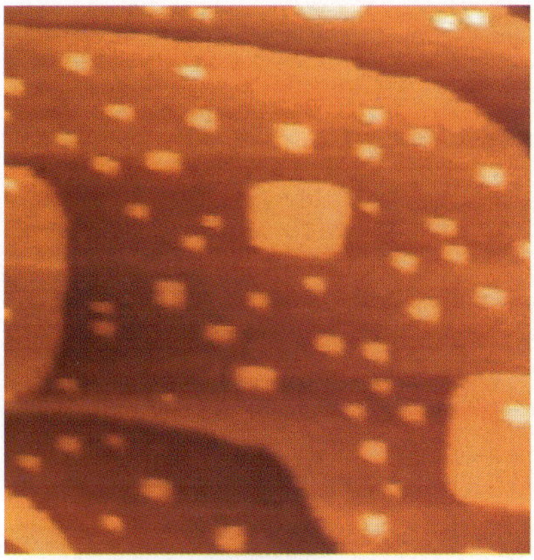

Time = 0s

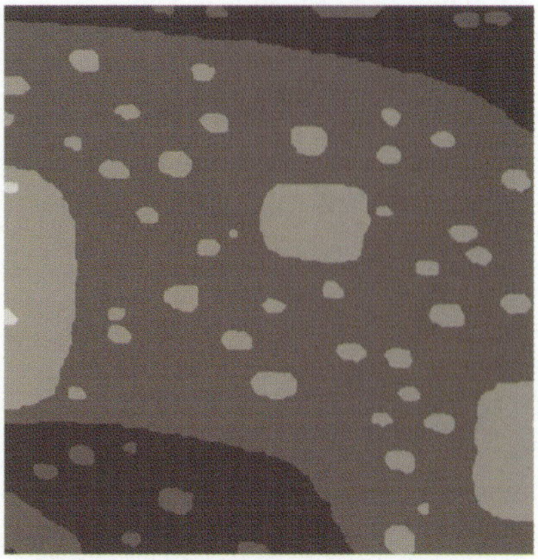

Time = 0s

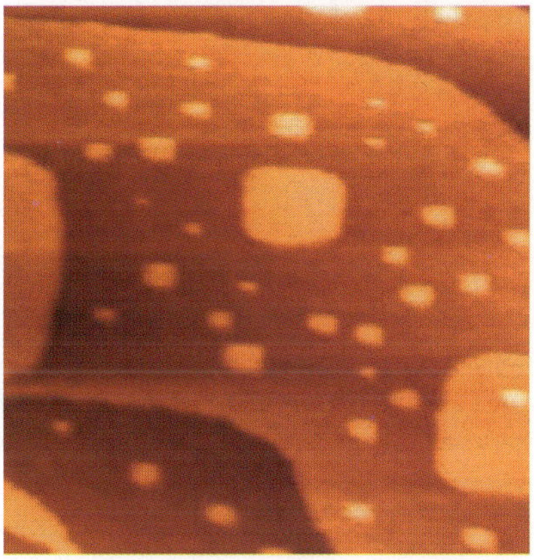

Time = 3180s

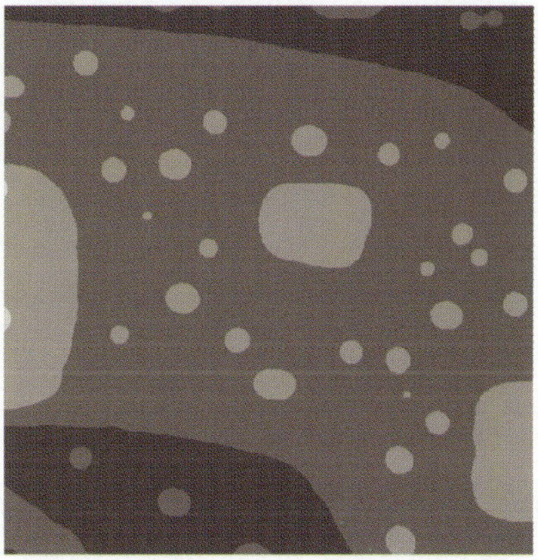

Time = 853s

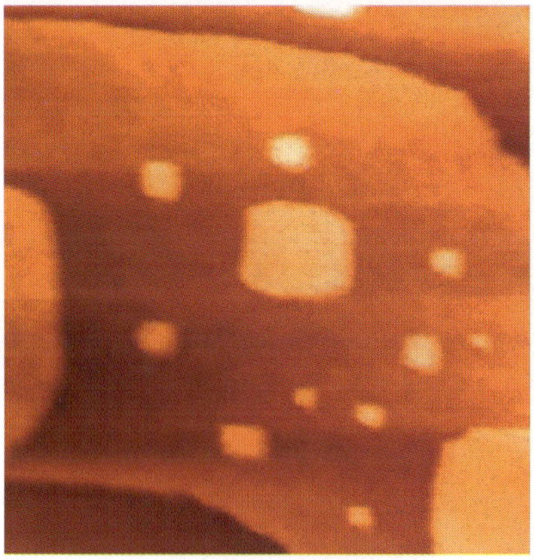

Time = 10260s

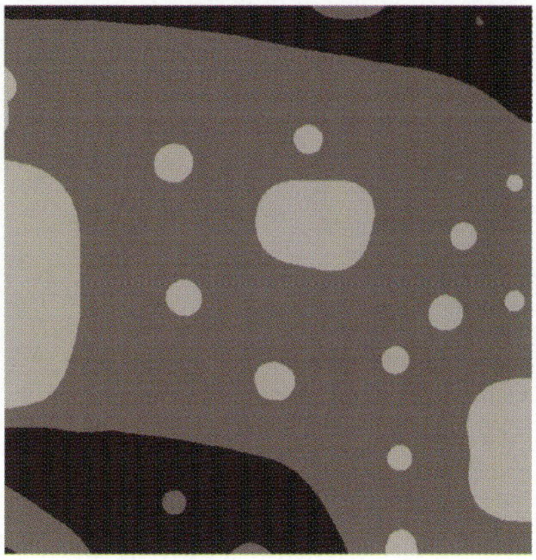

Time = 5500s

Figure 2.31: Time sequence of annealing TiN(002) at 800°C [30] compared with computed solution

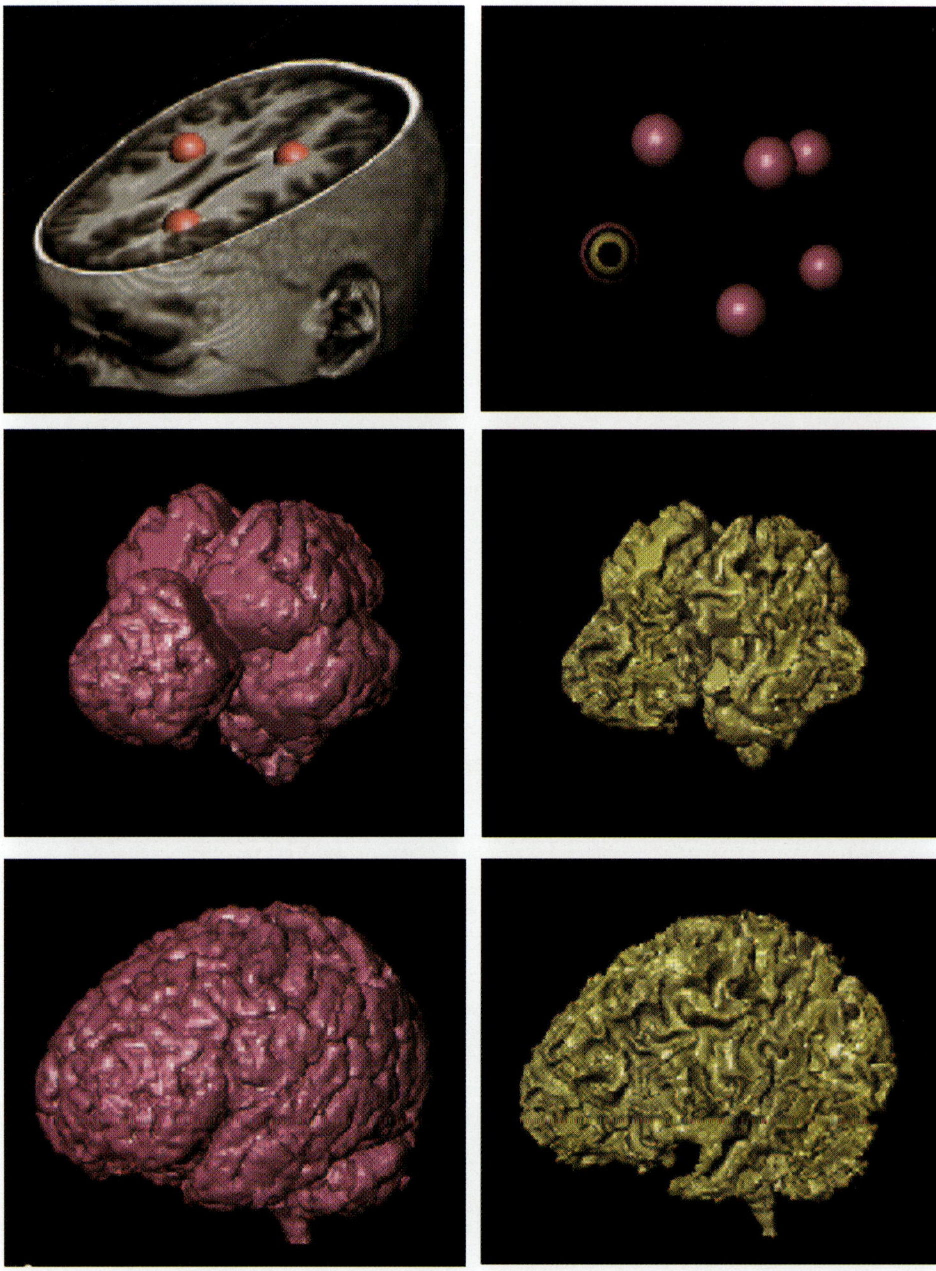

Figure 3.4: Propagation of the outer (pink) and inner (yellow) bounding surfaces. **Top Left**: embedded sphere sets as initializations shown in unedited 3-D MR brain volume. **Top Right**: outer (pink) and inner (yellow) bounding spheres. **Middle Left**: intermediate step in GM surface propagation. **Middle Right**: intermediate step in WM surface propagation. **Bottom Left**: final result of the segmented GM/CSF surface. **Bottom Right**: final result of the segmented WM/GM surface (Courtesy of Xiaolan Zeng, R2 Technology, Inc.).

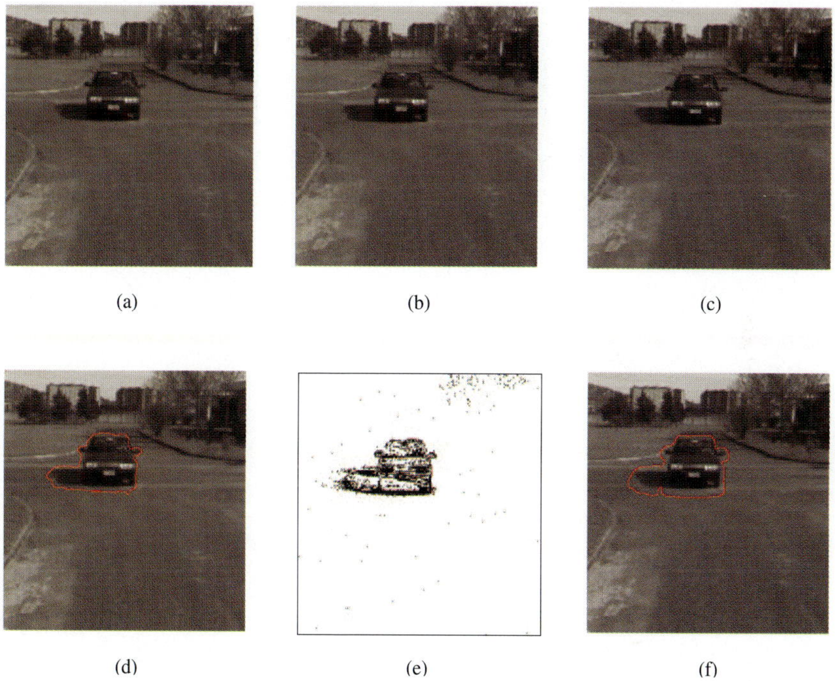

Figure 4.11: Segmentation results for the "moving car sequence". **Top Left**: Frame number 7. **Top Middle**: Frame number 8. **Top Right**: Frame number 9. **Bottom Left**: Result of the method of Paragios *et al.* [108]. **Bottom Middle**: Result of the method of Grimson *et al.* [107]. **Bottom Right**: Result of Zhang *et al.*'s [114] method (Reproduced with permission from IEEE).

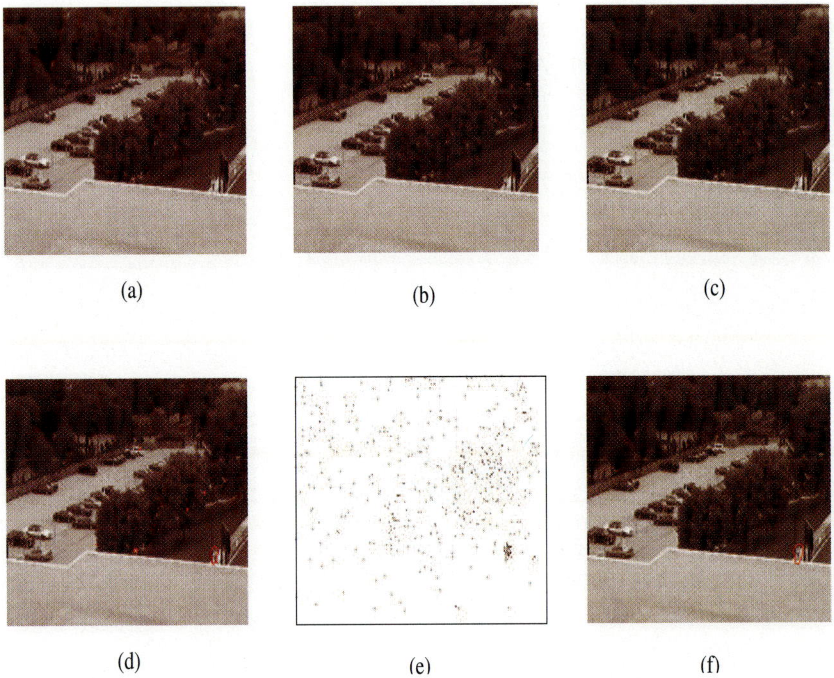

Figure 4.12: Segmentation of an "outdoor sequence". **Top Left**: Frame number 601. **Top Middle**: Frame number 602. **Top Right**: Frame number 603. **Bottom Left**: Result of the method of Paragios *et al.* [108]. **Bottom Middle**: Result of the method of Grimson *et al.* [107]. **Bottom Right**: Result of Zhang *et al.*'s [114] method (Reproduced with permission from IEEE).

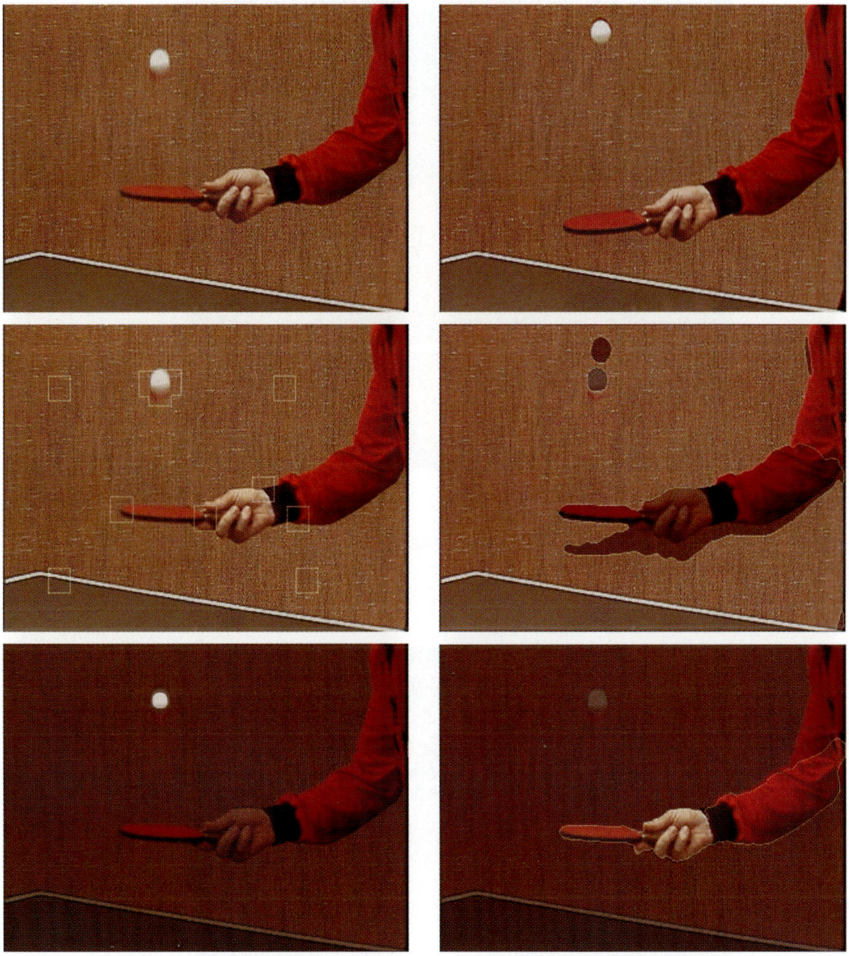

Figure 4.13: Segmentation results of the "*ping-pong* sequence" using PDE implemented in the level set framework. **Top Left**: Frame 30 of the "*ping-pong* sequence". **Top Right**: Frame 40 of the "*ping-pong* sequence". **Middle Left**: Initial segmentation: Three squares are associated with one region and there are three regions: background, ball and hand. Each of these square boundaries is the zero level set function corresponding to the respective regions. **Middle Right**: Final segmentation of the background. **Bottom Left**: Final segmentation of the ball. **Bottom Right**: Final segmentation of the hand (Courtesy of Abdol-Reza Mansouri, INRS Telecommunications, Montreal, Quebec, Canada).

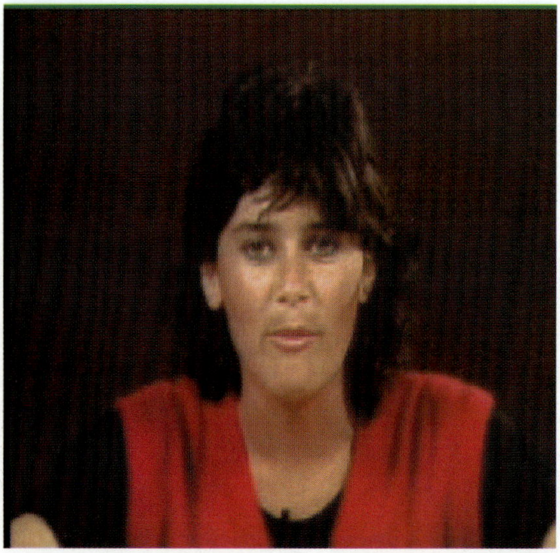

(a) Original Frame

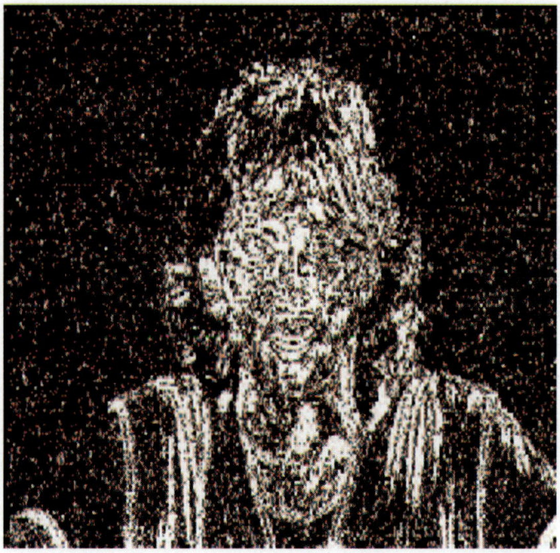

(b) Outlier of Background

Figure 5.4: Adaptive Background Detection for Missa Sequence.

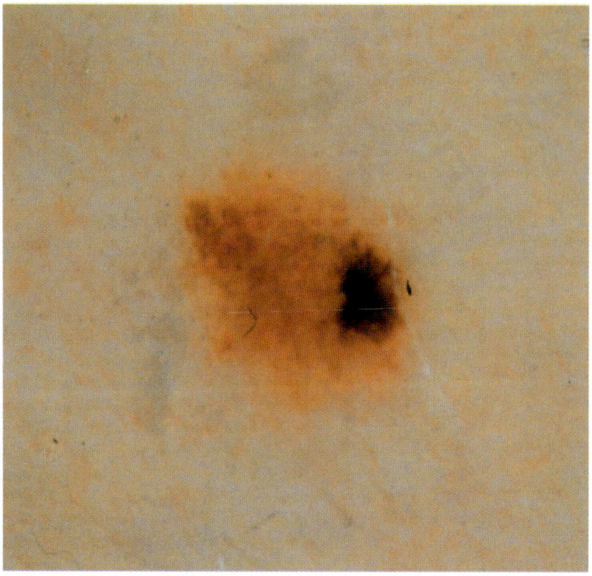

(a) Original Image (924x748)

(b) Segmentation Result (2 clusters)

Figure 5.6: Image Segmentation for Skin Lesion 1.

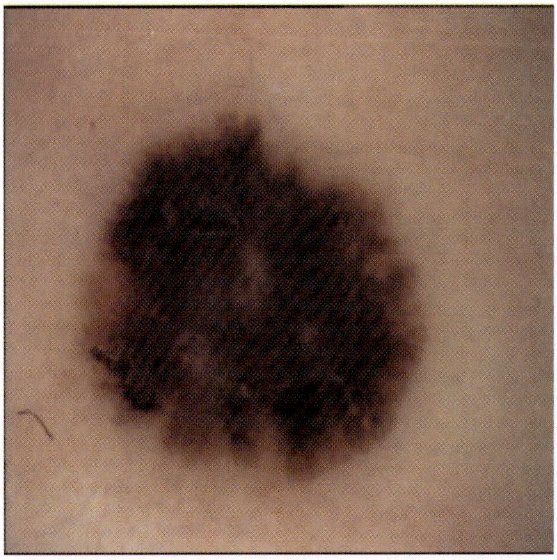

(a) Original Image

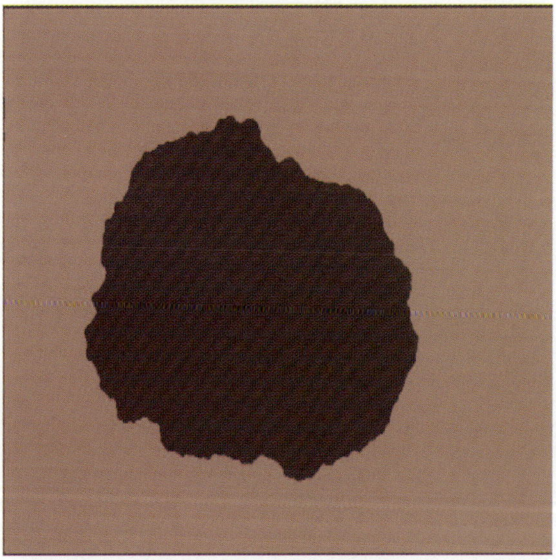

(b) Segmentation Result

Figure 5.7: Image Segmentation for Skin Lesion 2.

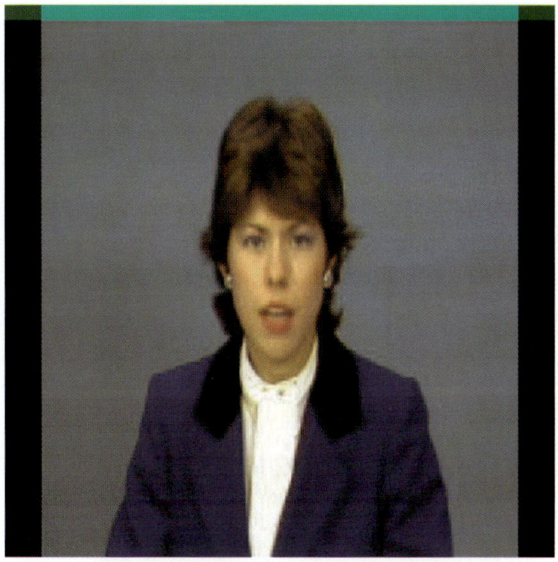

(a) One Frame of Claire Sequence

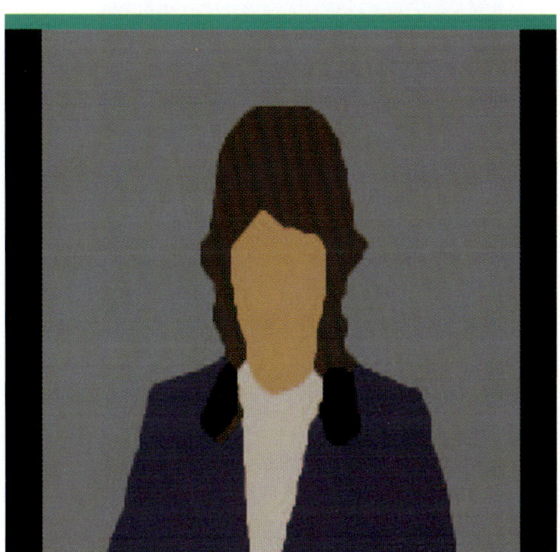

(b) Segmentation Result (7 clusters)

Figure 5.8: Image Segmentation for One Frame of Claire Sequence.

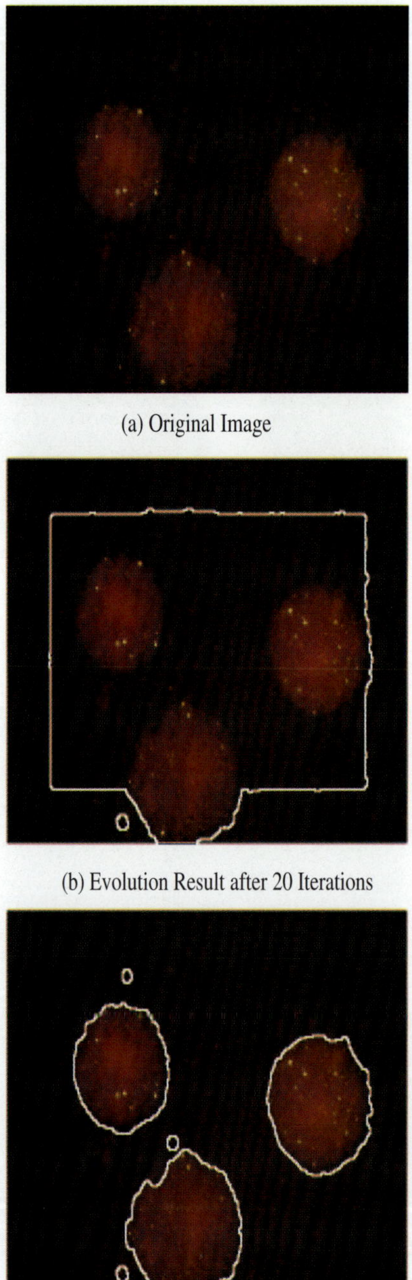

(a) Original Image

(b) Evolution Result after 20 Iterations

(c) Evolution Resolution after 100 Iterations

Figure 5.15: Color Snake with the Splitting of Curves.

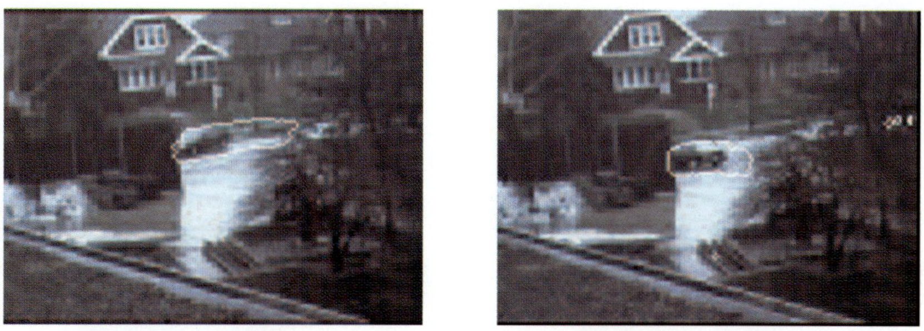

Figure 6.6: Segmentation Results for the Outdoor Sequence.

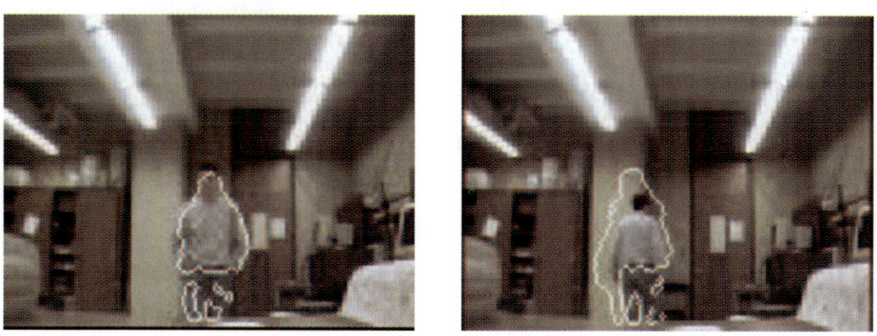

Figure 6.7: Segmentation Results for the Indoor Sequence.

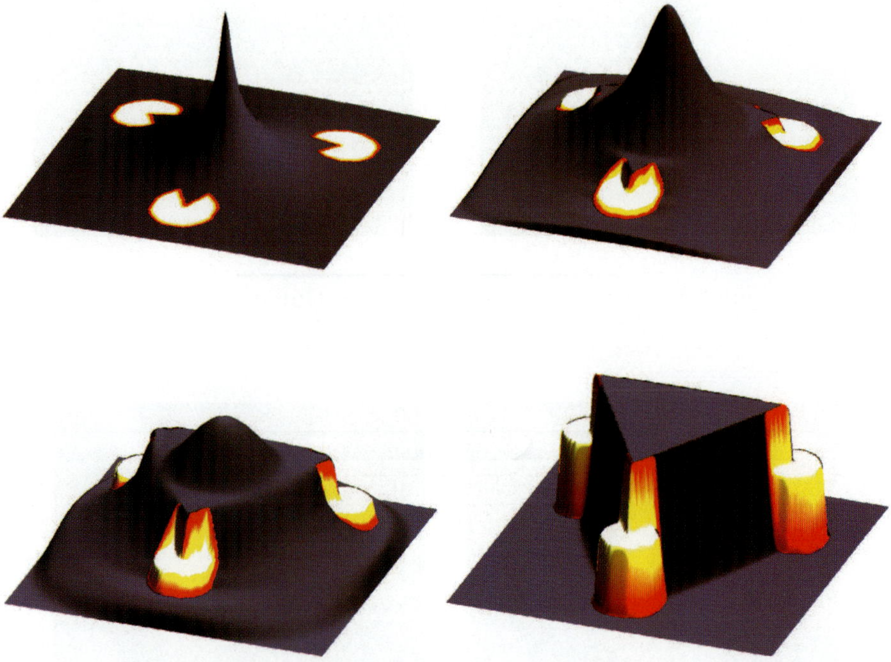

Figure 8.10: Four time frames showing the evolution of the point-of-view surface (upper left) towards the subjective surface (bottom right). In this visualization the original image has been texture mapped onto the surface.

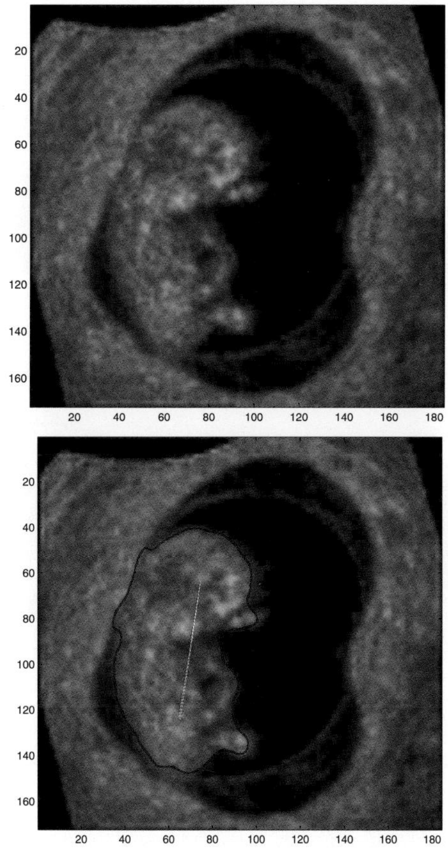

Figure 8.20: Fetal echography presenting the shape of a baby (left) and segmentation of the baby with the level set $\bar{u} = \{\max(u) - \varepsilon\}$ of the subjective surface (right).

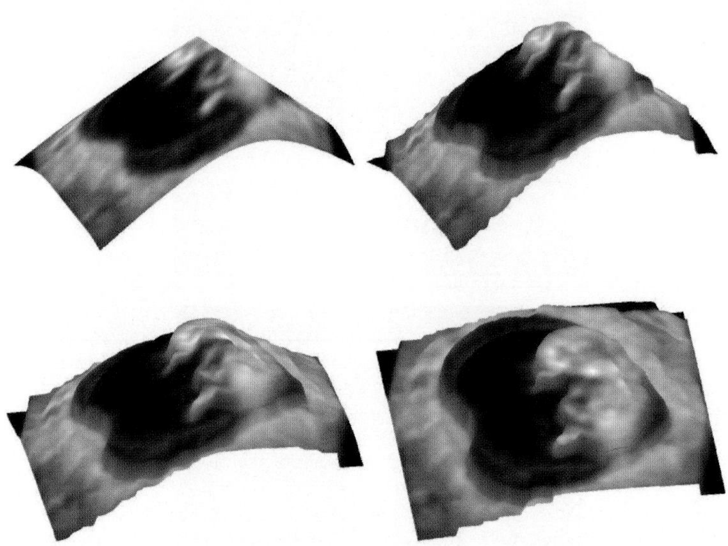

Figure 8.21: Evolution of the graph towards the subjective surface segmenting the fetus.

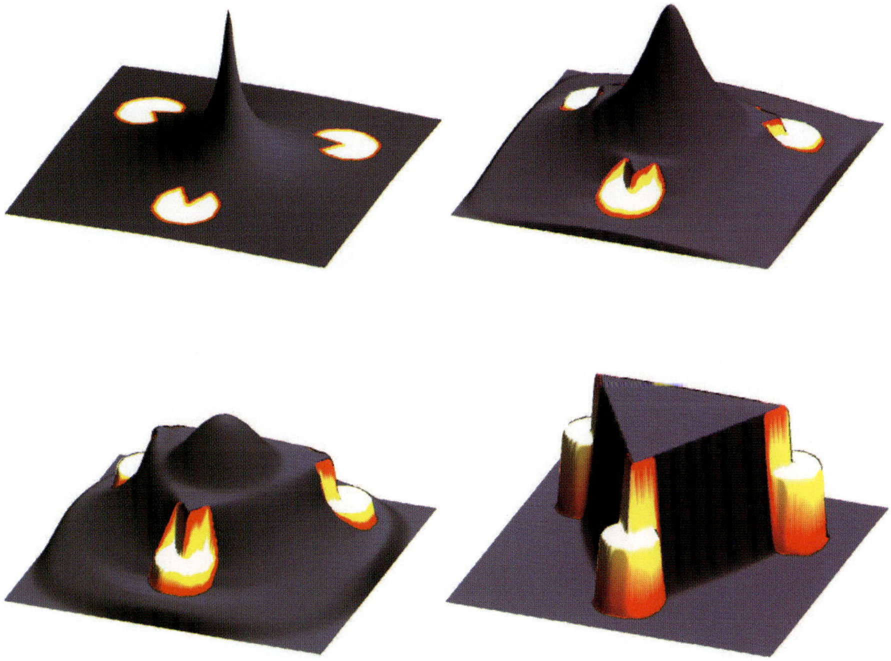

Figure 8.24: COLOR PLATES. Four time frames showing the evolution of the point-of-view surface (upper left) towards the subjective surface (bottom right). In this visualization the original image has been texture mapped onto the surface.

the grid point (x, y). In this time, the surface $T(x, y)$ satisfies the equation: $||\nabla T|| \,.\, V = 1$. By approximation, the solution to the Eikonal Equation is:

$$\begin{aligned} [\textbf{max}\ (\ \textbf{max}(D^{-x}\,T, 0), -\textbf{min}(D^{+x}\,T, 0)\ )]^2 + \\ [\textbf{max}\ (\ \textbf{max}(D^{-y}\,T, 0), -\textbf{min}(D^{+y}\,T, 0)\ )]^2 = \frac{1}{{V^2}_{xy}}, \end{aligned} \tag{4.5}$$

where ${V^2}_{xy}$ is the square of the speed at location (x, y) and $D^{-x}\,T$, $D^{+x}\,T$, $D^{-y}\,T$ and $D^{+y}\,T$ are the backward and forward differences in time, given as:

$$\begin{cases} D^{+x}\,T = \frac{T(x+1,y)-T(x,y)}{2} & \& \quad D^{-x}\,T = \frac{T(x,y)-T(x-1,y)}{2}, \\ D^{+y}\,T = \frac{T(x,y+1)-T(x,y)}{2} & \& \quad D^{-y}\,T = \frac{T(x,y)-T(x,y-1)}{2}. \end{cases} \tag{4.6}$$

There are efficient schemes for solving the Eikonal Equation (4.3). For details, see Sethian [88], Cao *et al.* [89] and Chen *et al.* [90].

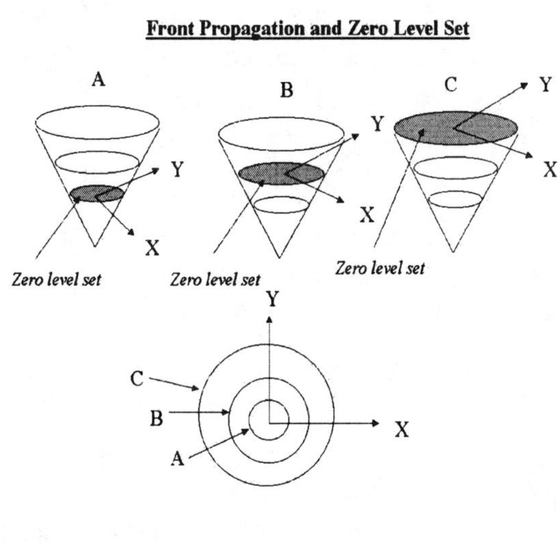

Figure 4.2: Front propagation of the *zero level set.* Top: Filled circles in figures (A), (B) and (C) show the position of the *zero level curve* as the front propagates. **Bottom**: These three projected circles are seen.

Having discussed the fundamentals of level sets, curve evolution and the Eikonal Equation, we will now discuss the PDE and level set application for image denoising.

4.3 Diffusion Imaging: Image Smoothing and Restoration Via PDE

The presense of noise in images is unavoidable. This could be introduced by the image formation process in MR, CT, X-ray or PET images, or image recording or even an image transmission process. Several methods such as morphological smoothing, linear, non-linear, geometric have been presented in noise removal and smoothing, but this Chapter focuses on "noise removal" or "noise diffusion" using PDE. This has been used for quite some time but recently, robust techniques for image smoothing have been developed (see Perona *et al.* [18], [19], Gerig *et al.* [20], Alvarez *et al.* [21], [22], Kimia *et al.* [25], [26], Sapiro *et al.* [28], Caselles *et al.* [33], Weickert [34], Black *et al.* [35], Arridge *et al.* [36], Bajla *et al.* [37], Olver *et al.* [38], Scherzer *et al.* [39], Romeny *et al.* [42], [40] and Nielsen *et al.* [41]). This section covers these articles in the following way: The fundamental diffusion equation is given in sub-section 4.3.1. Sub-section 4.3.2 presents multi-channel anisotropic diffusion imaging. Tensor non-linear anisotropic diffusion is discussed in sub-section 4.3.3. Anisotropic diffusion based on PDE and the Tukey/Huber weight function is discussed in sub-section 4.3.4. Image denoising using the curve evolution approach is presented in sub-section 4.3.5. Image denoising and histogram modification using PDE is presented in sub-section 4.3.6. Finally, the section concludes with non-linear image denoising in sub-section 4.3.7.

4.3.1 Perona-Malik Anisotropic Image Diffusion Via PDE (Perona)

One of the first papers on diffusion was from Perona and Malik [18], called Perona-Malik Anisotropic Diffusion (PMAD) (also called edge-based diffusion). PMAD's idea was based on one of the earlier papers by Witkin [17]. Perona *et al.* [18] gave the fundamental PDE-based diffusion equation for image smoothing as:

$$I_t = div(\mathcal{D}^t(x,y)\,\nabla I)\,, \tag{4.7}$$

where "*div*" was the divergence (also defined as $I_t = \nabla\cdot(\mathcal{D}^t(x,y)\,\nabla I))$ operator, I_t was the rate of change of image I, $\mathcal{D}^t(x,y)$ was the diffusion constant at location (x,y) at time t and ∇I was the gradient of the image I. Applying the divergence operator, the PDE diffusion equation was re-writtten as:

$$I_t = \mathcal{D}^t(x,y)\,\Delta I + \nabla\mathcal{D}^t(x,y).\nabla I\,, \tag{4.8}$$

where ΔI was the Laplacian operator, $\nabla\mathcal{D}^t(x,y)$ was the gradient of the diffusion constant at location (x,y) for time t. The diffusion constant was the key factor in the smoothing process. Perona *et al.* gave two expressions for the diffusion constants: $\mathcal{D}^t(x,y) = e^{-(\frac{||\nabla I^t||}{K})^2}$ and $\mathcal{D}^t(x,y) = \frac{1}{1+(\frac{||\nabla I^t||}{K})^2}$, where $||\nabla I^t||$ was the absolute value of the gradient of the image I at time t and K was a constant which was either manipulated manually for some fixed value or computed using a "noise estimator" as described by Canny [23]. Using the finite difference method, Eq. (4.8) was discretized to:

$$\begin{aligned} I^{t+1}(x,y) \;=\;& I^t(x,y) + \lambda\,\{\mathcal{D}^t{}_e(x,y)(I(x+1,y) - I(x,y)) + \\ & \mathcal{D}^t{}_w(x,y)(I(x-1,y) - I(x,y)) + \mathcal{D}^t{}_n(x,y)(I(x,y-1) - I(x,y)) \\ & +\mathcal{D}^t{}_s(x,y)((I(x,y+1) - I(x,y))\}\,, \end{aligned} \tag{4.9}$$

where $\mathcal{D}^t{}_n(x,y)$, $\mathcal{D}^t{}_s(x,y)$, $\mathcal{D}^t{}_e(x,y)$ and $\mathcal{D}^t{}_w(x,y)$ were the finite difference diffusion constants for time t in four different directions (north, south, east and west) given the central location (x,y). The values of these constants were chosen either exponentially or as a ratio as discussed above. To see the performance of the PMAD, we took three sets of examples: In case one, we took a simple two petal flower image, then added the Gaussian noise and finally applied the PMAD over it. The results of the input/ouput operation can be seen in Figure 4.3. We took a more complex image of a flower image with eight petals, added the same Gaussian noise and applied the PMAD over it. The results can be seen in Figure 4.4. In the same figure, we compare the PMAD with Pollak *et al.*'s inverse diffusion method (IDM). Pollak *et al.* [24] proposed a diffusion method which was different from PMAD in two respects: first, discontinuing the inverse flow function and second, merging the regions during diffusion. The first feature made the diffusion stable. Every local maximum was decreased and every local minimum was increased. The second feature made the algorithm fast and unique. In the third example, we applied the PMAD and Pollak *et al.*'s IDM over noisy functional MRI data of the brain. The results can be seen in Figure 4.5. Recently, Perona [19] also defined the angular or orientational diffusion based on the magnetic concept of attracting objects. This research is out of the scope of this Chapter.

Pros and Cons of PMAD Using PDE: The main advantage of the PMAD was its relatively low execution time and a good starting point on scale-space and anisotropic diffusion for image denoising. The following were the weaknesses of this method: first, the PMAD method brought blurring at small discontinuities and had a property of sharpening edges (see Gerig *et al.* [20]). Second, the PMAD method did not incorporate convergence criteria (see Gerig *et al.* [20]). Third, the method was not robust at handling large amounts of noise. The method did not preserve the discontinuities between regions. Fourth, the method needed to adjust tuning constants such as K and lastly, the method did not take into account inhomogeneity in data sampling.

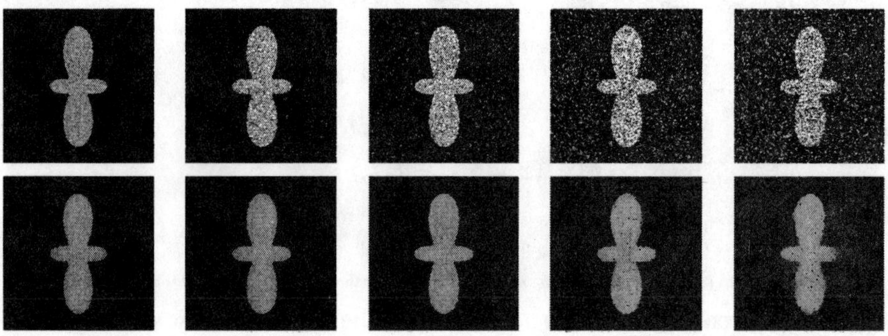

Figure 4.3: Two petal flower with Gaussian noise added and PMAD applied to it. <u>**TopRow**</u> (left to right): Noisy images with 20, 10, 5, 3 and 1 db. <u>**BottomRow**</u> (left to right): PMAD-PDE diffusion results from the above noisy images. The diffusion constant used was: $\mathcal{D}^t(x,y) = \frac{1}{1+(\frac{\|\nabla I^t\|}{K})^2}$, where K was chosen as 10, the time step as 1 and the total number of iterations were 200.

4.3.2 Multi-Channel Anisotropic Image Diffusion Via PDE (Gerig)

Recently, Gerig *et al.* [20] developed the non-linear diffusion system for smoothing or noise reduction in MR brain images. This method was called multi-channel since the processing involved three different kinds of scans: T_1-, T_2- and PD-weighted MR data sets. It was named coupled since the diffusion coefficient was coupled between two different MR data sets. Keeping PMAD's diffusion in mind, the multi-channel anisotropic image diffusion was given as:

$$\begin{pmatrix} \frac{\partial I_1(x,y,t)}{\partial t} \\ \frac{\partial I_2(x,y,t)}{\partial t} \end{pmatrix} = \begin{pmatrix} div(D_c(x,y,t)\nabla I_1{}^t) \\ div(D_c(x,y,t)\nabla I_2{}^t) \end{pmatrix}, \tag{4.10}$$

where the coupled diffusion coefficient D_c was computed from multi-channel data sets I_1 and I_2. $\frac{\partial I_1}{\partial t}$ and $\frac{\partial I_2}{\partial t}$ were the rate of change of multi-channel images. The coupled diffusion was given as: $\mathcal{D}^t{}_c(x,y,t) = e^{-(\frac{||(\nabla I_1^t)^2+(\nabla I_2^t)^2||}{K})^2}$ and $\mathcal{D}^t{}_c(x,y,t) = \frac{1}{1+(\frac{||(\nabla I_1^t)^2+(\nabla I_2^t)^2||}{K})^2}$, where $||(\nabla I_1^t)^2 + (\nabla I_2^t)^2||$ was the absolute value of the gradient of the multi-channel images I_1 and I_2 and K was a constant as used by PMAD. Note, if discontinuities were detected in both channels, then the combined diffusion coefficient was larger than any single component and the significance of local estimations was increased. On the other hand, if a discontinuity was detected only in one of the channels, the combined coefficient responded to the discontinuity and halted the diffusion.

Pros and Cons of Multi-Channel Anisotropic Diffusion: This technique had two major advantages: first, it showed efficient noise reduction in homogeneous regions and also preserved the object contours, boundaries between different tissues and small structures such as vessels. Second, filtered images appeared clearer and boundaries were better defined, leading to an improved differentiation of adjacent regions of similar intensity characteristics. The major weaknesses of this technique were: first, the Chapter did not show how the PDE flow behaved and how the convergence would become affected if the "coupled PDE diffusion" was computed. Second, the number of iterations in the smoothing process was selected by visual comparison. Thus the convergence to steady-state and stopping criteria were fuzzy. Third, there was no discussion on the computation time for 3-D filtering for non-isotropic (a volume whose three dimensions are not same) volumes; and lastly, selection of the parameter K was not automatic.

4.3.3 Tensor Non-Linear Anisotropic Diffusion Via PDE (Weickert)

To combat the problems of PMAD, Weickert [34] proposed a truly anisotropic diffusion, called Tensor Non-Linear Anisotropic Diffusion (TNAD) and was

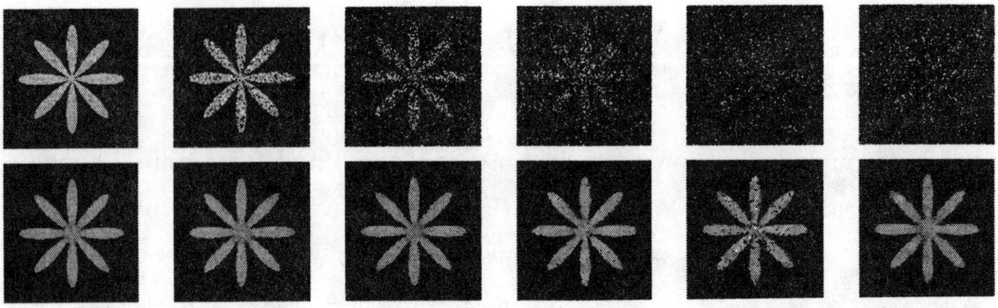

Figure 4.4: This flower image has a larger set of petals compared to Figure ?? and convolutions. **TopRow** (left to right): Noisy images with 20, 10, 5, 3, 1 and 1 db. **BottomRow** (left to right): PMAD-PDE diffusion results from the above noisy images. The diffusion constant used was: $\mathcal{D}^t(x,y) = \frac{1}{1+(\frac{||\nabla I^t||}{K})^2}$, where K was chosen as 10, the time step as 1 and the total iterations were 200. Note, the last image (right most) in the bottom row is the result due to Pollak *et al.*'s IDM [24]. The number of iterations used was 500.

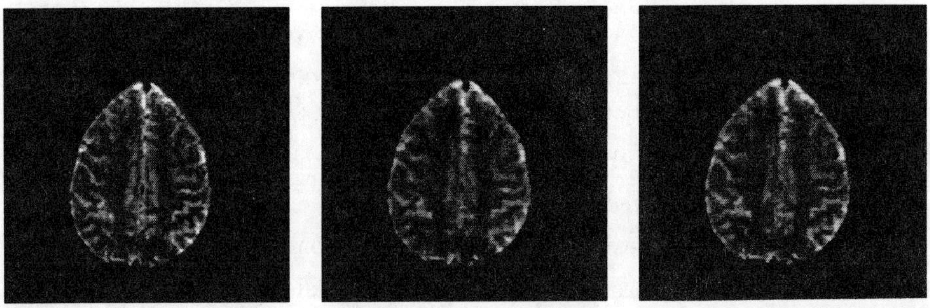

Figure 4.5: Noisy fMRI images with PMAD and Pollak *et al.*'s IDM applied to them. **Left**: fMRI noisy brain axial slice. **Middle**: PMAD-PDE diffusion results. The diffusion constant used was: $\mathcal{D}^t(x,y) = \frac{1}{1+(\frac{||\nabla I^t||}{K})^2}$, where K was chosen as 10, the time step as 0.1 and the total iterations were 200. **Right**: Pollak *et al.*'s IDM with time step 0.1 and number of iterations 500. As seen in this figure, Pollak *et al.*'s method does the best in removing the noise and highlighting the gray matter/white matter interface (for details on the importance of WM/GM interface, see Suri *et al.* [5]).

mathematically given as:

$$\frac{\partial I(x,y,t)}{\partial t} = div[\mathcal{D}(\nabla I)\,\nabla I]\,, \tag{4.11}$$

where $\mathcal{D}$ was the diffusion tensor having eigenvectors e_1 and e_2 and defined in a way such that: $\underbrace{e_1 \,||\, \nabla I}$ and $\underbrace{e_2 \perp \nabla I}$. Weickert suggested choosing the eigenvalues λ_1 and λ_2 such that: $\lambda_1 = g(||\nabla I||)$ and $\lambda_2 = 1$. The sample results of this technique can be seen in Figure 4.6 (see Weickert *et al.* [120]). Details on this method can be seen in the book by Weickert [34]. Other authors who did work in non-linear anisotropic diffusion were: Schnörr [13], [14] and Catte *et al.* [15], [16].

Pros and Cons of Tensor Non-Linear Anisotropic Diffusion: Besides being robust, the method was applied to a variety of images. The method did not taken into consideration, however, the inhomogeneity in data sampling.

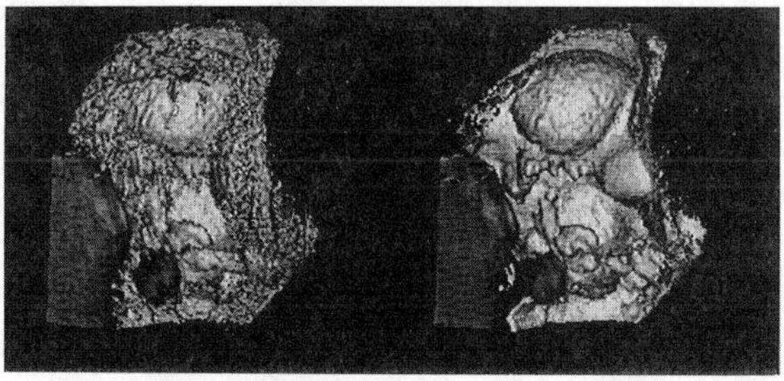

Figure 4.6: Tensor image diffusion on a 3-D ultrasound image. **Left**: Rendering of a 3-D ultrasound data set of a 10-week old human fetus. **Right**: Rendering after denoising by Tensor Non-Linear Anisotropic Diffusion (TNAD) filtering (see Weickert *et al.* [120]). Courtesy of Professor Weickert, Computer Vision, Graphics and Pattern Recognition Group, Department of Mathematics and Computer Science, University of Mannheim, Mannheim, Germany.

4.3.4 Anisotropic Diffusion Using the Tukey/Huber Weight Function (Black)

Black *et al.* [35] recently showed a comparative study between Perona-Malik Anisotropic Diffusion (PMAD) based on a combination of PDE and Tukey's bi-weight estimator, known as Black *et al.* 's Robust Anisotropic Diffusion (BRAD).

In this image smoothing process (estimating piecewise constant), the goal was to minimize I that satisfied:

$$\min_{I} \sum_{s \in I} \sum_{p \in \eta_s} \rho(I_p - I_s, \sigma), \tag{4.12}$$

where s was the pixel location, p took one of the four neighbours and η_s was the set of four neighbours of s. ρ was the error norm function (called a robust estimator, see Meer *et al.* [43]) and σ was the scale parameter. The relationship between ρ and PMAD was expressed as under: If PMAD was given by the function $g(x)$, where $g(x) = \frac{1}{1+(\frac{x}{K})^2}$, then $g(x) = \frac{\rho'}{x}$, the derivative of the error norm function. Black *et al.* used Tukey's Biweight and the Huber min-max function for error norm. This Tukey function was given as: $\rho(x, \sigma) = (\frac{x^2}{\sigma^2} - \frac{x^4}{\sigma^4} + \frac{x^6}{3\sigma^6})$, if $|x| \leq \sigma$ and $\rho(x, \sigma) = \frac{1}{3}$, if $|x| > \sigma$. The Huber's min-max for error norm was $\rho(x, \sigma) = (\frac{x^2}{2\sigma} + \frac{\sigma}{2})$, if $|x| \leq \sigma$ or $|x|$, if $|x| > \sigma$. Note that σ was computed as: $\sigma = 1.4 \times$ median $(||\nabla I - med_I(||\nabla I||)||)$. Black *et al.* used gradient descent for solving the image smoothing minimization problem. Thus the discrete solution of BRAD was:

$$I_s^{t+1} = I_s^t + \frac{\lambda}{\eta_s} \sum_{p \in \eta_s} \rho'(I_p - I_s^t, \sigma), \tag{4.13}$$

where ρ' was the derivative of error norm, σ. The whole idea of bringing the robust statistics was to remove outliers and preserve shape boundaries. Thus BRAD = PMAD + Huber/Tukey's Robust estimator. Figure 4.7 compares Perona-Malik's Anisotropic Diffusion (PMAD) with Black *et al.* 's Tukey function (BRAD). This figure shows the results for 100 and 500 iterations. As you can see, the results of Tukey are far superior compared to PMAD. Also at infinity, the PMAD will make the image go flat and the Tukey will not[6]. Readers interested in the application of Huber's weight function in medical application can see the detailed work by Suri, Haralick and Sheehan [44]. Here, the goal was to remove the outlier longitudinal axes of the Left Ventricle (LV) for ruled surface estimation to model the movement of the LV of the heart.

Pros and Cons of Anisotropic Diffusion Based on Robust Statistics: The following were the main advantages of the BRAD method: In comparison to PMAD, BRAD was more robust. The method was also stable for a large

[6]Personal communication with Professor Sapiro.

number of iterations and the image did not get flat when t was infinity. The major disadvantage of the system was that it did not show how to compute the σ for the design of the Huber's weight function. Secondly, the system did not discuss the timing issues.

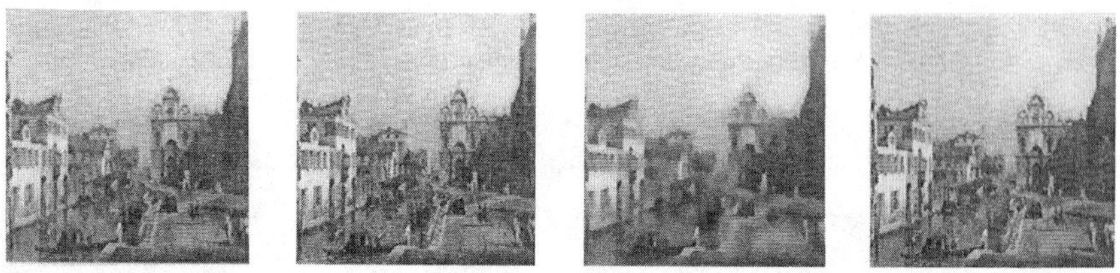

Figure 4.7: Comparison of the Perona-Malik function and Tukey function after 100 and 500 iterations. Results of Perona-Malik PDE and Black *et al.*'s Tukey methods. **Left Most**: PMAD with number of iterations set to 100. **Left Middle**: Tukey function with number of iterations set to 100. **Right Middle**: PMAD with number of iterations set to 500 iterations. **Right Most**: Tukey function with number of iterations set to 500 (Courtesy of Professor Sapiro, Department of Electrical and Computer Engineering, University of Minnesota, Minneapolis, MN, source: Black *et al.* [35]).

4.3.5 Image Denoising Using PDE and Curve Evolution (Sarti)

Recently, Sarti *et al.* [85] presented an image denoising method based on the curve evolution concept. Before we discuss what Sarti *et al.* did, we will just present the fundamental equation presented by Kichenassamy *et al.* [74] and Yezzi *et al.* [75]. They presented the curve evolution model by introducing an extra stopping term. This was expressed mathematically as:

$$\frac{\partial \phi}{\partial t} = c(\mathbf{x})(\kappa + V_0)\,|\nabla \phi| \;\; + \underbrace{(\nabla c . \nabla\, \phi)}\; . \tag{4.14}$$

Note that $(\nabla c . \nabla\, \phi)$ denoted the projection of an attractive force vector on the normal to the curve. This force was realized as the gradient of a potential field c. This potential field c for the 2-D and 3-D case was given as: $c(x, y) = -|\nabla(G_\sigma \otimes I(x, y))|$ and $c(x, y, z) = -|\nabla(G_\sigma \otimes I(x, y, z))|$, respectively, where ∇ was the gradient operator, $G_\sigma \otimes I(x, y)$ and $G_\sigma \otimes I(x, y, z)$ were the Gaussian convolution operations, respectively. Note that Equation (4.14) is similar to

Equation 7 given by Malladi *et al.* in [77]. Malladi *et al.* called the equation as an additional constraint on the surface motion ϕ_t. Rewriting Equation 7 of Malladi *et al.* [77] as:

$$\phi_t + c(\mathbf{x})(\epsilon\,\kappa + V_0)\,|\,\nabla\phi\,| - \beta\,(\nabla c.\nabla\,\phi) = 0\,, \tag{4.15}$$

where β was the edge strength constant, V_0 was a constant (1 as used by Malladi *et al.*), κ was the curvature dependent speed, ϵ was the constant term controlling the curvature dependent speed and $(\nabla c.\nabla\,\phi)$ was the same as defined above. Having presented the level set equation in terms of speed functions and constants, Sarti *et al.*'s method changed the above equation by removing the constant propagation force V_0 and simply solved the remaining equation for image denoising. The smoothing worked in the following way: If $|\nabla(G * I_0(\mathbf{x}))|$ was large, the flow was slow and the exact location of the edge was retained. If $|\nabla(G * I_0(\mathbf{x}))|$ was small, then the flow tended to be fast, thereby increasing the smoothing process. The filtering model was reduced to mean curvature flow when $c(\mathbf{x})$ was an equation to unity. Thus, the data consistency term $c(\mathbf{x})$ served as an edge indicator. The convolution operation simply eliminated the influence of spurious noise. Sarti *et al.* thus solved Eq. (4.14) iteratively and progressively smoothed it over time. The edge indicator function c became smoother and smoother over time and depended less and less on the spurious noise. Note that the minimal size of the detail was related to the size of the Gaussian kernel, which acted like a scale parameter. The variance of $G_\sigma(\mathbf{x})$ was taken as $\frac{1}{C_\sigma e^{-(\frac{|\mathbf{x}|^2}{4\sigma})}}$ which corresponded to the dimension of the smallest structure that had to be preserved. The sharpening of the edge information was due to the hyperbolic term $(\nabla c.\nabla\,\phi)$.

Pros and Cons of Image Denoising Using PDE and Curve Evolution: The main merits of the system were its simple extension from the basic curve evolution method and the ability to sharpen the image edges due to its hyperbolic term $(\nabla c.\nabla\,\phi)$. The drawbacks of the system were: first, there was not much discussion on the scale-space parameter, the variance of $G_\sigma(\mathbf{x})$, which was one of the critical pieces in the image denoising. Second, there was not much discussion on the stopping method for the PDE. Since constant force played a critical role as will be seen ahead as a "regularizer force" in segmentation modeling, we feel that constant force could have been used more efficiently rather than plain removal in the image denoising process.

4.3.6 Image Denoising and Histogram Modification Using PDE (Sapiro)

A description on diffusion would be incomplete if references from Sapiro were missed. Recently, Sapiro *et al.* [27], [28] and [29] developed the ensemble of two different algorithms in one PDE. This method used histogram modification (or histogram equalization) and image denoising in one PDE. This was called edge preservation anisotropic diffusion. The idea was to smooth the image only in the direction parallel to the edges, achieving this via curvature flows. This was done using the following flow equation:

$$\frac{\partial \phi}{\partial t} = \frac{1}{1 + ||\nabla(G \otimes \phi)||} \left(\phi_x^2 \phi_{yy} - 2\phi_x \phi_y \phi_{xy} + \phi_y^2 \phi_{xx}\right)^{\frac{1}{3}} ||\nabla \phi||\,, \tag{4.16}$$

where ϕ was the level set function which evolved according to the affine heat flow for planar shape smoothing with the velocity given by $\frac{1}{1+||\nabla(G\otimes\phi)||}$, where $\otimes$ was the convolution operator. The histogram equalization flow was given as:

$$\frac{\partial \phi}{\partial t} = (N^2 - H[\phi(x,y,t)]) - \mathcal{A}\left[(v,w) : \phi(v,w,t) >= \phi(x,y,t)\right], \tag{4.17}$$

where image $\phi(x,y,t) : [0,N]^2 \to [0,M]$ and $\mathcal{A}$ represented the area (or number of pixels). Combining Eq. (4.16) and Eq. (4.17) yielded a joint PDE as:

$$\begin{aligned} \frac{\partial \phi}{\partial t} &= \alpha \frac{1}{1 + ||\nabla(G \otimes \phi)||} \left(\phi_x^2 \phi_{yy} - 2\phi_x \phi_y \phi_{xy} + \phi_y^2 \phi_{xx}\right)^{\frac{1}{3}} ||\nabla \phi|| + \\ & (N^2 - H[\phi(x,y,t)]) - \mathcal{A}\left[(v,w) : \phi(v,w,t) >= \phi(x,y,t)\right]. \end{aligned} \tag{4.18}$$

Here, H was defined as: If the density function of image $I(x,y)$ is $h(n)$, where $n = 0...M$, then $H(n) = \sum_{i=0}^{n}(h(n))$, like a "cumulated" density function. Here, α was the weighting factor. There has been some research which relates anisotropic diffusion, curve evolution and segmentation. Interested researchers can see Sapiro [31] and Shah [32].

Pros and Cons of Image Denoising and Histogram Modification Via PDE: The paper took advantage of how different components were diffused together. The demerit of the system was that it was only able to smooth the edges in the direction of the edges. Besides that, there was no discussion about how to select the parameter α.

4.3.7 Image Denoising Using Non-linear PDEs (Rudin)

Rudin *et al.* [131] recently developed a denoising algorithm which could be interpreted as a first step of moving each level set of the image normal to itself with velocity equal to the curvature of the level set divided by the magnitude of the gradient of the image. The second step in this algorithm was to project the image back onto the constrain set. This problem was posed as a constrained minimization problem where the goal was to minimize over I the following: minimize $\int_\Omega \sqrt{(\frac{\partial u}{\partial x})^2 + (\frac{\partial u}{\partial y})^2}\, dx\, dy$. This was subjected to the linear and non-linear constraints given as: $\int_\Omega u\, dx\, dy = \int_\Omega u_0\, dx\, dy$ and $\int_\Omega \frac{(u-u_0)^2}{2}\, dx\, dy = \sigma^2$. This equation was changed into an Euler-Lagrange formulation and then into a PDE framework as:

$$u_t = \frac{\partial}{\partial x}\left(\frac{u_x}{\sqrt{u_x + u_y}}\right) + \frac{\partial}{\partial y}\left(\frac{u_y}{\sqrt{u_x + u_y}}\right) - \lambda\,(u - u_0)\,, \tag{4.19}$$

where u_t was the rate of change of u with respect to t, u_x and u_y were the partial derivatives $\frac{\partial u}{\partial x}$ and $\frac{\partial u}{\partial y}$, respectively. This was valid for t greater than 0 for every $x, y \in \Omega$. The value of λ was computed as:

$$\lambda = \frac{-1}{2\sigma}\int [\sqrt{u_x^2 + u_y^2} - (\frac{(u_0)_x\, u_x}{\sqrt{u_x + u_y}} + \frac{(u_0)_y\, u_y}{\sqrt{u_x + u_y}})dx\, dy]\,. \tag{4.20}$$

Here, we briefly present the numerical solution to Equations (4.19) and (4.20).

$$\begin{aligned} u_{ij}^{n+1} &= u_{ij}^n + \frac{\Delta t}{h}\,\{\mathcal{D}_x^-(\frac{\mathcal{D}_x^+ u_{ij}^n}{((\mathcal{D}_x^+ u_{ij}^n)^2 + (m(\mathcal{D}_y^+, \mathcal{D}_y^-))^2)^{\frac{1}{2}}}) + \\ &\quad \mathcal{D}_y^-(\frac{\mathcal{D}_y^+ u_{ij}^n}{((\mathcal{D}_y^+ u_{ij}^n)^2 + (m(\mathcal{D}_x^+, \mathcal{D}_x^-))^2)^{\frac{1}{2}}})\} + \Delta t\, \lambda^n\, (u_{ij}^n - u_0(ih, jh))\,, \end{aligned} \tag{4.21}$$

where $x_i = ih$, $y_j = jh$, $i, j = 1, ..., N$ with $Nh = 1$. h is the step size. $t_n = n\Delta t$, $n = 0, 1, ...,$ $u_{ij}^n = u(x_i, y_j, t_n)$ and $u_{ij}^0 = u_0(ih, jh) + \sigma\phi(ih, jh)$. $\mathcal{D}_x^\pm = \pm(u_{i\pm1,j} - u_{ij})$; $\mathcal{D}_y^\pm = \pm(u_{i\pm1,j} - u_{ij})$; $m(a, b) = \mathbf{minmod}(a, b) = (\frac{\mathbf{sgn}(a)+\mathbf{sgn}(b)}{2})\min(|a|, |b|)$ and

$$\begin{aligned} \lambda^n &= -\frac{h}{2\sigma^2}\{\sigma_{i,j}(\sqrt{(\mathcal{D}_x^+ u_{ij}^n)^2 + (\mathcal{D}_y^+ u_{ij}^n)^2} - \frac{(\mathcal{D}_x^+ u_{ij}^0)(\mathcal{D}_x^+ u_{ij}^n)}{\sqrt{(\mathcal{D}_x^+ u_{ij}^n)^2 + (\mathcal{D}_y^+ u_{ij}^n)^2}} \\ &\quad - \frac{(\mathcal{D}_x^+ u_{ij}^0)(\mathcal{D}_x^+ k u_{ij}^n)}{\sqrt{(\mathcal{D}_x^+ u_{ij}^n)^2 + (\mathcal{D}_y^+ u_{ij}^n)^2}})\} \end{aligned} \tag{4.22}$$

where $\mathcal{D}_x^\pm$ and $\mathcal{D}_y^\pm$ were the same as defined above. Note that the step size restriction was imposed for stability, i.e., $\frac{\Delta t}{h^2} \le c$, where c was a constant.

Pros and Cons of Non-linear PDEs for Image Denoising: The following were the major advantages of the non-linear image denoising method: first, the method introduced the constrain while solving the PDEs. As a result, the regularizer term λ improved the smoothing effect. Second, such a method was applied in techniques for sub-pixel accuracy. Third, this algorithm converged to the steady-state at $t \to \infty$, which was the denoised image. The following were the weaknesses of this method: First, the paper did not discuss the stability issues such as the ratio $\frac{\triangle t}{h^2}$ and secondly, the method introduced the λ term which needed extra computations.

Having discussed the different image diffusion techniques based on PDE, and their pros and cons, interested readers can go into more detail on behavioral analysis on anisotropic diffusion in image processing (see You *et al.* [30]). Also, see knowledge-based tensor anisotropic diffusion for cardiac MRI by Sanchez-Ortiz *et al.* [45]. A detailed review on PDE-based diffusion and a comparison between different smoothing techniques using PDE, scale-space mathematical morphology and inverse diffusion techniques can be seen by Suri *et al.* [46]. Next, we will discuss image segmentation in still images via PDE and the level set framework.

4.4 Segmentation in Still Imagery Via PDE/Level Set Framework

Dominance of PDE in the level set framework for image/volume segmentation has been tremendous. The following institutions are the major players: (**1**) UCLA, University of California, Los Angeles, CA, USA, (**2**) INRIA, Institut National de Recherche en Informatique et Automatique, Sophia-Antipolis, France, (**3**) IRISA, Institut de recherche en informatique et systemes aleatories, Rennes Cedex, France, (**4**) Technion, Israel Institute of Technology, Haifa, Israel, (**5**) MIT, Massachusetts Institute of Technology, Cambridge, MA, USA, (**6**) MGH, Massachusetts General Hospital, Harvard Medical School, Boston, MA, USA, (**7**) JHU, Johns Hopkins University, Baltimore, MD, USA, (**8**) UT, University of Toronto, Toronto, Canada, (**9**) LBNL, Lawrence Berkeley National Labs., Berkeley, CA, USA, (**10**) MNI, Montreal Neurological Institute, McGill University, Montreal, Canada, (**11**) Yale, Image Processing and Analysis Group, Yale University, New Haven, CT, USA, (**12**) MMS, Marconi Medical

Systems, Inc., Cleveland, OH, USA, (**13**) UF, University of Florida, Gainesville, FL, USA, (**14**) UM, University of Minnesota, Minneapolis, MN, USA and (**15**) UW, University of Wisconsin, Milwaukee, WI, USA. Since it is difficult to cover all level sets based techniques for segmentation, an attempt was made by Suri *et al.* [6] to design a level set survey paper which covered the state-of-the-art segmentation methods for medical imaging. This section will focus on the core PDE application for segmentation of still imagery. This section presents five systems which follow the generic segmentation modeling method. The layout of this section is as follows: The PDE-based example of fusing the fuzzy pixel classification in the level set framework is presented in sub-section 4.4.1. Application of Bayes' method in the PDE/level set framework for segmentation is discussed in sub-section 4.4.2. Vasculature segmentation in the PDE/level set framework is discussed in the sub-section 4.4.3. Sub-section 4.4.4 presents the PDE/level set application using inverse variational criterion. Finally, this section concludes by presenting the Bayesian-based regularizer for segmentation in sub-section 4.4.5.

4.4.1 Embedding of the Fuzzy Model as a Bi-Directional Regional Regularizer for PDE Design in the Level Set Framework (Suri/Marconi)

This sub-section shows how the fuzzy regularizers are embedded in the curve evolution or level sets and model the segmentation process in the level set framework using the PDE. The level set equation will then be derived by embedding the region statistics into the parametric classical energy model. Part of this sub-section has been taken from Chapter 8 of the book by Suri *et al.* [4]. Part of that derivation will be discussed here with a few of the implementation details. To start with, the standard dynamic classical energy model as given by Kass *et al.* [91] was:

$$\gamma \frac{\partial \mathbf{X}}{\partial t} = \frac{\partial}{\partial s}(\alpha \frac{\partial \mathbf{X}}{\partial s}) - \frac{\partial^2}{\partial s^2}(\beta \frac{\partial^2 \mathbf{X}}{\partial s^2}) + F_{ext}(\mathbf{X}), \tag{4.23}$$

where $\mathbf{X}$ was the parametric contour, and α, β were the elastic constants. $F_{ext}(\mathbf{X})$ was the external force and γ was the damping coefficient. Since the second derivative term did not affect significantly the performance of the active geometric snakes (see Caselles *et al.* [33]), that term was dropped and replaced with a new pressure force term, given as: $F_p(\mathbf{X}) = w_p(\mathbf{X})\mathcal{N}(\mathbf{X})$. This yielded the new parametric active contour, given as:

$$\gamma \frac{\partial \mathbf{X}}{\partial t} = \frac{\partial}{\partial s}(\alpha \frac{\partial \mathbf{X}}{\partial s}) + \underbrace{w_p(\mathbf{X})\mathcal{N}(\mathbf{X})} + F_{ext}(\mathbf{X}) \,. \tag{4.24}$$

Note that to make Eq. (4.24) invariant to changes in the parameterization of $\mathbf{X}$, Suri *et al.* considered s as a parameter of arc-length and w_p was the spatial-varying function. Readjusting the terms by defining $\epsilon = \frac{\alpha}{\gamma}$, $\frac{\partial}{\partial s}(\frac{\partial \mathbf{X}}{\partial s})$ to be the curvature term κ, $V_p = \frac{w_p(\mathbf{X})}{\gamma}\mathcal{N}(\mathbf{X})$, and $V_{ext} = \frac{F_{ext}}{\gamma}$, Eq. (4.24) was rewritten as:

$$\frac{\partial \mathbf{X}}{\partial t} = (\epsilon \kappa + V_p + V_{ext} \, . \mathcal{N}) \, \mathcal{N} \,. \tag{4.25}$$

From the definition of curve evolution first given by Sethian, this resulted in:

$$\frac{\partial \phi}{\partial t} = V(\kappa)\mathcal{N} \,. \tag{4.26}$$

Comparing Eqs. (4.25) and (4.26), and using the definition of normal as: $\mathcal{N} = -\frac{\nabla \phi}{|\nabla \phi|}$ and considering only the normal components of the internal and external forces: $\frac{\partial}{\partial s}(\alpha \frac{\partial \mathbf{X}}{\partial s}).\mathcal{N} = (\alpha\kappa)$, the level set function (ϕ) was obtained as:

$$\frac{\partial \phi}{\partial t} = (\epsilon \, \kappa + V_p) \, |\nabla \phi| - V_{ext}.\nabla \phi \,, \tag{4.27}$$

where V_p was a regional term. An example of such a term was defined as $\frac{w_R}{\gamma R}$, where w_R was the weighting factor and R was the region indicator term which was a function of the fuzzy membership and ranged between 0 and 1. The results of running the above algorithm can be seen in Figure 4.8. The raw contour deforms towards the topology of WM/CSF interface (for details, see Suri [1]). Other authors who performed the embedding of regional statistics into the boundary estimation framework were Pavlidis *et al.* [92], Zhu *et al.* [93] and Suri [94].

Pros and Cons of Geometric Boundary Fused with Clustering: The above system is one of the latest state-of-the-art systems which had the following advantages: first, in the above system, the fuzzy clustering acted as a regularizer for navigating the geometric geodesic snake. Since it was a pixel-classification procedure, one could easily estimate boundaries for different structures in the brain MRI data such as WM, GM, ventricles, etc. Second, the key characteristic of this system was that it was based on region, so the local noise or edge did not distract the growth process. Third, the technique was non-local and thus the local noise could not distract the final placement of the contour or the diffusion growth process. Fourth, the technique was very suitable for medical organ segmentation since it could handle any of the cavities, concavities, convolutedness, splitting or merging. Fifth, the technique was extendable to multi-phase, which meant that if there were multiple level set functions, then they automatically merged and split during the course of the segmentation process. The major weakness of such a system was in the computational expense of the fuzzy membership computation, however it is compensated by the fast level sets implementations (see Suri [1]). Besides that, although the system has a minimum number of coefficients compared to parametric snakes, it were not totally independent of image characteristics.

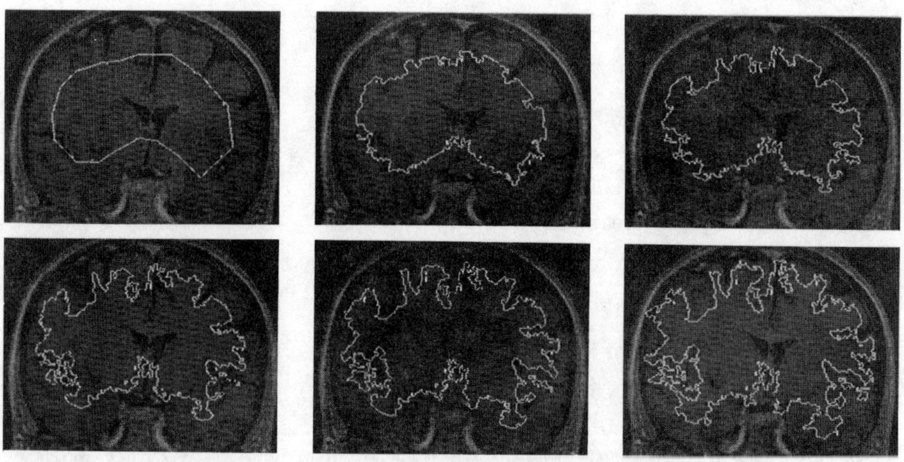

Figure 4.8: The above images (left to right, top row to bottom row) show the growth of the *zero level curve* to segment the white matter in human brain MR images. The narrow band width was 25 pixels on either side of the *zero level curve*, with the land mines at five pixels wide. Note, the deformation process had the ability to move in and out during the growth process (Courtesy of Dr. Jasjit Suri, Marconi Medical Systems, Inc.).

4.4.2 Embedding of the Bayesian Model as a Regional Regularizer for PDE Design in the Level Set Framework (Paragios/INRIA)

Paragios *et al.* [98] very recently added a Bayesian model as a regional term to redesign the PDE to improve Zhu *et al.*'s method [93]. Paragios *et al.* [98] implemented the fusion of region-based and boundary-based PDE in the level set framework. This meant incorporating the region statistics for PDE along with the boundary information of the PDE and solving the fused segmentation model in the level set framework. This will next be explained here. The classical deformable model for boundary estimation was originally given by Kass *et al.* [91] as:

$$E(C) = \underbrace{\alpha \int |C'(s)|^2\, ds + \beta \int |C''(s)|^2\, ds}_{Internal-Energy-Term} + \lambda \underbrace{\int |\nabla I(C(s))|\, ds}_{External-Energy-Term}, \tag{4.28}$$

where $E(C)$ was the classical energy of the snake or parametric contour. α, β were the elastic constants for smoothing and λ was the external energy constant. Note, the sum $\alpha \int |C'(s)|^2 ds + \beta \int |C''(s)|^2 ds$ was the smoothing energy term which was a function of the first and second partial derivative of the parametric curve along s. The term $\lambda \int |\nabla I(C(s))| ds$ was the external energy term as a function of image gradient ∇I. Following the derivation as proposed by Caselles *et al.* [33], the above was changed to the curve evolution form as: $\frac{\partial C}{\partial t}(t) = g(I)\kappa\mathcal{N} - (\nabla g \cdot \mathcal{N})\mathcal{N}$, where $\frac{\partial C}{\partial t}(t)$ was the rate of change of curve evolution, $g(I)$ was the edge detector, κ was the curvature and $\mathcal{N}$ was the surface outward unit normal. Using the reasoning as discussed by Caselles *et al.* [33], the above equation was given in terms of energy as:

$$E(u) = \int g(X)\, |\nabla u|\, dX\,. \tag{4.29}$$

Note, this was still in the boundary mode and the region term was still not integrated. In terms of the derivative operator, this can be given as:

$$E(\partial R) = \int g(\partial R_X(x))\, |\partial R_X(x)|\, dx\,. \tag{4.30}$$

If the image was composed of, say, two classes, $\mathcal{A}$ and $\mathcal{B}$, then using Zhu *et al.*'s [93] method of introducing the regional force with the boundary, was:

$$E(\partial R) = \underbrace{- \sum_{x \in \mathcal{A},\mathcal{B}} \alpha \int\int log(p_r, x(I(x,y))dx\, dy +}_{Region-Term} \underbrace{\sum_{x \in \mathcal{A},\mathcal{B}} (1-\alpha) \int\int g(p_b, x(I(\partial R(c_x)))) \, |\partial R_x(c_x)| \, dc_x,}_{Boundary-Term}, \tag{4.31}$$

where α was the smoothing constant, p_r and p_b were the regional and boundary probabilities. The Eulerian representation of the boundary model as given by Caselles *et al.* [33] was:

$$\frac{\partial \phi}{\partial t} = (g(I)\kappa + \nabla g(I).\frac{\nabla \phi}{|\nabla \phi|})\, |\nabla \phi| \,, \tag{4.32}$$

where $\nabla \phi$ was the gradient of the level set function. Thus, the level set framework for region term fused with boundary was given as:

$$\frac{\partial \phi_i}{\partial t}(u) = \underbrace{\alpha \left[r_i(u) - r_{o_{i(u)}} \right] |\nabla \phi_i(u)|}_{Regional-Force} + \underbrace{(1-\alpha) \left[b_i(u)\kappa_i(u) + \nabla b_i(u).\frac{\nabla \phi_i(u)}{|\nabla \phi_i(u)|} \right] |\nabla \phi_i(u)|}_{Boundary-Force}, \tag{4.33}$$

where r_i/r_o was a function that "captured" the inside/outside region features of the different classes and was given as: $\mathcal{R} \times \mathcal{R} \rightarrow \mathcal{R}, i \in [1, N]$, where N were the total number of regions. Similarly, b_i was a function that "captured" the boundary features of the different classes and had the range: $\mathcal{R} \times \mathcal{R} \rightarrow \mathcal{R}, i \in [1, N]$. $\kappa_i(u)$ was the curvature information of the boundary. $\nabla b_i(u)$ is the gradient at the boundary and $\frac{\nabla \phi_i(u)}{|\nabla \phi_i(u)|}$ was the outward/inward normal of the propagating contour. Note that the above contour had two parts: regional force and the boundary force, and i varied from 1 to N. Paragios *et al.* modified Eq. (4.33) by introducing the penalty function for the pixels that either did not belong to a region or which belonged to multiple regions. Interested reader can explore Paragios *et al.* [98] on this.

Pros and Cons of Paragios *et al.*'s Technique: Since the system took the region-based statistics into the geometric deformable model, the system had an advantage of being robust to noise. Second, the algorithm had the flexibility of putting multiple initial contours (multi-phase curve propagation) just like the bubble technique by Tek *et al.* [99]. Third, the algorithm was validated by taking three applications: texture segmentation, motion segmentation and tracking. The following were the major weaknesses of Paragios *et al.*'s technique: first, the methodology was able to segment texture well, but the results did not show that the segmented boundary was able to penetrate the convoluted shapes. For example in Figure 4.9 (left), we see that the final boundary was not able to go deep between the legs of the zebra. This problem was addressed by Xu *et al.* [100] and solved using gradient vector flow. Another solution would be to use a fuzzy regularizer rather than a Bayesian regularizer in this framework. This has been recently shown by Suri [1]. Second, like all region-based methods, this method was also computationally expensive.

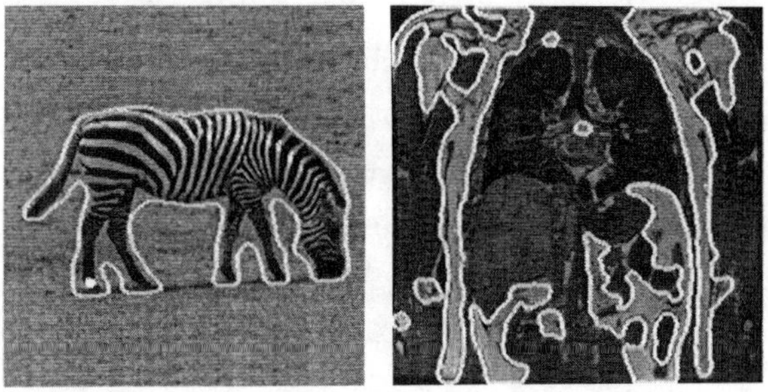

Figure 4.9: Segmentation results of Paragios *et al.*'s method. **Left**: zebra image showing the segmented contour around the zebra. **Right**: CT image of the chest showing the segmented results (Courtesy of Nikos Paragios, Siemens Corporate Research, Princeton, NJ).

4.4.3 Vasculature Segmentation Using PDE (Lorigo/MIT)

Recently, Lorigo *et al.* [95] presented an algorithm for brain vessel reconstruction based on curve evolution in 3-D, also known as "co-dimension two" in geodesic active contours. This method used two components: (i) mean curvature flow (MCF) and (ii) the directionality of vessels. The mean curvature flow component was used to derive the Eulerian representation of the level set equation. If ϕ was the signed distance transform (SDT) and $\lambda(\nabla\phi(\mathbf{x},t), \nabla^2\phi(\mathbf{x},t))$ was the eigenvalues of the projection operator: $\mathcal{P}_{\nabla\phi}\nabla^2\phi\,\mathcal{P}_{\nabla\phi}$, where $\mathcal{P} = I - \frac{qq^T}{|q|^2}$ and q was a non-zero vector and T represented the transpose. Using these eigenvalues, the Eulerian representation of the curve evolution was given by Lorigo *et al.* as: $\frac{\partial \phi}{\partial t} = \lambda(\nabla \phi(\mathbf{x}, t), \nabla^2 \phi(\mathbf{x}, t))$. The second component was the normal of these vessels projected onto the plane and was given as the product of $\nabla \phi$ with the projection vector d. This projection vector was computed using the Hessian H of the intensity image, I and was given as: $\frac{g'}{g}(H \frac{\nabla I}{|\nabla I|})$, where g was the edge detector operator. Adding these two components, the complete level set equation was:

$$\frac{\partial \phi}{\partial t} = \underbrace{\lambda(\nabla \phi(\mathbf{x}, t), \nabla^2 \phi(\mathbf{x}, t))}_{mean-curvature-force} + \underbrace{D \times S \times \frac{g'}{g}(H \frac{\nabla I}{|\nabla I|})}_{angular-balloon-force}, \tag{4.34}$$

where D was the directionality term which was the dot product of $\nabla \phi$ and ∇I which was the angle between these two vectors. S was the scale term. Note that the second term was like an angular balloon force which navigated the deformation process. The results of running the above algorithm can be seen in Figure 4.10 which shows the results in axial, coronal and sagittal directions, respectively.

Pros and Cons of Lorigo *et al.*'s Technique: The major advantages of this technique were: first, the method successfully demonstrated the segmentation of vessels of the brain. Second, the method used the directional component in the level set framework, which was necessary for segmenting twisted, convoluted and occluded vessels. Third, the technique was used to compute vessel radii, a clinically useful measurement. The weaknesses of Lorigo *et al.*'s work were: first, not much discussion was available on the computation of the scale factor S. Second, the method did not show the analytical model, since the output of the system showed relatively thinner vessels compared to maximum intensity projection (MIP). The MIP is a popular algorithm and an example can be seen by Suri *et al.* [97]. Third, there was no comparison made between segmented results and the ground truth hence, the system needed to be validated.

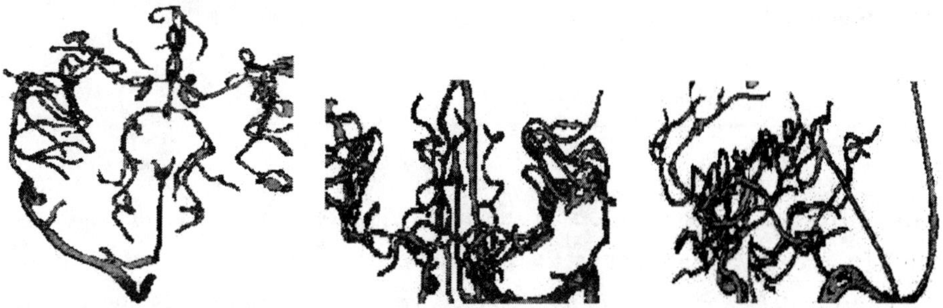

Figure 4.10: Segmentation results using Lorigo *et al.*'s technique [95], [96]. **Left**: Axial results. **Middle**: Coronal results. **Right**: Sagittal results (Courtesy of Professor Grimson, MIT, Cambridge, MA).

4.4.4 Segmentation Using Inverse Variational Criterion (Barlaud/CNRS)

Curve evolution as an inverse problem was first attempted by Santosa [102] and then by Barlaud and co-workers from CNRS (Center National Dela Recherche Scientifique, Cedex, France, see Amadieu *et al.* [101]). Here, segmentation method was developed using variational criterion of an inverse problem. The equation given by Barlaud and his co-workers was:

$$\frac{\partial \phi}{\partial t} + \alpha(x,t)\,||\nabla\phi|| = 0\,, \tag{4.35}$$

where $\frac{\partial \phi}{\partial t}$ was the rate of change of the level set function ϕ, $\alpha(x,t)$ was the rate at which the curve evolved, and $||\nabla\phi||$ was the gradient of ϕ. They applied this equation on images which consisted of binary objects represented as I_{in} and the image background as I_{out}, thus I was a *piecewise* constant function. If the image model was given as $g(x,y) = A(I(x,y)) + \eta$, where A was the operator over image I, η was the Gaussian perturbation, then the speed term $\alpha(x,t)$ was modeled as a function of discontinuities between regions and was expressed as the difference of the square of the background residual and foreground residual. This was mathematically expressed as: $\alpha(x,t) = [(AI_{out} - g(x,y))^2 - (AI_{in} - g(x,y))^2]$. They also added the length penalty ϵ to the curvature term κ. Thus, the complete PDE equation was:

$$\frac{\partial \phi}{\partial t}+[\underbrace{(A(I_{out}(x,y))-g(x,y))^2-(A(I_{in}(x,y))-g(x,y))^2}_{region}+\underbrace{\epsilon\kappa}_{curvature}\ ]\ ||\nabla\phi||=0\,. \tag{4.36}$$

Note here that the key factors in the PDE equation were the terms $I_{in}(x,y)$ and $I_{out}(x,y)$, which acted as the constants. Since the assumption was that $I_{in}(x,y)$ and $I_{out}(x,y)$ values were known from the binary objects and $g(x,y)$ was the observational pixel intensity, one could compute the discontinuity as the difference between $(A(I_{out}(x,y))-g(x,y))^2$ and $(A(I_{in}(x,y))-g(x,y))^2$. If the difference was zero, then the pixel was at the boundary.

Pros and Cons of Barlaud *et al.*'s Method: The technique was successfully presented to show the usage of regional term in PDE-framework which detected the boundary of the objects. The major weaknesses of this technique were: first, the paper did not present the application of the technique on gray scale images. One of the major drawbacks of this technique was the *a priori* information needed for the terms $I_{in}(x,y)$ and $I_{out}(x,y)$. Second, the model was too simple for complex gray scale medical imagery.

4.4.5 3-D Regional Geometric Surface: Fusion of the Level Set with Bayesian-Based Pixel Classification Regularizer (Barillot/IRISA)

Barillot and his co-workers (see Baillard *et al.* [104], [105] and [106]) recently designed the brain segmentation system based on the fusion of region into boundary/surface estimation. This algorithm was quite similar in approach to Suri *et al.*'s method discussed previously in sub-section 4.4.1. This algorithm was another instance where the propagation force V_0 in the fundamental level set segmentation equation $\frac{\partial \phi}{\partial t}=c(\mathbf{x})(\kappa+V_0)\ |\nabla\phi|$ was changed into a regional force. There were in all three changes made to this equation by Barillot and co-workers. The first change was in the propagation force V_0, the second was in the data consistency term or stopping term $c(\mathbf{x})$ and the third change was on the step size Δt. These equations and their interpretation will be briefly discussed next.

4.4.5.1 Design of the Propagation Force Based on the Probability Distribution

The key idea was to utilize the probability density function inside and outside the structure to be segmented. The pixel/voxel in the neighbourhood of the segmenting structure was responsible for creating a pull/push force on the propagating front. This was expressed in the form of the probability density function to be estimated inside the structure, $p_i(u)$, the probability density function to be estimated outside the structure, $p_e(u)$ and the prior probability for a voxel to be inside the structure. Note here, u was the intensity value of a voxel at location (x, y, z). Using the above concept, this bi-directional propagation force was estimated as:

$$V_0 = \mathbf{sgn}\{\alpha_i \, p_i(u) - (1 - \alpha_i) \, p_e(u)\}, \tag{4.37}$$

where $\mathbf{sgn}(x)$ was 1 if $x \geq 0$ and was -1 if $x < 0$. The second modification was to the data consistency term (also called stopping term) that changed from the gradient term into the extended gradient term. This term was changed from $c(\mathbf{x}) = \frac{1}{1+|\nabla[G_\sigma(\mathbf{x})*I(\mathbf{x})]|}$ to a term which was based on the transitional probability of going from inside to outside the object to be segmented. This was mathematically given as: $c(\mathbf{x}) = g[p_T(x|I, C)]$, where $g[x]$ was $1 - 4x^3$ if $x < 0.5$ and was $4(1 - x)^3$, if $x \geq 0.5$. The term p_T was computed based on these three parameters: α_i, $p_i(u)$ and $p_e(u)$, and mathematically estimated if the probability of a pixel/voxel class C belonged to a set inside and outside the object. If the class C was inside the region, then p_T was given as $\frac{(1-\alpha_i)\, p_e(I(x))}{\alpha_i\, p_i(I(x))+(1-\alpha_i)\, p_e(I(x))}$, while it was $\frac{(\alpha_i)\, p_i(I(x))}{\alpha_i\, p_i(I(x))+(1-\alpha_i)\, p_e(I(x))}$ if C was outside, derived from the simple Bayesian rule.

Pros and Cons of Baillard/Barillot's Technique: The major advantages of this technique were: (**1**) The paper provided an excellent example of the fusion of region-based information into the boundary/surface. (**2**) The results are very impressive; however, it would have been valuable to see an enlarged version of the results. (**3**) The algorithm was adaptive since the data consistency term ($c(\mathbf{x})$) and the step size (Δt) were adaptively estimated in every iteration of the front propagation. This provided a good trade-off between convergence speed and stability. (**4**) This method used stochastic-EM (SEM) instead of expectation-minimization (EM), which is a more robust and accurate method for estimation of probability density function parameters. (**5**) The method had successfully been successfully applied to various brain structures and to various imaging modalities such as ultrasound. (**6**) The algorithm hardly needed any tuning parameters and thus, it was very efficient. Both methods (Suri's and Baillard *et al.*'s) were designed to control the propagation force using region-based analysis. Suri *et al.*'s method used regional-force computed using pixel-classification based on fuzzy clustering, while Baillard *et al.*'s method uses pixel-classification based on Bayesian-statistics.

4.5 Segmentation in Motion Images Via PDE/Level Set Framework

Segmentation and tracking in motion imagery are very critical in several applications of computer vision. Here, we will discuss two different techniques of segmenting objects in an image sequence based on PDE and the level sets. In sub-section 4.5.1, we discuss a technique for segmenting objects in the motion sequence based on global motion compensation and robust frame differencing utilizing the PDE and level sets. Sub-section 4.5.2 presents object segmentation in the motion sequence using region competition based on PDE and level set framework.

4.5.1 Motion Segmentation Using Frame Difference Via PDE (Zhang/UW)

Recently, Zhang and his coworkers (see Zhang *et al.* [113], [114] and Gao [112]) proposed an object segmentation in motion imagery that consisted of: (**1**) fast global motion compensation; (**2**) robust frame differencing and (**3**) level set based curve evolution. The algorithm segments the objects in the temporal sequence with a moving background using the fast global motion estimation. The robust frame differencing method was adapted in order to detect motion in a sequence by calculating the 3-D structural tensor in the spatial-temporal domain. The curve evolution based on level set was used to segment the different moving objects.

4.5.1.1 Eigenvalue Based-PDE Formation for Segmentation in Motion Imagery

Zhang *et al.* 's [114] fast method of global motion estimation and compensation was in spirit of Zhang *et al.* 's [109] method. Zhang *et al.* 's method [114] was fast as it used only used hundreds of pixels rather than the whole frame for estimating the motion parameters for an affine model. In this sub-section, we present the mathematical formalism for eigenvalue computation given the image sequence. Motion compensation is out of the scope of this Chapter (for details on motion compensation, see Zhang *et al.* [114]).

The robust motion segmentation method based on frame differencing and level set based curve evolution was the key to success in Zhang *et al.* 's technique (see Zhang *et al.* [114]). The main idea in the frame differencing technique was to calculate the 3-D structural tensor in the spatial-temporal domain (see Jahne *et al.* [110]). For an image sequence $f(\mathbf{x},t)$, where $\mathbf{x} = \{x_1, x_2\}$, the 3-D structural tensor (a 3×3 matrix) was computed as the convolution of the product of gradient of f and its transpose by the Gaussian function h. This was mathematically given as:

$$\mathbf{R}(\mathbf{x},t) = \underbrace{\int h(\mathbf{x}-\mathbf{x}', t-t') \underbrace{\nabla f(\mathbf{x}',t')}_{3\times 1} \underbrace{\nabla f(\mathbf{x}',t')^T}_{1\times 3} \, d\mathbf{x}' \, dt'}_{convolution-operation} , \tag{4.38}$$

where $h(\mathbf{x},t)$ was a spatial-temporal Gaussian function and ∇ was the gradient operator and T represented the transpose operation. The eigenvector associated with the smallest eigenvalue of $\mathbf{R}(\mathbf{x},t)$ depicted the direction of motion for the pixel at $(\mathbf{x},t)$. This eigenvalue was denoted by $\lambda_3(\mathbf{x},t)$ (for details on the tensor calculation, see Jahne's book [130]). The discrete representation of Tensor Eq. (4.38) at location (x_1, x_2, t) was:

$$R(x_1,x_2,t) = h(x_1,x_2,t) \otimes \underbrace{R'(x_1,x_2,t)}_{3\times 3} , \tag{4.39}$$

where $\otimes$ was the convolution operator and $R'(x_1,x_2,t) = [f_{x_1} f_{x_2} f_t] \times [f_{x_1} f_{x_2} f_t]^T$, where f_{x_1}, f_{x_2} and f_t were the partial derivatives for sequence f in the spatial and temporal directions. $\lambda_3(x_1,x_2,t)$ was the smallest eigenvalue of $R(x_1,x_2,t)$. It was found that compared to the simple frame differencing, the eigen-based method was more robust to noise.

Zhang *et al.* 's algorithm used the curve evolution to segment out the moving objects based on the smallest eigenvalue of $\mathbf{R}(\mathbf{x},t)$, i.e., $\lambda_3(\mathbf{x},t)$. If $C = C(s)$, $s \in [0,1]$, was the closed curve, then the curve evolution equation amounts to evolving C over time $\mathbf{C}_t$ by using the following PDE:

$$\mathbf{C}_t = [g(\lambda_3)(V_0 + \kappa) - (\nabla g(\lambda_3) \cdot \vec{\mathbf{N}})]\vec{\mathbf{N}}\,, \tag{4.40}$$

where $g(v)$ was a monotonically decreasing function that approached zero when v was large, and was associated with the external force; V_0 was a constant that made the curve move inward or outward; κ was the curvature of the evolving curve, that made the curve smooth; ∇ was the gradient operator; and $\vec{\mathbf{N}}$ was the normal[7] to the curve. The first term in this speed function decreased to zero and stopped from evolving when the curve hit the motion boundaries. The second term, $(\nabla g(\lambda_3) \cdot \vec{\mathbf{N}})$, was used to track object boundaries.

4.5.1.2 The Eulerian Representation for Object Segmentation in Motion Imagery

Zhang and his co-workers (see Zhang *et al.* [114] and Gao [112]) implemented the curve evolution by embedding curve C in a surface $u(\mathbf{x};t)$. Specifically, at $t = 0$, the curve was the level set given by $\{\mathbf{x}|u(\mathbf{x};0) = 0\}$. The evolved curve was obtained from the level set $\{\mathbf{x}|u(\mathbf{x};T) = 0\}$, when the evolution of $u(\mathbf{x};t)$ stopped at $t = T$. The evolution equation for the surface $u(\mathbf{x};t)$ was derived from the PDE Eq. (4.40) as:

$$\frac{\partial u}{\partial t} = [\,g(\lambda_3)(V_0 + \kappa) - (\nabla g(\lambda_3) \cdot \frac{\nabla u}{|\nabla u|})\,]\,|\nabla u|\,. \tag{4.41}$$

The initial curve in this method was the largest possible curve, which contained all moving objects. As this initial curve evolved, it moved towards the moving objects. The initial surface, $u(\mathbf{x};0)$, which embedded the initial curve, was given by the minimum distance between the location $\mathbf{x}$ and the initial curve. This distance was assigned a negative sign if the location $\mathbf{x}$ was inside the curve. Zhang *et al.* 's method used the narrow-band approach, originally developed by Sethian [111].

Two examples were taken from Zhang *et al.* 's work (see Zhang *et al.* [114]) to show the representative results. In the first example (see Figure 4.11), a surveillance sequence that consisted of a moving car (known as the "moving

[7]The normal computation is the same as previously discussed in sub-section 4.4.1, however the symbols are different. Sometimes $\mathcal{N}$ is used instead of $\vec{\mathbf{N}}$.

car sequence") was taken as frame numbers 7, 8 and 9, as shown in Figure 4.11-(a, b and c). Note here, the movement of the car is towards the viewer. Figure 4.11-f shows the segmented result using Zhang *et al.*'s algorithm [114]. The image sequence contained low noise, clutter and had high object-background contrast. As a result, it was relatively easy to segment. In the second representative example (see Figure 4.12) of object segmentation in the moving "outdoor sequence", the goal was to detect the walking person near the bottom right in the scene. The frames used in this sequence were 601, 602 and 603, as shown in Figure 4.12-(a, b and c). This sequence contained the moving objects and random motions due to trees. Figure 4.12-f shows the segmented results from this "outdoor sequence" using Zhang *et al.*'s technique. As seen in this figure, the sequence was primarily hard to segment for two reasons: first, it had a lot of noise and second, there was random motion due to the trees. A simple technique such as frame difference had difficulty differentiating between these two types of motion. However, the tensor based frame-differencing embedded in PDE and the level set framework technique were effective in suppressing both the noise and the trees' random motion.

Zhang *et al.* [114] compared their technique with Paragios *et al.*'s [108] and Grimson *et al.*'s [107] approach. Paragios *et al.*'s [108] technique of curve evolution applied the frame difference images associated with an image sequence to achieve the segmentation. To enhance the frame difference images, a non-linear transform was used, which was motivated by statistical analysis in the boundary area. If the frame difference was large at a pixel position and not too large at some of its neighboring positions, then the pixel was considered as a point on a moving object boundary. This technique worked well when the noise level was low and the contrast was high. On the image sequence in Figure 4.11, Paragios *et al.*'s technique produced good results. However, when the noise level was high and the contrast was low, or when there was a random motion, Paragios *et al.*'s method did not perform well. This can be seen in Figure 4.12-d, where Paragios *et al.*'s technique produced several false moving objects in the scene.

The technique by Grimson *et al.* [107] used an adaptive background estimation method using simple frame differencing. Intuitively, this worked by dynamically maintaining estimating background images. Every pixel $f(x_1, x_2, t)$ in the current frame was compared to the pixel in the same position for the estimated background images. This set of background images was denoted by $\pi_i(x_1, x_2, t)$, where $i = 1...k$ and k was the total number of estimated background images. The pixel in location (x_1, x_2, t) was identified as a moving "object point", if it was not similar to all of the estimated background images $\pi_i(x_1, x_2, t)$. If the pixel was similar to one of the estimated background images, then the background image pixel $\pi_i(x_1, x_2, t)$ was updated by this current pixel location $f(x_1, x_2, t)$. To measure the similarities between the current pixel at (x_1, x_2, t) and the background image pixel $\pi_i(x_1, x_2, t)$, the probability $P(x_1, x_2, t|i)$ was computed based on the Gaussian assumption. As seen in Figures 4.11-e and 4.12-e, post-processing is usually needed to link such "object points" into connected meaning objects. The advantages of this technique were their simplicity and speed: each pixel in the background image was estimated by a first-order recursive filter in time. The disadvantage was that the background images estimated were not always accurate near object boundaries. Also, the objects estimated tended to be noisy since each pixel was processed independently from its neighbors. Readers interested in segmentation of color image sequences, the extension of Zhang *et al.*'s technique, can be found in Gao [112] and Zhang *et al.* [114].

Pros and Cons of Zhang *et al.*'s Technique: The following were the major advantages of Zhang *et al.*'s technique: **(1)** It was insensitive to noise and global motion. This was due to the combination of successfully using three techniques: global motion compensation, robust frame differencing and level set based curve evolution. **(2)** It produces all segmented moving objects simultaneously. **(3)** Due to the fast marching method of curve evolution and fast global motion compensation, the whole system was relatively fast. **(4)** It was simple and straightforward to compute the tensor and eigenvalues. The following were the major weaknesses of Zhang *et al.*'s technique: **(1)** If there were several motions with large varying speeds, this technique encountered a problem. Since the λ_3 had a large range of values, it was very difficult to set the parameters, such as constant V_0, and selection of g on the curve evolution equation, to segment out all of the moving objects in the same frame. **(2)** Furthermore, since this was a method based not only on motion, the boundary of segmentation was not exact on the boundary of motion. Having discussed the frame difference method for object segmentation, we will next present a different approach for object segmentation in motion imagery, based on region

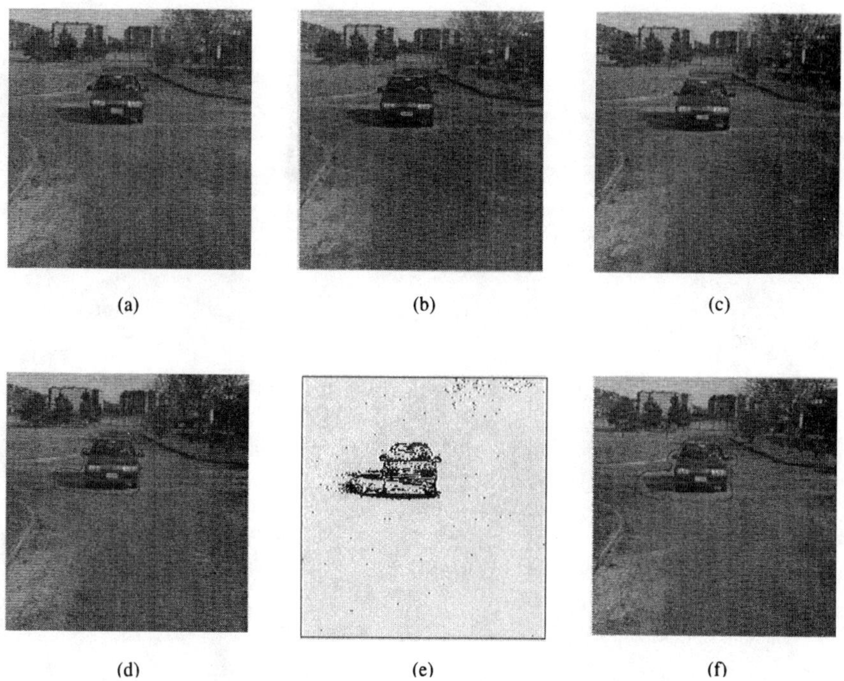

Figure 4.11: Segmentation results for the "moving car sequence". **Top Left**: Frame number 7. **Top Middle**: Frame number 8. **Top Right**: Frame number 9. **Bottom Left**: Result of the method of Paragios *et al.* [108]. **Bottom Middle**: Result of the method of Grimson *et al.* [107]. **Bottom Right**: Result of Zhang *et al.*'s [114] method (Reproduced with permission from IEEE). *(See color insert)*

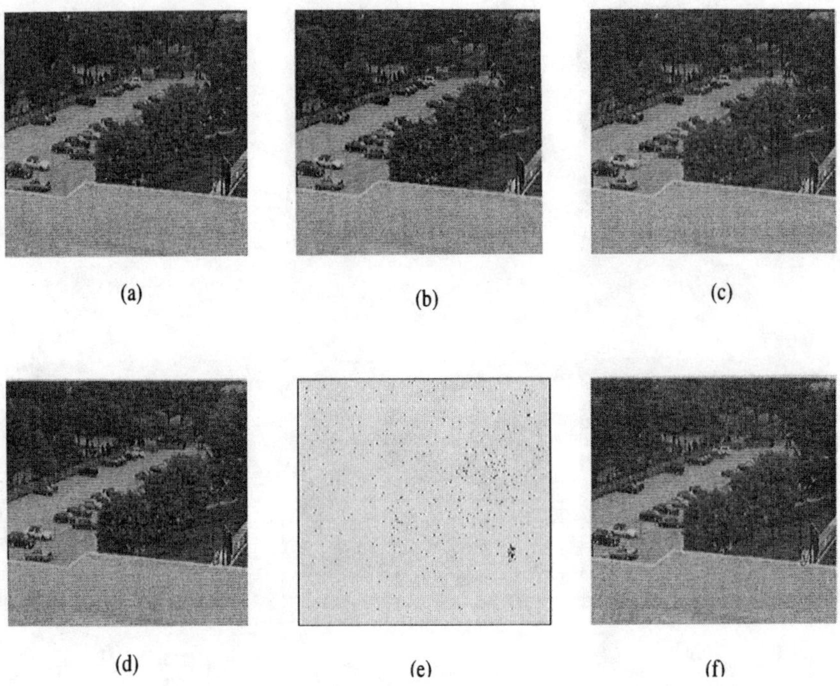

Figure 4.12: Segmentation of an "outdoor sequence". **Top Left**: Frame number 601. **Top Middle**: Frame number 602. **Top Right**: Frame number 603. **Bottom Left**: Result of the method of Paragios *et al.* [108]. **Bottom Middle**: Result of the method of Grimson *et al.* [107]. **Bottom Right**: Result of Zhang *et al.*'s [114] method (Reproduced with permission from IEEE). *(See color insert)*

competition.

4.5.2 Motion Segmentation Via PDE and Level Sets (Mansouri/INRS)

Mansouri *et al.* [116] recently demonstrated an algorithm for motion segmentation in image sequence, based on the region competition approach originally developed by Zhu and Yullie (see Zhu *et al.* [115]). The goal was to partition each frame of the sequence into regions of distinct motion. Although the results demonstrated by Mansouri *et al.* were illustrated using affine motion models, the proposed algorithm can accommodate any motion model. Motion segmentation was formulated in the two-motion case (moving object on a fixed or moving background) as a Bayesian estimation, and subsequently, energy minimization. The Euler-Lagrange descent equations corresponding to this energy minimization problem resulted in a curve evolution equation, which was then translated into the corresponding level set partial differential equation. Generalization to the multiple motion case (many moving objects) was done by analyzing the level set PDE in the two-motion case. Thus, this work was an excellent example of the fusion of regional information with the PDE and the level set framework. This research work had three characteristics: (**1**) The segmentation formulation used "region competition" in the PDE and the level set framework. (**2**) The motion segmentation algorithm was based purely on motion, unlike other techniques which also relied on intensity boundaries to refine motion boundaries. Nevertheless, the algorithm was extendable to have the capability of using intensity boundaries. (**3**) The motion segmentation algorithm could accommodate any motion model.

In the two-motion case, i.e., where there is a moving object on a fixed or moving background, PDE was as follows: If $\mathcal{C}$ represented the closed curve, then the flow of the curve, represented as the rate of change $\frac{d\mathcal{C}(s)}{dt}$ of $\mathcal{C}$ with time, was given by a partial differential equation consisting of three terms: regional energy, curvature energy and gradient energy. Thus the PDE equation was given as:

$$\frac{d\mathcal{C}(s)}{dt} = -[\underbrace{\mathcal{R}_o^2(\mathcal{C}(s)) - \mathcal{R}_b^2(\mathcal{C}(s))}_{regional-energy} + \underbrace{\lambda_L \, \kappa_{\mathcal{C}}(s)}_{curvature-energy} - \underbrace{\lambda_I \, (H_I \frac{\nabla I}{||\nabla I||})}_{gradient-energy}] \cdot \mathcal{N}(s)\,, \tag{4.42}$$

where H_I was the Hessian of the image function I, $\mathcal{N}$ was the outward-pointing unit normal to $\mathcal{C}$, $\mathcal{R}_o^2 - \mathcal{R}_b^2$ represented the regional velocity term. This term was the difference between the squared motion residuals which was given as: $\mathcal{R}_o^2 - \mathcal{R}_b^2$ was actually given in terms of $\mathcal{R}(\mathbf{T}_o, \mathbf{X})_o^2 - \mathcal{R}(\mathbf{T}_b, \mathbf{X})_b^2$, where $\mathbf{T}_o$ and $\mathbf{T}_b$ were the transformations for the object and background regions, respectively. $\mathbf{X}$ represented the point with coordinates (x, y). of the object ($\mathcal{R}_o^2$) and the background ($\mathcal{R}_b^2$). The curvature velocity was given by $\kappa_{\mathcal{C}}(s)$, pre-multiplied by λ_L, the smoothing constant. This curvature velocity of the closed contour followed directly from the prior on $\mathcal{C}$ which minimized curve length (as had been popular to do so). The last term was the velocity due to the image gradient and favored alignment of motion boundaries with intensity boundaries. This was given as $-H_I \frac{\nabla I}{||\nabla I||}$, pre-multiplied by the constant λ_I. The interpretation is as follows: **(1)** A boundary point $\mathcal{C}(s)$ undergoing the same motion as the object would satisfy $\mathcal{R}_o^2(\mathcal{C}(s)) \leq \mathcal{R}_b^2(\mathcal{C}(s))$, i.e., its motion residual will be smaller (in absolute value) for object motion than for background motion. Neglecting the contribution of curvature and intensity boundaries, this would induce a velocity vector $\frac{d\mathcal{C}(s)}{dt}$ in the direction of the outward normal $\mathcal{N}$, growing the curve $\mathcal{C}$ so as to englobe the point $\mathcal{C}(s)$. **(2)** If $\mathcal{C}(s)$ was a point undergoing the same motion as the background, then, neglecting the effect of curvature and intensity boundaries, $\frac{d\mathcal{C}(s)}{dt}$ would be oriented opposite to the normal $\mathcal{N}$, and curve $\mathcal{C}$ would shrink, relinquishing the point $\mathcal{C}(s)$. **(3)** The term $\kappa_{\mathcal{C}}(s)$ would tend to straighten out the curve, by pulling in convexities ($\kappa_{\mathcal{C}} > 0$), and pushing out concavities ($\kappa_{\mathcal{C}} < 0$). The Eulerian level set representation of Eq. (4.42) was given by:

$$\frac{\partial u}{\partial t}(\mathbf{X}) = -\underbrace{\underbrace{[\mathcal{R}_f^2(\mathbf{X}) - \mathcal{R}_{\mathbf{b}}^2(\mathbf{X})}_{regional-term} + \underbrace{\lambda_L \, \kappa_{\mathcal{C}}(\mathbf{X})}_{curvature-term} \; \underbrace{- \lambda_I \, (H_I \frac{\nabla I}{||\nabla I||})}_{gradient-term}]}_{\textbf{velocity}} \, ||\nabla \mathbf{u}|| \, . \tag{4.43}$$

Note that Eq. (4.43) can be compared to the standard equation by Sethian: $\frac{\partial u}{\partial t} = V(\kappa) \, || \, \nabla u \, ||$, where $V(\kappa)$ was the velocity with which the curve propagated in the direction of the gradient of the level set function u.

Figure 4.13 shows the result of motion segmentation using Mansouri *et al.* 's [116] algorithm on frames 30 and 40 of the "*ping-pong* sequence", using affine motion models with $\lambda_L = 2500$ and $\lambda_I = 0$. These motion models were computed prior to the segmentation, using point correspondences and clustering in affine parameter space (see Mansouri *et al.* [116] for details). A total of three distinct motion classes were found: The first, corresponding to the (still) background; the second, to the ball, having an upwards direction of motion; and finally, the third motion class was that of the hand and was a rotational motion around the elbow in the counter-clockwise direction. The top-left and top-right pictures show frames 30 and 40 of "*ping-pong* sequence", respectively. In the middle-left picture, the initial zero level set curves are shown. The final segmentation is shown in the remaining pictures. In each of them, for ease of viewing, the region segmented is shown without alteration, while the remaining regions have been dimmed. The middle-right picture shows the background region; note that in addition to the ball and the hand, the occlusion regions have also been excluded from the background. The bottom-left picture shows the ball region, and finally, the bottom-right picture shows the hand region. Note that all these regions have been very precisely estimated, despite the fact that no use was made of intensity boundaries in this segmentation.

Pros and Cons of Region Competition in PDE/Level Set Framework for Segmentation in Motion Imagery: The major advantages of this technique were as follows: (**1**) Although Mansouri *et al.*'s [116] algorithm has the capability to rely on intensity boundaries to guide the motion segmentation, it did not need to. Indeed, the vast majority of their results have been obtained through segmentation based on motion alone, which demonstrated that very accurate motion segmentation can be obtained, even where intensity boundaries were hardly visible. (**2**) The algorithm can be combined with any motion detection algorithm. All that was needed for this to work successfully was the number of distinct motion classes and their parameters. (**3**) Initial conditions for the proposed level set PDE were quite arbitrary, and the initial level set functions need not be in the vicinity of the solution. The major weakness of Mansouri *et al.*'s algorithm was the computational burden of the algorithm grew linearly with the number of motion classes. Thus, the larger the number of distinct motion classes, the slower the resulting segmentation. Recently, Aubert and his co-workers (see Besson *et al.* [103]) also developed a segmentation and tracking method for the motion sequence based on the scheme presented in sub-section 4.4.4. Interested readers can explore this method further.

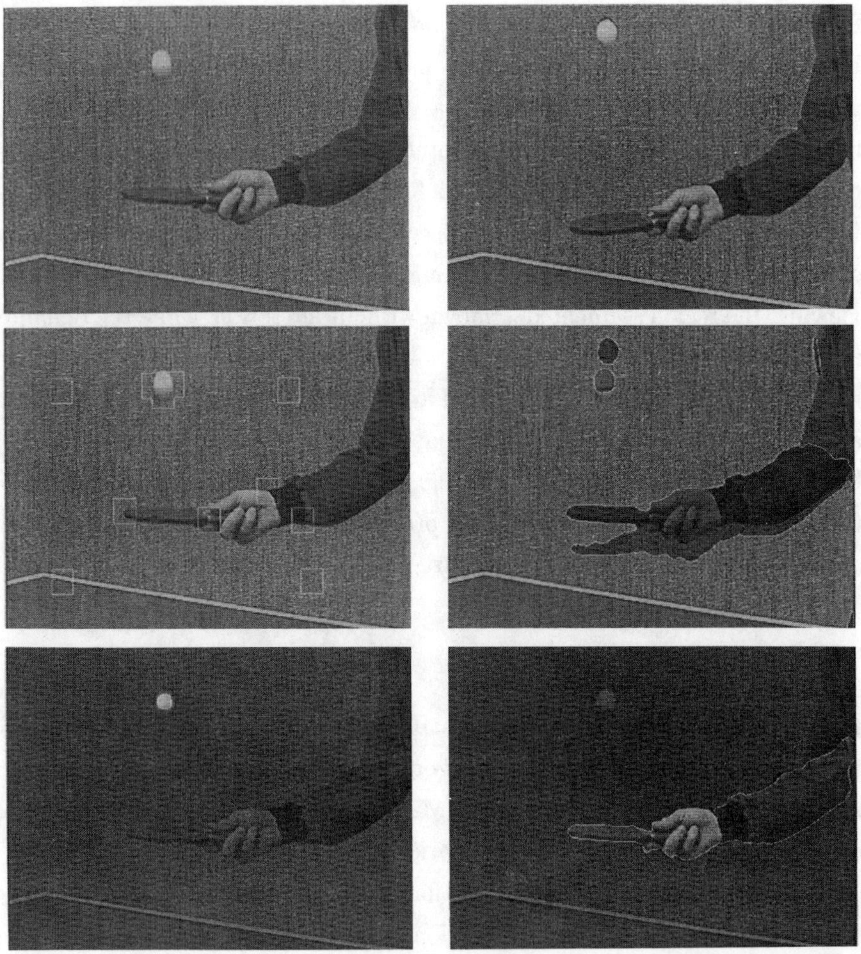

Figure 4.13: Segmentation results of the "*ping-pong* sequence" using PDE implemented in the level set framework. **Top Left**: Frame 30 of the "*ping-pong* sequence". **Top Right**: Frame 40 of the "*ping-pong* sequence". **Middle Left**: Initial segmentation: Three squares are associated with one region and there are three regions: background, ball and hand. Each of these square boundaries is the zero level set function corresponding to the respective regions. **Middle Right**: Final segmentation of the background. **Bottom Left**: Final segmentation of the ball. **Bottom Right**: Final segmentation of the hand (Courtesy of Abdol-Reza Mansouri, INRS Telecommunications, Montreal, Quebec, Canada). *(See color insert)*

4.6 Miscellaneous Applications of PDEs in Image Processing

This section presents additional applications of PDE-based approaches. In sub-section 4.6.1, we discuss the PDE-based approach for filling missing information. Sub-section 4.6.2 presents the mathematical morphology implementation using the PDE-based approach. Sub-section 4.6.3 presents the low pass filtering operation.

4.6.1 PDE for Filling Missing Information for Shape Recovery Using Mean Curvature Flow of a Graph

Sarti *et al.* [126] recently fused the local and global information in PDE/level set framework to estimate the missing edge information. If c was the edge extractor or edge indicator function, ϕ the level set function, then the flow equation derived by Sarti *et al.* was as under: If $S : (x, y) \to (x, y, \phi)$ was defined in the same domain M of the image I, then the differential area of the graph S in the Euclidean space was given as $dA_E = \sqrt{1 + \phi_x^2 + \phi_y^2}\, dx\, dy$. Applying the edge indicator function or data consistency term, $c(x, y)$ to this and then computing the area A_c under the surface was given as:

$$A_c = \int_M c(x, y) \sqrt{1 + \phi_x^2 + \phi_y^2} dx\, dy, \qquad (4.44)$$

where M was the domain. Note, this comes about from the *mean curvature flow* which was the steepest descent of the *area functional.* This equation was minimized using the steepest descent by applying multivariate calculus to obtain the flow equation as:

$$\frac{\partial \phi}{\partial t} = c(x, y) \frac{(1 + \phi_x^2)\, \phi_{yy} - 2\phi_x\, \phi_y\, \phi_{xy} + (1 + \phi_y^2)\, \phi_{xx}}{1 + \phi_x^2 + \phi_y^2} + (c_x \phi_x + c_y \phi_y)\, , \qquad (4.45)$$

where c_x and c_y are the edges in the x and y directions, respectively. Figure 4.14 shows the results of running the above algorithm. Other work of Sarti in the area of level sets can also be explored (see Sarti *et al.* [127], [128], [129]).

Pros and Cons of Sarti *et al.*'s Method (**1**) Sarti *et al.*'s method did not compute the flow of the surface using the *geometry of the levels*, but it did compute the flow depending upon the *geometry of the surface itself.* (**2**) The above equation was the *weighted mean curvature flow of a graph*, while Sarti *et al.*'s work [85] was the *level set flow* on a 3-D volume.

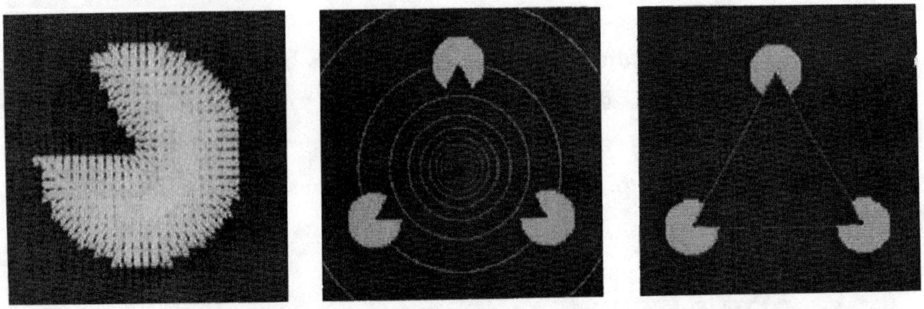

Figure 4.14: Filling missing information for shape recovery. **Left**: Kanizsa Triangle initial image. **Middle**: Evolution process. **Right**: Final triangle boundary with missing information completed (Courtesy of A. Sarti, Mathematics Department, LBNL, University of California, Berkeley and DEIS, University of Bologna, Italy).

4.6.2 Mathematical Morphology Via PDE

The mathematical morphology field has been used for shape analysis and shape quantification for some time (see Sapiro *et al.* [65], Arehart *et al.* [66], Catte *et al.* [67] and Sochen *et al.* [68]). It was in the early 1990's when the role of level sets started to move into mathematical morphology. Here, we will just show the dilation transformation modeling. Let some shape $\mathcal{C}(s,t)$ evolved by a mathematical morphology operation (say, dilation), by some structuring element $\mathcal{B}(\lambda)$ of size λ, to a new shape $\mathcal{C}(s,t+\lambda)$. This evolution was represented as $\mathcal{C}(s,t+\lambda)$-$\mathcal{C}(s,t) = \Gamma(s,t,\lambda)\mathcal{N}(s,t)$, where Γ was the distance along $\mathcal{N}$ that a point on the boundary moved in a dilation operation with a structuring element of size λ. Since $\Gamma(s,t,0)$=0:

$$\frac{\partial \mathcal{C}}{\partial t} = lim_{\lambda\to 0}\frac{\Gamma(s,t,\lambda)-\Gamma(s,t,0)}{\lambda}\mathcal{N}. \tag{4.46}$$

The above equation was written as:

$$\frac{\partial \mathcal{C}}{\partial t} = \frac{\Gamma(s,t,\lambda)}{\partial\lambda}\mathcal{N}. \tag{4.47}$$

The above equation was simply $\beta(s,t)\mathcal{N}$, where β was the differential deformation of a shape $\mathcal{S}$ at a point P due to the dilation with a convex structuring element. This was also the maximal projection of the structuring element onto the normal $\mathcal{N}$ of the boundary at P. Note that β depended on the orientation of the target to the tangent shape $\mathcal{T}(s,t)$. This led to the evolution of the equation as:

$$\begin{cases} \frac{\partial \mathcal{C}}{\partial t} & = & \beta(\mathcal{T}(s,t))\mathcal{N} \\ \mathcal{C}(s,0) & = & \mathcal{C}_0(s) \, . \end{cases} \tag{4.48}$$

We can similarly model the erosion process (for details, see Sochen *et al.* [68]).

4.6.2.1 Erosion with a Straight Line Via PDE

If I was the original image, then the erosion of image I with the straight line segment was given as:

$$I_e = |\hat{n}.\nabla I| \, , \tag{4.49}$$

where $\hat{n}$ was the vector representing the direction vector $(cos(\theta)\, sin(\theta))$ and θ was the angle between the given line segment and the x-axis. The above equation was written as:

$$I_e = ||\hat{n}|| \; ||\nabla I|| \; cos(\alpha) \, , \tag{4.50}$$

where α was the angle between $\hat{n}$ and ∇I. Since $||\nabla I||$ was computed in the level set bed as it was a PDE, thus the morphologic erosion was solved via PDE. Note, here α was computed by taking the inverse of the tangent of the ratio of the y and x components and then subtracted by θ.

4.6.3 PDE in the Frequency Domain: A Low Pass Filter

Banks [117] showed the interpretation of the finite difference method (FDM) for the PDE as a low pass filter (LPF). This was shown using the frequency domain analysis. We will discuss this key derivation of PDE as a LPF using the Fast Fourier Transform (FFT) method (for details, see Bloor *et al.* [118] and Brown *et al.* [119]). The ability to model the fitting problem into a PDE using the Euler-Lagrange method and then applying the finite difference method (FDM) to solve the PDE was one of the key characteristics of the PDE-based methods. The smoothing problem was posed as a surface fitting problem or minimization of the surface ϕ to the data points, say P_k. This was posed as a Least Squares problem where they minimized the function I as under:

$$I = \alpha \underbrace{\sum_{k=1}^{N_p} [\phi(u_k, v_k) - P_k]^2}_{closeness} + \beta \int_{v_1}^{v_n+1} \int_{u_1}^{u_n+1} \underbrace{||\frac{\partial^n \phi(u,v)}{\partial u^n}||^2 + ||\frac{\partial^n \phi(u,v)}{\partial v^n}||^2 \, du\, dv}_{smoothness} , \tag{4.51}$$

where α, β are the smoothing constants. n was the degree of the surface and $\frac{\partial^n \phi(u,v)}{\partial u^n}$ was the nth derivative of the surface ϕ with respect to the variable u and $\frac{\partial^n \phi(u,v)}{\partial v^n}$ was the nth derivative of the surface ϕ with respect to the variable v. N_p was the total limit. Note, the surface fitting consisted of two terms: an error or closeness term which reduced the fitting error between the data points and the surface passing through them, and the second term was the smoothness term reducing the variations of the surface. Note the smoothness term was also the curvature reduction term. The second term was the smoothness term and we will focus on that. The second term can be expressed as a function of the derivatives of u and v. Taking the simplest case n=1, the smoothing function (given as L) was given as: $L = \phi_u^2 + \phi_v^2$. The Euler-Lagrange Eq. is thus given as: $\frac{\partial^2 \phi}{\partial u^2} + \frac{\partial^2 \phi}{\partial v^2}$=0, and we know the finite difference solution of this PDE. Now to show the PDE to be a LPF, imagine a continuous surface $f(u)$ being sampled at N intervals on a regularly spaced grids $u = ih$, where $i = 0, ...(N-1)$. By taking the Fourier Transform of the sampled signal f_n with frequency k, this is given as:

$$\hat{f}_k = \sum_{n=0}^{N-1} f_n \, exp(\frac{-2\pi \, i \, n \, k}{N}) \, . \tag{4.52}$$

If $\phi_{i,j}$ was the discrete function and we sample it into M points in two directions u and v, then the discrete Fourier Transform of $\phi_{m,n}$ was given as:

$$\hat{\phi}_{k,l} = \sum_{n=0}^{N-1} \sum_{m=0}^{M-1} \phi_{m,n} \, exp(-2\pi i [\frac{mk}{M} + \frac{nl}{N}]) \, . \tag{4.53}$$

We know that using the finite difference method, the value of the Euler-Lagrange Eq. was given as:

$$[\phi_{i+1,j} - 2\phi_{i,j} + \phi_{i-1,j} + \phi_{i,j+1} - 2\phi_{i,j} + \phi_{i,j-1}] - \lambda \phi_{i,j} = -\lambda P_{i,j} \, . \tag{4.54}$$

Substituting $\phi_{m,n}$ into the above equation and equating the coefficients of the (k,l) frequency mode, we get:

$$\hat{\phi}_{k,l} \, \frac{-\lambda \, \hat{P}_{k,l}}{[sin^2(\frac{\pi k}{M}) + sin^2(\frac{\pi l}{N}) + \frac{\lambda}{4}]} \, . \tag{4.55}$$

Eq. (4.54) can be interpreted as an input-output with a transfer function $\frac{-\lambda \hat{P}_{k,l}}{[sin^2(\frac{\pi k}{M})+sin^2(\frac{\pi l}{N})+\frac{\lambda}{4}]}$. The output $\hat{\phi}_{k,l}$ was being smoothed in the sense that the amplitudes of the high frequency modes have been reduced with respect to low frequency, which is simply the LPF.

4.7 Advantages, Disadvantages, Conclusions and the Future of 2-D and 3-D PDE-Based Methods in Medical and Non-Medical Applications

This section is divided into the following parts: Sub-section 4.7.1 presents a general purpose PDE/level set framework where most of the image segmentation issues fit in. Sub-section 4.7.2 presents an example demonstrating the segmentation application using PDE and the level set framework. Sub-section 4.7.3 discusses the advantages of PDE in conjunction with level sets. Sub-section 4.7.4 presents the disadvantages of the PDE in the level set framework. Finally, sub-section 4.7.5 presents a discussion on the conclusions and the future for PDE and level set based approaches.

4.7.1 PDE Framework for Image Processing: Implementation

Figure 4.15 shows a general purpose PDE and level set based image processing segmentation system, where given the data set and the raw contour, one can model the segmentation by primarily computing the regional statistics term (called statistical modeling), gradient term and curvature analysis of the moving contour. An example of such an implementation can be seen by Suri *et al.* [3], [4], [5] and [6]. They are all fused into one model and the segmentation problem can be solved as an energy minimization problem. This was used to frame the PDE equation which was solved in the level set framework to estimate the converged boundary. Thus, the PDE and level set framework have the following abilities: first, to transform a segmentation modeling problem into a partial differential equation and to embed the regularizers into these models; second, solving these partial differential equations using the finite difference methods; third, linkage between the partial differential equations and the level set framework for implementing the finite difference methods; and fourth, the ability to extend the PDE framework from 2-D to 3-D or higher dimensions. Having presented the abstract framework, we will next present a segmentation example using a finite difference method and then summarize the advantages/disadvantages of the PDE and the level set based segmentation modeling issue in sub-sections 4.7.3 and 4.7.4.

4.7.2 A Segmentation Example Using a Finite Difference Method

Here, speed control functions and their integration in terms of the level set function ϕ to estimate the ϕ over time are presented (for details, see Suri [1] and [3]). The time step restrictions for solving the partial differential equation will not be discussed here (the reader can refer to the work by Osher and Sethian [47] and the recent work by Barillot and his co-workers [104]). Using the finite difference method (see also Sethian [88]), the level set Eq. (4.27) was given in terms of time n as (for details, see Suri [2] and [3]):

$$\phi_{x,y}^{n+1} = \phi_{x,y}^{n} - \Delta t \, \{ \, V_{reg}(x,y) + V_{grad}(x,y) - V_{cur}(x,y) \, \}, \tag{4.56}$$

where $\phi_{x,y}^{n}$ and $\phi_{x,y}^{n+1}$ were level set functions at pixel location (x, y) at times n and $n+1$, Δt was the time difference, and $V_{reg}(x,y)$, $V_{grad}(x,y)$ and $V_{cur}(x,y)$ were the regional, gradient and curvature speed terms, respectively. Now, these terms are presented as follows: First, the regional speed term expressed in terms of the level set function (ϕ) was given as: $V_{reg}(x,y) = \mathbf{max}(V_p(x,y),0)\ \nabla^+ + \mathbf{min}(V_p(x,y),0)\ \nabla^-$, where terms $V_p(x,y)$, ∇^+ and ∇^- were given as: $V_p(x,y) = \frac{w_R}{\gamma\, R_{ind}(x,y)}$, $R_{ind} = 1 - 2\,u(x,y)$, $\nabla^- = [\nabla_x^- + \nabla_y^-]^{\frac{1}{2}}$ and $\nabla^+ = [\nabla_x^+ + \nabla_y^+]^{\frac{1}{2}}$.

$$\begin{cases} \nabla_x^+ & = & [\mathbf{max}(D^{-x}(x,y),0))^2 + \mathbf{min}(D^{+x}(x,y),0))^2] \\ \nabla_y^- & = & [\mathbf{max}(D^{-y}(x,y),0))^2 + \mathbf{min}(D^{+y}(x,y),0))^2], \end{cases} \tag{4.57}$$

where $u(x,y)$ took a value between 0 and 1. This could be coming from, say, a fuzzy membership function or any other clustering technique. R_{ind} was the region indicator function that was in the range between -1 to +1. Second, the gradient speed term, called the edge strength of the object boundaries, was expressed in terms of the level set function (ϕ) as the x and y components of

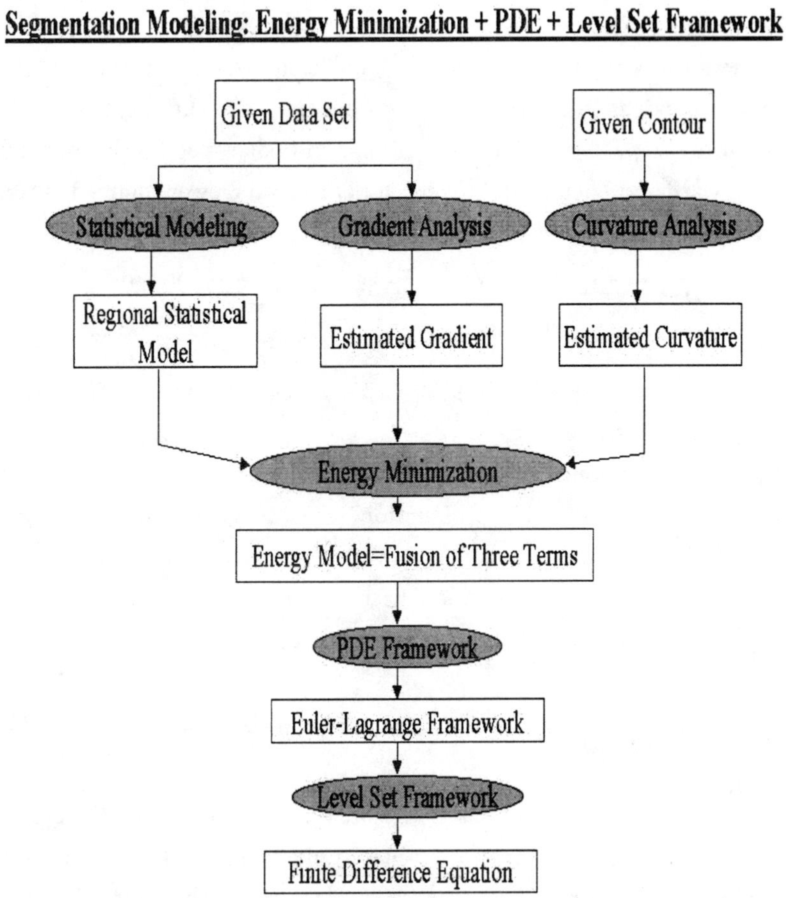

Figure 4.15: The generic level set framework consists of three stages: (i) energy minimization; (ii) PDE formation and (iii) implementation in the level set framework. The input to the energy minimization algorithm consists of three terms: (a) design of the regularizer or statistical modeling; (b) gradient estimation technique and (c) the curvature analysis.

the gradient speed as: $V_{grad}(x,y) = V_{gradx}(x,y) + V_{grady}(x,y)$, where:

$$\begin{cases} V_{gradx}(x,y) &= \mathbf{max}(p^n(x,y),0)\ D^{-x}(x,y) + \mathbf{min}(q^n(x,y),0)\ D^{+x}(x,y) \\ V_{grady}(x,y) &= \mathbf{max}(q^n(x,y),0)\ D^{-y}(x,y) + \mathbf{min}(q^n(x,y),0)\ D^{+y}(x,y) \\ p^n(x,y) &= \nabla_x(w_e\ \nabla(G_\sigma * I))\ \&\ q^n(x,y) = \nabla_y(w_e\ \nabla(G_\sigma * I)), \end{cases} \tag{4.58}$$

where w_e was the weight of the edge and was also a fixed constant. $p^n(x,y)$ and $q^n(x,y)$ were defined as the x and y components of the gradient strength at a pixel location (x,y). Note that the regional and edge speed terms depended upon the forward and backward difference operator which were defined in terms of the level set function ϕ, defined as:

$$\begin{cases} D^{-x}(x,y) = \frac{(\phi(x,y)-\phi(x-1,y))}{\triangle x} & \&\ \ D^{+x}(x,y) = \frac{(\phi(x+1,y)-\phi(x,y))}{\triangle x} \\ D^{-y}(x,y) = \frac{(\phi(x,y)-\phi(x,y-1))}{\triangle y} & \&\ \ D^{+y}(x,y) = \frac{(\phi(x,y+1)-\phi(x,y))}{\triangle y}, \end{cases} \tag{4.59}$$

where $\phi(x,y)$, $\phi(x-1,y)$, $\phi(x+1,y)$, $\phi(x,y-1)$, $\phi(x,y+1)$ were the level set functions at pixel locations (x,y), $(x-1,y)$, $(x+1,y)$, $(x,y-1)$, $(x,y+1)$, being the four neighbours of (x,y). Third, the curvature speed term expressed in terms of the level set function (ϕ) was given as: $V_{cur}(x,y) = \epsilon\,\kappa^n(x,y)\,[\,(D^{0x}(x,y))^2 + ((\,D^{0y}(x,y))^2\,]^{\frac{1}{2}}$, where ϵ was a fixed constant, $\kappa^n(x,y)$ was the curvature at a pixel location (x,y) at n^{th} iteration as: $\kappa^n(x,y) = \frac{\phi_{xx}^2\,\phi_y^2 - \phi_x^2\,\phi_y^2\,\phi_{xy}^2 + \phi_{yy}^2\,\phi_x^2}{(\phi_x^2+\phi_y^2)^{\frac{3}{2}}}$ and $D^{0x}(x,y)$ and $D^{0y}(x,y)$ were defined as:

$$D^{0x}(x,y) = \frac{(\phi(x+1,y)-\phi(x-1,y))}{2\,\triangle x}\ \ \&\ \ D^{0y}(x,y) = \frac{(\phi(x,y+1)-\phi(x,y-1))}{2\,\triangle y}. \tag{4.60}$$

Thus, to numerically solve Eq. (4.56), all that was needed was: (i) the gradient speed values (p,q), (ii) the curvature speed κ at pixel location (x,y) and (iii) the membership function $u(x,y)$ for a particular class K. In the next sub-section, we will discuss the advantages of PDE in the level set framework.

4.7.3 Advantages of PDE in the Level Set Framework

The PDE based method in the level set framework offers a large number of advantages. Since the number of advantages is large, we will present them in a list format as follows: **(1)** *Capture Range*: The greatest advantage of this technique is that this algorithm increases the capture range of the "field flow", which increases the robustness of the initial contour placement. **(2)** *Effect of Local Noise*: When the regional information is integrated into the system, then the local noise or edge does not distract the growth process. This technique is non-local and thus the local noise cannot distract the final placement of the contour or the diffusion growth process. (**3**) *No Need of Elasticity Coefficients*: These techniques are not controlled by the elasticity coefficients, unlike the classical parametric contour methods. There is no need to fit the tangents to the curves and compute the normals at each vertex. In this system, the normals are embedded in the system using the divergence of the field flow. These methods have the ability to model the incremental deformations in the shape. (**4**) *Suitability for Medical Image Segmentation*: These techniques are very suitable for medical organ segmentation since they can handle any of the cavities, concavities, convolutedness, splitting or merging. (**5**) *Finding the Local and Global Minima*: There is no problem finding the local minima or global minima issues, unlike the optimization techniques of parametric snakes. (**6**) *Normal Computation*: These techniques are less prone to the normal computational error which is very easily incorporated in the "classical balloon force" snakes for segmentation. (**7**) *Automaticity*: It is very easy to extend this model from semi-automatic to completely automatic because the region is determined on the basis of prior information. (**8**) *Integration of Regional Statistics*: These techniques are based on the propagation of curves (just like the propagation of ripples in the tank or propagation of the fire flames) utilizing the region statistics. (**9**) *Flexible Topology*: These techniques adjust to the topological changes of the given shape such as joining and breaking of the curves. (**10**) *Wide Applications*: This technique can be applied to unimodal, bimodal and multimodal imagery, which means it can have multiple gray scale values in it. These PDE/level set based methods have a wide range of applications in 3-D surface modeling. (**11**) *Speed of the System*: These technique can be implemented using the fast marching methods in the narrow band and thus can be easily optimized. (**12**) *Extension*: This technique is an easy extension from 2-D to 3-D. (**13**) *Incorporation of Regularizing Terms*: This can easily incorporate other features for controlling the speed of the curve. This is done by adding an extra term to the region, gradient and curvature speed terms. (**14**) *Handling Corners*: The system takes care of the corners easily unlike the classical parametric curves, where it needs special handling at the corners of the boundary. (**15**) *Resolution Changes*: This technique is extendable to multi-scale resolutions, which means that at lower resolutions, one can compute regional segmentations. These segmented results can then be used for higher resolutions. (**16**) *Multi-phase Processing*: These techniques are extendable to multi-phase, which means that if there are multiple level set functions, then they automatically merge and split during the course of the segmentation process. (**17**) *Surface Tracking*: Tracking surfaces are implemented using level sets very smoothly. (**18**) *Quantification of 3-D Structures*: Geometrical computations can be done in a natural way, for example, one can compute the curvature of 3-D surfaces directly while performing normal computations. (**19**) *Integration of Regularization Terms*: Allows easy integration of vision models for shape recovery such as fuzzy clustering, Gibbs model, Markov Random Fields and Bayesian models (see Paragios *et al.* [62]). This makes the system very powerful, robust and accurate for medical shape recovery. One can segment any part of the brain depending upon the membership function of the brain image. So, depending upon the number of classes estimated, one can segment any shape in 2-D or 3-D. (**20**) *Concise Descriptions*: One can give concise descriptions of differential structures using level set methods. This is because of the background mesh resolution controls. (**21**) *Hierarchical Representations*: The level set offers a natural scale space for hierarchical representations. (**22**) *Reparameterization*: There is no need for reparameterization for curve/surface estimation during the propagation, unlike in the classical snakes model. (**23**) *Modeling in a Continuous Domain*: One can model the segmentation process in a continuous domain using PDEs. Thus the formalism process is greatly simplified which is grid independent and isotropic. (**24**) *Stability Issues*: With the help of research in numerical analysis, one can achieve highly stable segmentation algorithms using PDEs. (**25**) *Existence and Uniqueness*: Using PDEs, one can derive not only successful algorithms but also useful theoretical results, such as existence and uniqueness of solutions (see Alvarez *et al.* [22]).

4.7.4 Disadvantages of PDE in Level Sets

Even though level sets have dominated several fields of imaging science, these front propagation algorithms have certain drawbacks. They are as follows: (**1**) *Convergence Issue:* Although the edges will not be blurry when one performs the diffusion imaging, the issue of convergence always remains a challenge. In diffusion imaging, if the step size used is small, then it takes longer to converge. (**2**) *Design of the Constant Force:* The design of the constant force in the PDE is another challenge yet to be overcome. This involves computation of regional statistics in the region of the moving contour. There is a trade-off between the robustness of the regional design, computational time for the operation and the accuracy of the segmentation. The design of the model plays a critical role in segmentation accuracy and remains as a challenge. Another challenge occurs if the design force is internal or external (for details, see Suri *et al.* [6]). (**3**) *Stability Issues:* The stability issues in PDEs are also important during the front propagation. The ratio of $\frac{\triangle t}{\triangle x}$, called the CFL number (Courant number, named after the author Courant *et al.* [135]), is another factor which needs to be carefully designed. (**4**) *Initial Placement of the Contour:* One of the major drawbacks of the parametric active contours has been its initial placement. This does not have either enough capture range or enough power to grab the topology of the shapes. Both of these drawbacks are removed by level sets provided the initial contour has been placed symmetrically with respect to the boundaries of interest. This ensures that the level sets reach object boundaries almost at the same time. On the contrary, if the initial contour is much closer to the first portion of the object boundary compared to the second portion, then the evolving contour crosses over the first portion of the object boundary. This is because the stop function does not turn out to be zero. One of the controlling factors for the stop function is the gradient of the image. The relationship of the stop function to the gradient is its inverse and also depends upon the index power m in the ratio $\frac{1}{1+|\nabla G_\sigma * I(x,y)|^m}$. For stopping the propagation, the denominator needs to be large, which means the image forces due to the gradient need to be high. This means index m needs to be high. In other words, if m is high, then the gradient is high, which means the weak boundaries are not detected well and will be easily crossed over by the evolving curve. If m is low (low threshold), then the level set will stop at noisy or at isolated edges. (**5**) *Embedding of the Object:* If some objects (say, the inner objects) are embedded in another object (the outer object), then the level set will not capture all the objects of interest. This is especially true if the embedded objects are asymmetrically situated. Under such conditions, one needs multiple initializations of the active contours. This means there can be only one active contour per object. (**6**) *Gaps in the Object Boundaries:* This is one of the serious drawbacks of the level set method and has been pointed out by Siddiqi *et al.* [76]. Due to the gaps in the object, the evolving contour simply leaks through the gaps. As a result, the objects represented by incomplete contours are not captured correctly and fully. This is especially prominent in realistic images, such as in ultrasound and in multi-class MR and CT images. (**7**) *Problems Due to Shocks:* Shocks are among the most common problems in level sets. Kimia and co-workers in [123], [124], [125] developed such a framework by representing shape as the set of singularities (called shocks) that arise in a rich space of shape deformations as classified into the following four types: (i) first-order shocks are orientation discontinuities (corners) and arise from protrusions and indentations; (ii) second-order shocks are formed when a shape breaks into two parts during a deformation; (iii) third-order shocks represent bends; and (iv) fourth-order shocks are the seeds for each component of a shape. These shocks arise in level sets and can sometimes cause serious problems. (**8**) *Challenge in Segmentation:* Although the level set segmentation method succeeds in the object and motion segmentation, it has weakness in segmenting many other kinds of images. This can occur in images that do not have a homogeneous background; for example, when images are composed of many different regions, such as in natural scenery images (containing streets, mountains, trees, cars and people). The method based on curve evolution will not produce the correct regions as desired. Such a segmentation problem is a challenge yet to be overcome.

4.7.5 Conclusions and the Future in PDE-based Methods

The class of differential geometry, also called PDE in conjunction with level sets, has been shown to dominate image processing, in particular to medical imaging, in a major way. We still need to understand how the regularization terms can be integrated into the level sets to improve segmentation schemes. Even though the application of level sets has gone well in the fields of medical imaging, biomedicine, fluid mechanics, combustion, solidification, CAD/CAM, object tracking/image sequence analysis and device fabrication, we are still far away from achieving stable 3-D volumes and a standard segmentation in real-time. By standard, we mean that which can segment the 3-D volume with a wide variation in pulse sequence parameters (see Suri [136]). We will likely see in the near future the modeling of front propagation that takes into account the physical constraints of the problem, for example, minimization of variation geodesic distances, rather than simple distance transforms. We will likely also see more incorporation of likelihood functions and adaptive fuzzy models to prevent leaking of the curves/surfaces. A good example of integration of the low level processes into the evolution process could be given as: $\frac{\partial \phi}{\partial t} = L(x, y)\,(\beta_0 - \beta_1 \kappa)\,|\nabla\,\phi|$, where $L(x, y) = 1 - max(S_1, S_2, S_i, ..., S_n)$, where S_i is the low level process from edge detection, optical flow, stereo disparity, texture, etc. The better the $S_i(x, y)$, the more robust could be the level set segmentation process. We also hope to see more papers on level sets where the segmentation step does require a re-initialization stage (see Zhao *et al.* [121] and Evans *et al.* [122]). It would also, however, be helpful if we can incorporate a faster triangulation algorithm for isosurface extraction in 3-D segmentation methods.

We also see a massive effort by the computer vision community to integrate regularization terms to improve the robustness and accuracy of the 3-D segmentation techniques. In this Chapter, we have shown the role of PDE and level set method for image smoothing or image diffusion or image denoising. Also shown was how curve/surface propagation hypersurfaces based on differential geometry are used for the segmentation of objects in still imagery. We also have shown the relationship between the parametric deformable models and curve evolution framework; incorporation of clamping/stopping forces to improve the robustness of these topologically independent curves/surfaces. We have discussed considerably segmentation of an object in motion imagery based on PDE and the level set framework. In this Chapter, we have also presented research in the area of coupled PDEs for edge preservation and smoothing. Some coverage has also been given on PDE in miscellaneous applications. Finally, this Chapter concludes with the advantages and the disadvantages of segmentation modeling via geometric deformable models (GDM), PDE and level sets.

4.7.6 Acknowledgements

Thanks are due to Dr. Elaine Keeler and Dr. John Patrick from Marconi Medical Systems, Inc., Cleveland, OH, Dr. George Thoma, National Institutes of Health, Bethesda, MD, Professor Linda Shapiro, University of Washington, Seattle, WA, for their motivations. Thanks are also due to Abdol-Reza Mansouri, INRS Telecommunications, Montreal, Quebec, Canada, for his valuable suggestions on motion segmentation via PDE. Thanks go to Professor Eric Grimson, MIT, Cambridge, MA, for the vasculature images and Dr. Nikos Paragios, Siemens Corporate Research, Princeton, NJ, for the zebra and chest CT images. Special thanks go also to Marconi Medical Systems, Inc., for the MR data sets.

Bibliography

[1] Suri, J. S., Two Dimensional Fast MR Brain Segmentation Using a Region-Based Level Set Approach, Int. Journal of Engineering in Medicine and Biology, Vol. 20, No. 4, pp. 84-95, July/Aug. 2001.

[2] Suri, J. S., Leaking Prevention in Fast Level Sets Using Fuzzy Models: An Application in MR Brain, Inter. Conference in Information Technology in Biomedicine, pp. 220-226, Nov. 2000.

[3] Suri, J. S., White Matter/Gray Matter Boundary Segmentation Using Geometric Snakes: A Fuzzy Deformable Model, Proc. International Conference on Advances in Pattern Recognition, Lecture Notes in Computer Science (LNCS) No. 2013, Singh, S., Murshed, N. and Kropatsch, W. (Eds.), Springer-Verlag, Rio de Janeiro, Brazil, pp. 331-338, March 11-14, 2001.

[4] Suri, J. S., Setarehdan, S. K. and Singh, S., Advanced Algorithmic Approaches to Medical Image Segmentation: State-of-the-Art Applications in Cardiology, Neurology, Mammography and Pathology, ISBN 1-85233-389-8, First Eds., In Press, 2001.

[5] Suri, J. S., Singh, S. and Reden, L., Computer Vision and Pattern Recognition Techniques for 2-D and 3-D MR Cerebral Cortical Segmentation: A State-of-the-Art Review, Accepted for Publication In: Inter. Journal of Pattern Analysis and Applications, 2001.

[6] Suri, J. S., Singh, S., Laxminarayana, S., Zeng, X., Liu, K. and Reden, L., Shape Recovery Algorithms Using Level Sets in 2-D/3-D Medical Imagery: A State-of-the-Art Review, IEEE Trans. in Information Technology in Biomedicine (ITB), 2001 (In Press).

[7] Haker, S., Geometric PDEs in Computer Vision, Ph.D. Thesis, Department of Computer Science and Engineering, University of Minnesota, Minneapolis, MN, 1999.

[8] Chambolle, A., Partial Differential Equations and Image Processing, in Proc. First IEEE Int. Conf. on Image Processing, Austin, Texas, pp. 16-20, Nov. 1994.

[9] Morel, J. -M. and Solimini, S., Variational Methods in Image Segmentation, Boston, MA, Birkhauser, ISBN: 0-8176-3720-6, 1995.

[10] Sapiro, G., Geometric Partial Differential Equations and Image Analysis, Cambridge University Press, Cambridge, MA, ISBN 0-521-79075-1, 2001.

[11] Weickert, J., Fast segmentation methods based on partial differential equations and the watershed transformation, In Levi, P., Ahlers, R.-J., May, F., Schanz, M., (Eds.): Mustererkennung, Springer, Berlin, ISBN 3-519-02606-6, pp. 93-199, 1998.

[12] Weickert, J. and Schnörr, C., PDE-based preprocessing of medical images, Künstliche Intelligenz, No. 3, pp. 5-10, 2000, revised version of Technical Report 8/2000, Computer Science Series, University of Mannheim, Mannheim, Germany, Feb. 2000.

[13] Schnörr, C., Unique reconstruction of piecewise smooth images by minimizing strictly convex non-quadratic functions, J. Math. Imag. Vision, Vol. 4, No. 2, pp. 189-198, 1994.

[14] Schnörr, C., A study of a convex variational diffusion approach for image segmentation and feature extraction, J. Math. Img., Vision, Vol. 8, No. 3, pp. 271-292, 1998.

[15] Catte, F., Lions, P.-L., Morel, J. M. and Coll, T., Image selective smoothing and edge detection by nonlinear diffusion-I, SIAM J. Numer. Anal., Vol. 29, No. 1, pp. 182-193, 1992.

[16] Catte, F., Lions, P.-L., Morel, J. M. and Coll, T., Image selective smoothing and edge detection by nonlinear diffusion-II, SIAM J. Numer. Anal., Vol. 29, No. 3, pp. 845-866, 1992.

[17] Witkin, A., Scale-space filtering, In Int. Joint Conf. on Artificial Intelligence, pp. 1019-1022, 1983.

[18] Perona, P. and Malik, J., Scale-space and edge detection using anisotropic diffusion, IEEE Trans. in Pattern Analysis and Machine Intelligence, Vol. 12, No. 7, pp. 629-639, Apr. 1990.

[19] Perona, P., Orientation diffusions, IEEE Trans. on Image Processing, Vol. 7, No. 3, pp. 457-467, March 1998.

[20] Gerig, G., Kubler, O., Kikinis, R. and Jolesz, F. A., Nonlinear anisotropic filtering of MRI data, IEEE Trans. on Medical Imaging, Vol. 11, No. 2, pp. 221-232, 1992.

[21] Alvarez, L., Lions, P.-L. and Morel, J. M., Image selective smoothing and edge detection by nonlinear diffusion, SIAM J. Numer. Anal., Vol. 29, No. 3, pp. 845-866, 1992.

[22] Alvarez, L., Fuichard, F., Lions, P.-L. and Morel, J. M., Axioms and fundamental equations on image processing, Arch. Ration. Mech., Vol. 123, No. 3, pp. 199-257, 1993.

[23] Canny, J., A computational approach to edge detection, IEEE Trans. on Pattern Analysis and Machine Intelligence, Vol. 8, No. 6, pp. 679-698, 1986.

[24] Pollak, I., Willsky, A. S. and Krim, H., Image Segmentation and Edge Enhancement with Stabilized Inverse Diffusion Equations, IEEE Trans. on Image Processing, Vol. 9, No. 2, pp. 256-266, Feb. 2000.

[25] Kimia, B. B. and Siddiqi, K., Geometric heat equation and non-linear diffusion of shapes and images, in IEEE Computer Society Conference on Computer Vision and Pattern Recognition, pp. 113-120, 1994.

[26] Kimia, B. B. and Siddiqi, K., Geometric Heat Equation and Nonlinear Diffusion of Shapes and Images, Computer Vision and Image Understanding, Vol. 64, No. 3, pp. 305-322, 1996.

[27] Sapiro, G., Tannenaum, A., You, Y. L. and Kaveh, M., Experiments on geometric image enhancement, in Proc. First IEEE Int. Conference on Image Processing, Austin, TX, Nov. 1994.

[28] Sapiro, G. and Caselles, V., Histogram modification via differential equations, J. Differential Equations, Vol. 135, No. 2, pp. 238-268, 1997.

[29] Sapiro, G. and Caselles, V., Contrast Enhancement Via Image Evolution Flows, Graphical Models and Image Processing, Vol. 59, No. 6, pp. 407-416, 1997.

[30] You, Y. L., Xu, W., Tannenbaum, A. and Kaveh, M., Behavioral analysis of anisotropic diffusion in image processing, IEEE Trans. on Image Processing, Vol. 5, No. 11, pp. 1539-1553, 1996.

[31] Sapiro, G., From active contours to anisotropic diffusion: Connections between basic PDEs in image processing, in Proc. of IEEE Int. Conf. in Image Processing, Vol. 1, pp. 477-480, Sept. 1996.

[32] Shah, J., A common framework for curve evolution, segmentation and anisotropic diffusion, in Proc. of IEEE Proc. Conf. Computer Vision and Pattern Recognition, pp. 136-142, June 1996.

[33] Caselles, V., Kimmel, R. and Shapiro, G., Geodesic active contours, Int. J. of Computer Vision, Vol. 22, No. 1, pp. 61-79, 1997.

[34] Weickert, J., Anisotropic Diffusion in Image Processing, Teubner-Verlag, Stuttgart, Germany, ISBN 3-519-02606-6, 1998; see also the article: A review of nonlinear diffusion filtering, In Scale-Space Theory in Computer Vision, Utrecht, The Netherlands, pp. 3-28, 1997.

[35] Black, M., Sapiro, G., Marimont, D. and Heeger, D., Robust Anisotropic Diffusion, IEEE Trans. Image Processing, Vol. 7, No. 3, pp. 421-432, 1998.

[36] Arridge, S. R. and Simmons, A., Multi-spectral probabilistic diffusion using Bayesian classification, in Romeny, B. ter Haar, Florack, L., Koendernick, J., Viergever, M. (Eds.), Scale-Space Theory in Computer Vision, Lecture Notes in Computer Science, Springer, Berlin, Vol. 1252, pp. 224-235, 1997.

[37] Bajla, I. and Hollander, I., Nonlinear filtering of magnetic resonance tomograms by geometry-driven diffusion, Machine Vision and Applications, Vol. 10, No. 5-6, pp. 243-255, 1998.

[38] Olver, P. J., Sapiro, G. and Tannenbaum, A., Classification and uniqueness of invariant geometric flows, Comptes Rendus De L'Acadmie Des Sciences. / Srie I Mathmatique, Paris, 319, Serie I, pp. 339-344, 1994.

[39] Scherzer, O. and Weickert, J., Relations between regularization and diffusion filtering, J. Math. Imaging Vision, Vol. 12, No. 1, pp. 43-63, 2000.

[40] Romeny, B. ter Haar, Florack, L., Koendernick, J. and Viergever, M., Scale-Space Theory in Computer Vision, Lecture Notes in Computer Science, Springer, Berlin, Vol. 1252, 1997.

[41] Nielsen, M., Johansen, P., Olsen, O. F. and Weickert, J., Scale-Space Theories in Computer Vision, Lecture Notes in Computer Science, Springer, Berlin, Vol. 1682, 1999.

[42] Romeny, B. ter Haar, Geometry-Driven Diffusion in Computer Vision, ISBN 0-7923-3087-0, Kluwer, Boston, MA, 1994.

[43] Meer, P., Mintz, D., Rosenfeld, A. and Kim, D. Y., Robust regression methods for computer vision: A review, Int. Journal in Computer Vision, Vol. 6, No. 1, pp. 59-70, 1991.

[44] Suri, J. S., Haralick, R. M. and Sheehan, F. H., Left Ventricle Longitudinal Axis Fitting and LV Apex Estimation Using a Robust Algorithm and its Performance: A Parametric Apex Model, Proc. of the International Conference in Image Processing, Santa Barbara, CA, IEEE, Volume III of III, ISBN: 0-8186-8183-7/97, pp. 118-121, 1997.

[45] Sanchez-Ortiz, G. I., Rueckert, D. and Burger, P., Knowledge-based tensor anisotropic diffusion of cardiac magnetic resonance images, Medical Image Analysis, Vol. 3, No. 1, pp. 77-101, 1999.

[46] Suri, J. S. and Gao, J., Image Smoothing Using PDE, Scale-Space and Mathematical Morphology, Submitted for Int. Conf. in Visualization, Imaging and Image Processing, 2001.

[47] Osher, S. and Sethian, J., Fronts propagating with curvature-dependent speed: algorithms based on Hamilton-Jacobi formulations, J. Comput. Physics, Vol. 79, No. 1, pp. 12-49, 1988.

[48] Sethian, J. A., An Analysis of Flame Propagation, Ph.D. Thesis, Department of Mathematics, University of California, Berkeley, CA, 1982.

[49] Angenent, S., Chopp, D. and Ilmanen, T., On the singularities of cones evolving by mean curvature, Communications in Partial Differential Equations (CPDE), Vol. 20 (11 and 12), pp. 1937-1958, 1995.

[50] Chopp, D. L., Flow under curvature: Singularity formation, minimal surfaces and geodesics, Experimental Mathematics, Vol. 2, No. 4, pp. 235-255, 1993.

[51] Chopp, D. L., Numerical computation of self-similar solutions for mean curvature flow, Experimental Mathematics, Vol. 3, No. 1, pp. 1-15, 1993.

[52] Sethian, J. A., Numerical algorithms for propagating interfaces: Hamilton-Jacobi equations and conservation laws, J. of Differential Geometry, Vol. 31, No. 1, pp. 131-161, 1990.

[53] Sethian, J. A., Curvature flow and entropy conditions applied to grid generation, J. Computational Physics, Vol. 115, No. 1, pp. 440-454, 1994.

[54] Mulder, W., Osher, S. J. and Sethian, J. A., Computing interface motion in compressible gas dynamics, J. Computational Physics, Vol. 100, No. 1, pp. 209-228, 1992.

[55] Sussman, M., Smereka, P. and Osher, S. J., A level set method for computing solutions to incompressible two-phase flow, J. Computational Physics, Vol. 114, No. 1, pp. 146-159, 1994.

[56] Rhee, C., Talbot, L. and Sethian, J. A., Dynamical study of a premixed V-flame, J. of Fluid Mechanics, Vol. 300, pp. 87-115, 1995.

[57] Adalsteinsson, D. and Sethian, J. A., A unified level set approach to etching, deposition and lithography I: Algorithms and two-dimensional simulations, J. Computational Physics, Vol. 120, No. 1, pp. 128-144, 1995.

[58] Whitaker, R. T., Algorithms for Implicit Deformable Models, Int. Conference on Computer Vision (ICCV), pp. 822-827, June 1995.

[59] Whitaker, Ross, T., A Level-Set Approach to 3-D Reconstruction From Range Data, Int. J. of Computer Vision (IJCV), Vol. 29, No. 3, pp. 203-231, Oct. 1998.

[60] Whitaker, Ross T. and Breen, David E., Level-Set Models for the Deformation of Solid Objects, Proceedings of Implicit Surfaces, Eurographics/Siggraph, pp. 19-35, June 1998.

[61] Paragios, N. and Deriche, R., Geodesic Active Contours and Level Sets for the Detection and Tracking of Moving Objects, IEEE Transactions on Pattern Analysis and Machine Intelligence (PAMI), Vol. 22, pp. 266-280, March 2000.

[62] Paragios, N. and Deriche, R., Coupled Geodesic Active Regions for Image Segmentation: A level set approach, In the Sixth European Conference on Computer Vision (ECCV), Trinity College, Dublin, Ireland, Vol. II, pp. 224-240, 26th June-1st July, 2000.

[63] Kornprobst, P., Deriche, R. and Aubert, G., Image Sequence Analysis Via Partial Differential Equations, J. of Mathematical Imaging and Vision (JMIV), Vol. 11, No. 1, pp. 5-26, 1999.

[64] Faugeras, O. and Keriven, R., Variational principles, surface evolution, PDEs level set methods and the stereo problem, IEEE Trans on Image Proc., Vol. 7, No. 3, pp. 336-344, May 1998.

[65] Sapiro, G., Kimmel, R., Shaked, D., Kimia, B. B. and Bruckstein, A. M., Implementing continuous-scale morphology via curve evolution, Pattern Recognition, Vol. 26, No. 9, pp. 1363-1372, 1997.

[66] Arehart, A., Vincent, L. and Kimia, B. B., Mathematical Morphology: The Hamilton-Jacobi connection, In Int. Conference in Computer Vision (ICCV), pp. 215-219, 1993.

[67] Catte, F., Dibos, F. and Koepfler, G., A morphological scheme for mean curvature motion and applications to anisotropic diffusion and motion of level sets, in SIAM Jour. of Numerical Analysis, Vol. 32, No. 6, pp. 1895-1909, 1995.

[68] Sochen, N., Kimmel, R. and Malladi, R., A Geometrical Framework for Low Level Vision, IEEE Trans. on Image Processing, Vol. 7, No. 3, pp. 310-318, 1998.

[69] Malladi, R., Kimmel, R., Adalsteinsson, D., Sapiro, G., Caselles, V. and Sethian, J. A., A Geometric Approach to Segmentation and Analysis of 3-D Medical Images, Proc. of IEEE/SIAM Workshop on Mathematical Morphology and Biomedical Image Analysis (MMBIA), San Francisco, CA, pp. 244-252, June 1996.

[70] Malladi, R. and Sethian, J. A., Image Processing Via Level Set Curvature Flow, Proc. Natl. Acad. Sci. (PNAS), USA, pp. 7046-7050, 1995.

[71] Malladi, R. and Sethian, J. A., Image processing: flows under min/max curvature and mean curvature, Graphics Models Image Processing (GMIP), Vol. 58, No. 2, pp. 127-141, 1996.

[72] Malladi, R., Sethian, J. A. and Vemuri, B. C., A fast level set based algorithm for topology independent shape modeling, Journal of Mathematical Imaging and Vision, Special Issue on Topology and Geometry in Computer Vision, Eds., Rosenfeld, A. and Kong, Y., Vol. 6, No. 2 and 3, pp. 269-290, April 1996.

[73] Malladi, R. and Sethian, J. A., A Unified Approach to Noise Removal, Image-Enhancement and Shape Recovery, IEEE Trans. in Image Processing, Vol. 5, No. 11, pp. 1554-1568, Nov. 1996.

[74] Kichenassamy, S., Kumar, A., Olver, P., Tannenbaum, A. and Yezzi, A., Conformal curvature flows: from phase transitions to active vision, Arch. Rational Mech. Anal., Vol. 134, pp. 275-301, 1996.

[75] Yezzi, A., Kichenassamy, S., Kumar, A., Olver, P. and Tannenbaum, A., Snake model for segmentation of medical imagery, IEEE Tran. in Med. Imag., Vol. 16, No. 2, pp. 199-209, 1997.

[76] Siddiqi, K., Lauriere, Y. B., Tannenbaum, A. and Zucker, S. W., Area and length minimizing flows for shape segmentation, IEEE Trans. in Image Processing, Vol. 7, No. 3, pp. 433-443, 1998.

[77] Malladi, R. and Sethian, J. A., An O(N log N) algorithm for shape modeling, Applied Mathematics, Proc. Natl. Acad. Sci. (PNAS), USA, Vol. 93, No. 18, pp. 9389-9392, Sept. 1996.

[78] Gomes, J. and Faugeras, O., Level sets and distance functions, In Proc. of the 6th European Conference on Computer Vision (ECCV), pp. 588-602, 2000.

[79] Grayson, M., The heat equation shrinks embedded plane curves to round points, J. of Differential Geometry, Vol. 26, pp. 285-314, 1987.

[80] Sethian, J. A., Algorithms for tracking interfaces in CFD and material science, Annual Review of Computational Fluid Mechanics, 1995.

[81] Sethian, J. A. and Strain, J. D., Crystal growth and dentritic solidification, J. Computational Physics, Vol. 98, No. 2, pp. 231-253, 1992.

[82] Sapiro, G., Color Snakes, Computer Vision and Image Understanding (CVIU), Vol. 68, No. 2, pp. 247-253, 1997.

[83] Suri, J. S., Fast WM/GM Boundary Segmentation From MR Images Using the Relationship Between Parametric and Geometric Deformable Models, Chapter 8, in book edited by Suri, Setarehdan and Singh, titled Advanced Algorithmic Approaches to Medical Image Segmentation: State-of-the-Art Applications in Cardiology, Neurology, Mammography and Pathology, In Press, First Eds., to be published in Jan. 2001.

[84] Zeng, X., Staib, L. H., Schultz, R. T. and Duncan, J. S., Segmentation and measurement of the cortex from 3-D MR images using coupled-surfaces propagation, IEEE Trans. on Med. Imag., Vol. 18, No. 10, pp. 927-37, Sept. 1999.

[85] Sarti, A., Ortiz, C., Locket, S. and Malladi, R., A Geometric Model for 3-D Confocal Image Analysis, IEEE Trans. on Biomedical Engineering, Vol. 47, No. 12, pp. 1600-1609, Dec. 2000.

[86] Sethian, J. A., A review of recent numerical algorithms for hypersurfaces moving with curvature dependent flows, J. Differential Geometry, Vol. 31, pp. 131-161, 1989.

[87] Sethian, J. A., Theory, algorithms and applications of level set methods for propagating interfaces, Acta Numerica, Vol. 5, pp. 309-395, 1996.

[88] Sethian, J. A., Level Set Methods and Fast Marching Methods: Evolving interfaces in computational geometry, fluid mechanics, Computer Vision

and Material Science, Cambridge University Press, Cambridge, UK, 2nd Edition, ISBN: 0-521-64204-3, 1999.

[89] Cao, S. and Greenhalgh, S., Finite-difference solution of the Eikonal equation using an efficient, first-arrival, wavefront tracking scheme, Geophysics, Vol. 59, No. 4, pp. 632-643, April 1994.

[90] Chen, S., Merriman, B., Osher, S. and Smereka, P., A Simple Level Set Method for Solving Stefan Problems, Journal of Comput. Physics, Vol. 135, No. 1, pp. 8-29, 1997.

[91] Kass, M., Witkin, A. and Terzopoulos, D., Snakes: Active Contour Models, Int. J. of Computer Vision, Vol. 1, No. 4, pp. 321-331, 1988.

[92] Pavlidis, T. and Liow, Y., Integrating region growing and edge detection, IEEE Trans. on Pattern Analysis and Machine Intelligence, Vol. 12, No. 3, pp. 225-233, 1990.

[93] Zhu, S. and Yuille, A., Region Competition: Unifying Snakes, Region Growing and Bayes/MDL for multiband image segmentation, IEEE Trans. on Pattern Analysis and Machine Intelligence, Vol. 18, No. 9, pp. 884-990, 1996.

[94] Suri, J. S., Computer Vision, Image Processing and Pattern Recognition in Left Ventricle Segmentation: Last 50 Years, J. of Pattern Analysis and Applications, Vol. 3, No. 3, pp. 209-244, Sept. 2000.

[95] Lorigo, L. M., Faugeras, O., Grimson, W. E. L., Keriven, R., Kikinis, R. and Westin, Carl-Fredrik, Co-Dimension 2 Geodesic Active Contours for MRA Segmentation, In Proceedings of 16th Int. Conference of Information Processing in Medical Imaging, Visegrad, Hungary, Lecture Notes in Computer Science, Volume 1613, pp. 126-139, June/July 1999.

[96] Lorigo, L. M., Grimson, W. Eric L., Faugeras, O., Keriven, R., Kikinis, R., Nabavi, A. and Westin, Carl-Fredrick, Two Geodesic Active Contours for the Segmentation of Tubular Structures, In Proc. of the Computer Vision and Pattern Recognition (CVPR), pp. 444-451, June 2000.

[97] Suri, J. S. and Bernstein, R., 2-D and 3-D Display of Aneurysms from Magnetic Resonance Angiographic Data, 6th Int. Conference in Computer Assisted Radiology, pp. 666-672, 1992.

[98] Paragios, N. and Deriche, R., Geodesic Active Regions: A New Paradigm to Deal with Frame Partition Problems in Computer Vision, Journal of Visual Communication and Image Representation (JVCIR), Special Issue on Partial Differential Equations in Image Processing, Computer Vision and Computer Graphics (To appear).

[99] Tek, H. and Kimia, B. B., Deformable bubbles in the reaction-diffusion space, in Proc. of the 5th Int. Conference in Computer Vision (ICCV), Cambridge, MA, pp. 156-162, 1995.

[100] Xu, C. and Prince, J. L., Generalized gradient vector flow external forces for active contours, Int. Journal of Signal Processing, Vol. 71, No. 2, pp. 131-139, 1998.

[101] Amadieu, O., Debreuve, E., Barlaud, M. and Aubert, G., Inward and outward curve evolution using level set method, in Proc. IEEE Int. Conference in Image Processing, Vol. III, pp. 188-192, Oct. 1999.

[102] Santosa, F., A level set approach for inverse problems involving obstacles, ESAIM: Control, Optimisation and Calculus of Variations, European Series in Applied and Industrial Mathematics, Vol. 1, pp. 17-33, 1996.

[103] Besson, Stéphanie J., Barlaud, M. and Aubert, G., Detection and Tracking of Moving Objects Using a New Level Set Based Method, Int. Conference on Pattern Recognition, Barcelona, pp. 1112-1117, Sept. 2000.

[104] Baillard, C., Hellier, P. and Barillot, C., Segmentation of 3-D Brain Structures Using Level Sets, Research Report 1291, IRISA, Rennes Cedex, France, 16 pages, Jan. 2000.

[105] Baillard, C., Barillot, C. and Bouthemy, P., Robust Adaptive Segmentation of 3-D Medical Images with Level Sets, Research Report 1369, IRISA, Rennes Cedex, France, 26 pages, Nov. 2000.

[106] Baillard, C., Hellier, P. and Barillot, C., Cooperation between level set techniques and dense 3d registration for the segmentation of brain structures, In Int. Conference on Pattern Recognition, Vol. 1, pp. 991-994, Sept. 2000.

[107] Grimson, W. E. L., Stauffer, C., Romano, R., Lee, L., Viola, P. and Faugeras, O. D., Forest of sensors: using adaptive tracking to classify and monitor activities in a site, Proceedings of 1998 DARPA Image Understanding Workshop, Vol. 1, pp. 33-41, 1998.

[108] Paragios, N. and Deriche, R., PDE-based level-set approach for detection and tracking of moving objects, Proceedings of the Int. Conference in Computer Vision, pp. 1139-1145, 1998.

[109] Zhang, K. and Kittler, J., Global motion estimation and robust regression for video coding, ICIP'98, Vol. 3, pp. 944-947, Oct. 1998.

[110] Jahne, B., Haussecker, H., Spies, H., Schmundt, D. and Schurr, U., Study of dynamical processes with sensor-based spatiotemporal image processing techniques, European Conference in Computer Vision (ECCV), pp. 322-335, 1998.

[111] Sethian, J. A., Level Set Methods and Fast Marching Methods: Evolving interfaces in computational geometry, fluid mechanics, Computer Vision and Material Science, Cambridge University Press, Cambridge, UK, 2nd Edition, ISBN: 0-521-64204-3, 1999.

[112] Gao, J., Image Sequence Segmentation, Ph.D. Thesis, Department of Electrical Engineering and Computer Science, University of Wisconsin, Milwaukee, WI, 1999.

[113] Zhang, J. and Gao, J., Image sequence segmentation using curve evolution, Conference Record of the Thirty-Third Asilomar Conference on Signals, Systems and Computers, Vol. 2, pp. 1426 -1430, 1999.

[114] Zhang, J., Gao, J. and Liu, W., Image Sequence Segmentation Using 3-D Structure Tensor and Curve Evolution, IEEE Transactions on Circuits and Systems for Video Technology, 2001 (to appear).

[115] Zhu, S. C. and Yullie, A., Region Competition: Unifying snakes, region growing and Bayes/MDL for multiband image segmentation, IEEE Trans. Pattern Anal. Machine Intell., Vol. 18, No. 9, pp. 884-900, Sept. 1996.

[116] Mansouri, Abdol-Reza and Konrad, J., Multiple motion segmentation with level sets, IEEE Trans. in Img. Proc., 2001 (To Appear).

[117] Banks, S., Signal Processing, Image Processing and Pattern Recognition, Prentice-Hall, Englewood Cliffs, NJ, ISBN 0-13-812579-1, 1990.

[118] Bloor, M. I. G., Wilson, M. J. and Hagen, H., The smoothing properties of variations schemes for surface design, Computer Aided Geometric Design, Vol. 112, No. 4, pp. 381-394, 1995.

[119] Brown, J. M., Bloor, M. I. G., Bloor, M. S., Nowacki, H. N. and Wilson, M. J., Fairness of B-spline surface approximations to PDE surfaces using the finite-element method, in Bowyer Eds., Computer-Aided Surface Geometry and Design: The Mathematics of Surfaces IV, 1994.

[120] Weickert, J., Heers, J., Schnorr, C., Zuiderveld, K. J., Scherzer, O. and Stiehl, H. S., Fast parallel algorithms for a broad class of nonlinear variational diffusion approaches, Real-Time Imaging, Vol. 7, No. 1, pp. 31-45, Feb. 2001.

[121] Zhao, H. K., Chan, T., Merriman, B. and Osher, S., A variational level set approach to multiphase motion, J. Computational Physics, Vol. 127, No. 1, pp. 179-195, 1996.

[122] Evans, L. C. and Spruck, J., Motion of level sets by mean curvature: Part-I, J. of Differential Geometry, Vol. 33, pp. 635-681, 1991.

[123] Kimia, B. B., Tannenbaum, A. R. and Zucker, S. W., Shapes, shocks and deformations, I: The components of shape and the reaction-diffusion space, Int. Journal of Computer Vision (IJCV), Vol. 15, No. 3, pp. 189-224, 1995.

[124] Siddiqi, K., Tresness, K. J. and Kimia, B. B., Parts of visual form: Ecological and psychophysical aspects, Perception, Vol. 25, No. 4, pp. 399-424, 1996.

[125] Stoll, P., Tek, H. and Kimia, B. B., Shocks from images: Propagation of orientation elements, In Proceedings of Computer Vision and Pattern Recognition (CVPR), Puerto Rico, IEEE Computer Society Press, pp. 839-845, June 15-16, 1997.

[126] Sarti, A., Malladi, R. and Sethian, J. A., Subjective Surfaces: A Method for Completing Missing Boundaries, Proceedings of the National Academy of Sciences of the USA, Vol. 12, No. 97, pp. 6258-6263, 2000.

[127] Sarti, A., Mikula, K. and Sgallari, F., Nonlinear Multiscale Analysis of 3-D Echocardiographic Sequences, IEEE Trans. on Med. Imag., Vol. 18, No. 6, pp. 453-466, 1999.

[128] Sarti, A. and Malladi, R., A geometric level set model for ultrasounds analysis, LBNL-44442, University of California, Berkeley, CA, 1999.

[129] Sarti, A., Ortiz, C., Locket, S. and Malladi, R., A unified geometric model for 3-D confocal image analysis in cytology, Report Number: LBNL-41740, University of California, Berkeley, CA, April 1998.

[130] Jahne, B., Digital Image Processing: Concepts, Algorithms and Scientific Applications, 4th Edition, ISBN Number: 0-387-569-413, Springer Verlag, 1997.

[131] Rudin, L. I., Osher, S. and Fatemi, E., Nonlinear total variation based noise removal algorithms, Physica D, Vol. 60, pp. 259-268, 1992.

[132] Whitaker, R. T. and Pizer, S. M., A multi-scale approach to non-uniform diffusion, Computer Vision, Graphics and Image Processing: Image Understanding, Vol. 51, No. 1, pp. 99-110, 1993.

[133] Pauwels, E. J., Fiddelaers, P. and Van Gool, L. J., Shape-extraction for curves using geometry-driven diffusion and functional optimization, in Proc. ICCV, pp. 396-401, June 1995.

[134] Dibos, F., Koepfler, G., Image denoising through a level set approach, Proceedings International Conference on Image Processing, Vol. 3, pp. 264-268, 1998.

[135] Courant, R., Friedrichs, K. O. and Lewy, H., On the partial difference equations of mathematical physics, IBM Journal, Vol. 11, pp. 215-235, 1967.

[136] Suri, J. S., Complex 2-D and 3-D Segmentation Issues and Variational Methods in Medical Imagery, Under Submission in Int. Journal, 2002.

Chapter 5

Motion Imagery Segmentation Via PDE

Jianbo Gao[1], *Jun Zhang*[2] *and Jasjit S. Suri*[3]

5.1 Introduction

5.1.1 Why Image Sequence Segmentation?

In recent years, there has been considerable interest in the image sequence segmentation problem, due to its applications in a wide range of areas. With recent developments in communication technologies, applications such as the storage and transmission of digital video have been growing rapidly. These include high definition television (HDTV), digital TV, video conferencing, and video-on-demand (VOD), etc. Image sequence segmentation plays a key role in object-based video compression and representation (e.g., MPEG4 and MPEG7). Object-based video representation needs to decompose a scene into different objects. To decompose the scene, image sequence segmentation is the most important technique. Industrial and military applications in video surveillance and monitoring have grown rapidly over the past few years. Their uses for home property surveillance and school children monitoring are also growing. Automatic target detection and tracking, such as human face detection and recognition, are widely used. Their use in the analysis of medical and other scientific applications, such as cardiac imaging, will improve human health services. The key to these applications is how to separate moving objects from their background.

[1]KLA-Tencor, Milpitas, CA, USA
[2]University of Wisconsin-Milwaukee, Milwaukee, WI, USA
[3]Marconi Medical Systems, Inc., Cleveland, OH, USA

PDE & Level Sets: Algorithmic Approaches to Static & Motion Imagery
Edited by Jasjit Suri and Swamy Laxminarayan, Kluwer Academic/Plenum Publishers, 2002

5.1.2 What is Image Sequence Segmentation?

It is known that the role of still image segmentation is to separate an object from its background, such as lesion from the background skin [17]. Image sequence segmentation separates moving objects from the background by intensity, color, texture and motion. The main difference between them is that motion is introduced in the latter. This makes the segmentation more complicated and more interesting. One method is carrying out segmentation by identifying the different motions for all objects in the sequence. Of course, we can still use other image properties as we did in still image segmentation.

Let us look at an example of image sequence segmentation. Assume we have two successive frames, which are shown in Figs. 5.1.(a) and 5.1.(b). There is a moving object (tank) on the images with a textured background and noise. The estimated motion field should look like Fig. 5.1.(c). According to the motion field, we can get the moving object segmented as shown in Fig. 5.1.(d).

This is a very simple example. A more complicated situation is when the sequence has a moving background as well as moving objects. Sometimes the SNR (Signal Noise Ratio) of the image sequence is very low (such as in infrared sequences), and the lens may have non-linear distortions [79] which needs more sophisticated models. In this Chapter, we only consider the linear lens.

5.1.3 Basic Idea of Sequence Segmentation

Most previous work in image sequence segmentation can be classified into four classes. In the first class, intra-frame segmentation, is performed as in still image segmentation. After this, inter-frame tracking is used to match the same regions between consecutive frames. The difficult problem here is how to get an effective segmentation for still images of real world scenes. Furthermore, tracking objects between frames does not work well when there are too many regions and may fail because of the different shapes for the same objects between the frames. Alternatively if we have a good motion field, we can use motion field clustering to get the segmentation [71, 72]. The problem with this method is that it needs an accurate motion field estimation, which is not easy for real world image sequences. Recent research found that frame differencing is a good way to detect motion and moving objects because it is simple and computationally efficient. Many robust motion detection techniques have been

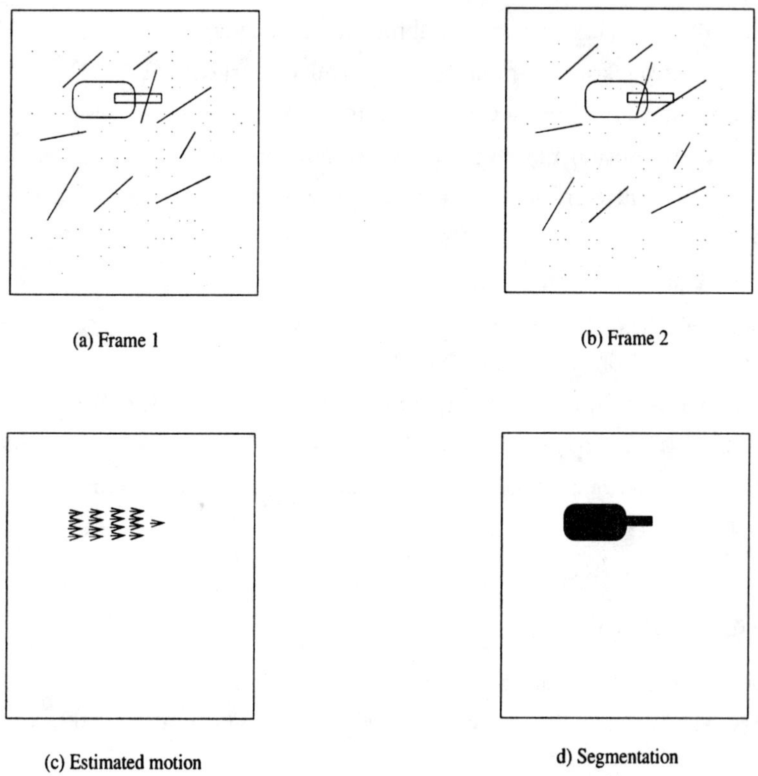

Figure 5.1: An Example of Image Sequence Segmentation.

studied. Besides the above automatic motion segmentation techniques, there is a semi-automatic segmentation approach. The basic idea of this approach is to manually give a good initial segmentation, and then follow this initial segmentation by getting the next frame's segmentation. The advantage of this method is that it may work well when there is a complicated background and object motion.

We have developed a new technique for color image segmentation, which can improve intra-frame segmentation performance because it can effectively segment images. This method combines many techniques such as multiresolution, MRF (Markov Random Field), mean field theory, EM (Expectation-Maximization) algorithm and multivariable analysis for color images. With a special multiresolution implementation, this algorithm is computationally efficient. Better intra-frame segmentation can improve the existing sequence segmentation techniques.

In this Chapter we have also developed a new approach for image sequence segmentation which belongs to the frame differencing category, and only segments the moving objects rather than the regions in the frame. Its main idea is: 1) using a fast global motion compensation to compensate for the background motion, 2) getting a robust frame differencing by a local structure tensor field, and 3) segmenting out whole objects by using level set based curve evolution.

5.1.4 Contributions of This Chapter

The main contributions of this Chapter are:

1. A new technique for color image segmentation by using multiresolution, the MRF, mean field theory, EM algorithm, and multivariable analysis, etc.

2. A new approach for robust frame differencing (motion detection) by local structure tensor field to eliminate the noise.

3. A new framework for sequence segmentation by a combination of frame differencing and curve evolution.

5.1.5 Outline of this Chapter

This Chapter is organized as follows. In Section 5.2, we will review the literature on image sequence segmentation. In Section 5.3, a new multiresolution technique in color image segmentation is detailed with the results of this method demonstrated. Our image sequence segmentation approach will be described in Section 5.4. Experimental results on TV and surveillance sequences will be presented in the end of this section. Conclusions and directions for future work will be given in Section 5.5.

5.2 Previous Work in Image Sequence Segmentation

The most difficult aspect for image sequence segmentation is how to classify a pixel into a moving object or the background. Sometimes the background is also moving, caused by the camera motion. The camera motion can be due to translation, rotation, and zooming.

Most previous work in image sequence segmentation can be classified into four approaches: 1) intra-frame (intensity) segmentation plus inter-frame tracking, 2) motion field clustering/segmentation, 3) frame differencing and 4) semi-automatic segmentation. Here we will give some discussions about these approaches.

5.2.1 Intra-Frame Segmentation with Tracking

It is straightforward to show that an image segmentation method can be used to segment an image sequence. In this approach (for example, see [43], [38]), two consecutive frames in an image sequence are segmented independently (i.e., intra-frame) into regions of homogeneous intensity or texture using traditional *image segmentation* techniques. We can use many different kinds of image segmentation methods for this, such as watershade [58], and image clustering [80]. Then the regions in the two frames are matched [38]. This works well if intra-frame segmentation produces a small number of regions closely related to real-world objects, because it will not take much time to do the matching, and the accuracy of the matching will be high. However, since image segmentation using intensity or texture remains a difficult problem, this approach often encounters problems since many image segmentation techniques produce over-segmentation. It is very hard to match a large number of regions for two reasons. One is that this is time consuming, and the other is that the same object in the two consecutive frames may not have the same shape. That may make the matching unsuccessful.

Smith's edge and corner feature extraction and matching [65, 66] are similar to this intra-frame segmentation method. His system extracts the corners and edges, then matches them between the frames. To make it in real-time, the system can only use corner matching. Another similar method was proposed by Meier *et al.* [44], which is based on edge features, and matches the edges of objects for tracking.

A significant extension is to treat the image sequence as a 3D image (with two spatial and one temporal dimension) and group the pixels along space and time. Because in an image sequence the resolutions in space and time are generally different, it is not suitable to treat the image sequence as a 3D image. In most cases, the spatial resolution is much greater than that in the temporal direction. Another reason is that because the camera, which is mounted on a helicopter or a missile, has rapid movement, the image sequence may be very shaky from frame to frame. This means the global motion may not be steady within several frames. To segment such a kind of image sequence will fail using 3D image segmentation. While some good results were demonstrated (e.g., in [63]), 3D segmentation is generally computation intensive, even when one segments several frames (e.g., 8) at a time.

Recently, we have developed a new multiresolution technique for color image segmentation which can be applied to image sequence segmentation of this approach. This algorithm can improve the intra-frame segmentation of regions. Then we can track the regions from frame to frame. Details of our image segmentation method will be introduced in the next section. Here is a brief introduction: We classify the color image pixels in different clusters based on MRF, mean field techniques, etc. The new multiresolution technique only updates the boundary area of regions, "Narrow Band", in the high resolution levels. This dramatically saves computation in the EM algorithm, makes the algorithm more efficient than the traditional multiresolution technique and single resolution methods. With a similar approach, we can still use this "Narrow Band" technique to carry out the segmentation from the previous frame to the current frame as the multiresolution does in the boundaries of areas from low resolution to high resolution. Image segmentation, which has accurate boundaries of regions, can also be integrated into the image sequence segmentation framework to improve the accuracy of motion boundaries of moving objects.

5.2.2 Segmentation Based on Dense Motion Fields

Originally motion estimation was used for image sequence coding. In MPEG-1 and MPEG-2, motion estimation is an essential technique for coding since motion compensated frame difference is coded. As an alternative to previous image sequence segmentation methods, a dense motion field is used for the sequence segmentation. This makes sense since pixels with similar motion vectors can be grouped into regions (e.g., see [9], [71], [61], [66], [3], [23]). Similarly, small regions generated from intra-frame segmentation can also be grouped based on the similarity of their motion vectors (e.g., see [15], [64], [4], [1], [76], [77]). This approach produces good results when a reliable motion field can be obtained from motion estimation.

There are many motion estimation algorithms. According to the motion models, we can classify them into 2-D motion estimation and 3-D motion estimation. In 2-D motion estimation, the algorithms can be also divided into optical flow methods, block-based methods, pel-recursive methods and Bayesian method.

5.2.2.1 2-D Motion Estimation

Because we use the block-matching technique in our global motion compensation method, we will discuss it in more detail in this sub-section.

Block Matching When people first studied video coding, block-matching was considered the most popular method of motion estimation due to its simplicity. As a result, most international video compression standards, such as MPEG-1, MPEG-2 and H.263, adopted block-matching for motion compensation. The model of block-matching is based on the translation of plane objects. There is no rotation or zooming in block-matching. The basic idea is illustrated in Fig. 5.2. Here, the image at time t is divided into blocks of equal size (such as 8×8) and the corresponding block is searched for in frame $t-1$ within a limited region, such as inside the dotted line. For each block in frame t, a search is done in the previous frame for the block that best matches the current block. The match is determined by minimizing a distortion criterion, and the most popular is the mean-squared-error. The connection vector between the

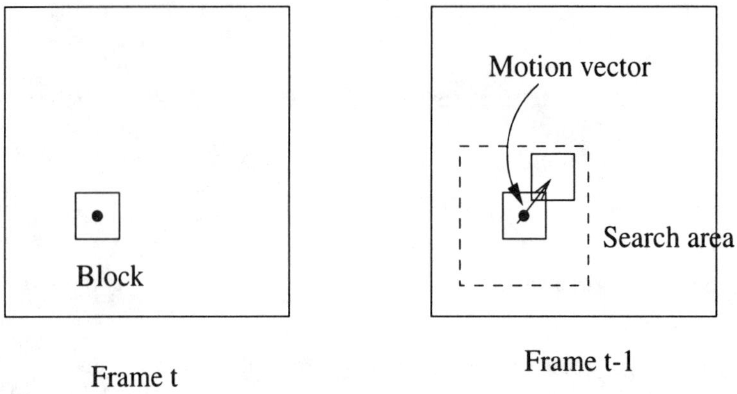

Figure 5.2: Block-matching.

two matched blocks is the motion vector. Although the block matching is simple and easy to implement, it can not model the true motion of an object. The block matching method can not precisely represent the object motion due to several reasons. One is that the object may not be a square object with a fixed size block. Another reason is that sometimes there may be several different motions within one object. Yet another reason is that moving objects can be a different surface other than a plane surface. Furthermore, the motion of the objects could be more complicated than translation, zooming, and rotation, etc.

To solve such kinds of problems, one method is to improve the block-matching with different sizes [11], the others include overlapping the block [68], and deforming block-matching [74].

In the block-matching, there are three general search procedures: full size search, three-step search and cross-search [20]. The latter two are the fast algorithms. If the motion is large, hierarchical (multiresolution) motion estimation is introduced [9]. The basic idea of hierarchical block-matching is to perform motion estimation at each level successively, starting with the lowest resolution level [6].

Optical Flow Method Horn *et al.* [29] proposed an optical flow method, which attempts to provide an estimation of the optical flow field in terms of spatio-temporal image intensity gradients. The optical flow equation is given as:

$$\frac{\partial I(\mathbf{x},t)}{\partial x}v_x(\mathbf{x}) + \frac{\partial I(\mathbf{x},t)}{\partial y}v_y(\mathbf{x}) + \frac{\partial I(\mathbf{x},t)}{\partial t} = 0, \tag{5.1}$$

where $I(\mathbf{x},t)$ is the image intensity for time t at spatial location $\mathbf{x} = (x,y)$, and $\mathbf{v} = (v_x, v_y)$ refers to the velocity vector. To solve this equation, a regularization method, with an enforced smoothness constraint, is used since it is an ill-posed problem. The problem with this method is that it can lead to over-smoothing at the motion edges since it assumes that the motion vector is smooth. To avoid this kind of problem, a number of robust models have been proposed by [27] and [48].

Other 2-D Motion Estimation Methods In pel-recursive methods, the motion estimates are found pixel by pixel based on a prediction from previously found neighborhood estimations. It can be written as [69]:

$$\hat{\mathbf{d}}_a(\mathbf{x},t;\delta t) = \hat{\mathbf{d}}_b(\mathbf{x},t;\delta t) + \mathbf{u}(\mathbf{x},t;\delta t), \tag{5.2}$$

where $\hat{\mathbf{d}}_a(\mathbf{x},t;\delta t)$ denotes the estimated motion vector at the location $\mathbf{x}$ and time t, $\hat{\mathbf{d}}_b(\mathbf{x},t;\delta t)$ denotes the predicted motion estimate, and $\mathbf{u}(\mathbf{x},t;\delta t)$ is the update term. The prediction step is generally considered as an implicit smoothness constraint.

Bayesian methods [81] have been shown to be a powerful alternative to the problem of 2-D motion estimation. The fundamental theory of this method is the Markov Random Field (MRF) model, which has a spatial constraint to make the segment smooth. This approach has been successfully applied in both motion estimation and motion segmentation for its accurate boundaries of regions. The problem with this method is that it is computationally expensive, since it obtains results iteratively.

5.2.2.2 3-D Motion Estimation

2-D motion estimation deals with the case of plane surface objects with the viewpoint directly at the object. In the real world, objects can be very complicated and the viewpoint is also very complicated. So, 3-D models should be considered to solve these kinds of problems. There are two main 3-D models which can be used in motion estimation. They are orthogonal and perspective.

In 3-D motion estimation, a plane object motion with an orthogonal system can be modeled as affine flow. The 6-parameter affine flow can be formulated as:

$$
\begin{aligned}
v_x &= a_1 + a_2 x + a_3 y \\
v_y &= a_4 + a_5 x + a_6 y,
\end{aligned}
\tag{5.3}
$$

where $\mathbf{a} = [a_1, a_2, a_3, a_4, a_5, a_6]$ are the affine parameters, and v_x and v_y represent the velocity in the x and y directions, respectively. Or we can write it in matrix form,

$$\mathbf{v} = \mathbf{\Lambda x} + \mathbf{d}, \tag{5.4}$$

where $\mathbf{v} = (v_x, v_y)$, $\mathbf{\Lambda}$ is the affine transformation matrix, $\mathbf{x} = (x, y)^T$, and $\mathbf{d}$ is the translational vector. T means transpose.

A more complicated quadratic flow model (8 parameters) is an exact model for the case of planar surface under perspective projection [73]. We can formulate it as:

$$
\begin{aligned}
v_x &= a_1 + a_2 x + a_3 y + a_7 x^2 + a_8 xy \\
v_y &= a_4 + a_5 x + a_6 y + a_7 xy + a_8 y^2,
\end{aligned}
\tag{5.5}
$$

where $\mathbf{a} = [a_1, a_2, a_3, a_4, a_5, a_6, a_7, a_8]$ are the perspective parameters, and v_x and v_y represent the velocity in the x and y directions as before, respectively.

In most cases, we can use affine model to approximate the real world imaging system. Weak perspective model can be an affine with scale or zooming [70] when the object is not close to the viewpoint. In this Chapter we will use affine model only to estimate the background motion. It is straightforward to extend applications to the perspective model.

However, most motion estimation techniques can not get a good "true" motion estimation, especially on real-world image sequences.

To solve this problem, recent hybrid techniques (simultaneous estimation and segmentation) that alternate between motion estimation and motion field grouping or segmentation have been proposed ([69], [67] and [26]). While these lead to some improvements in accuracy, they often require an excessive amount of computation.

5.2.3 Frame Differencing

5.2.3.1 Direct Frame Differencing

If there is no camera motion or global motion, the scenery will be changed only when there are moving objects. The easiest way is to check the difference between two consecutive frames. So in this approach, image segmentation is achieved *partially* through frame-differencing (see e.g., [69]) by a threshold. Here is the formulation:

$$d(\mathbf{x}, t) = |I(\mathbf{x}, t) - I(\mathbf{x}, t-1)|, \tag{5.6}$$

where $I(\mathbf{x}, t)$ and $I(\mathbf{x}, t-1)$ are two pixel values at position $\mathbf{x} = (x, y)$ at time t and $t-1$ respectively , $d(\mathbf{x}, t)$ is the frame difference value at position $\mathbf{x}$. If a pixel has a large frame difference d, which is larger than $\mathbf{T}$, it is linked to a moving object, where $\mathbf{T}$ is a predefined threshold. Otherwise, it is linked to the background. This approach, although extremely simple and computationally efficient, generally does not produce whole objects. Furthermore, it is very sensitive to noise, because sometimes the pixels with noise in the background can be larger than the specified threshold $\mathbf{T}$. Also, it will fail completely if there is a global motion.

5.2.3.2 Temporal Wavelet Filtering Frame Differencing

Recently, there have been efforts to make frame-differencing more robust to noise. These include temporal wavelets [14], wavelets related by Lie groups [39], adaptive background estimation [21], [33], and combined PDE optimization [37].

Temporal wavelets can remove noise in the temporal direction and are an extension of frame differencing. If we have several frames, $\mathbf{I}(\mathbf{x}, t) = \{I(\mathbf{x}, t+m), I(\mathbf{x}, t+m-1), ..., I(\mathbf{x}, t), ..., I(\mathbf{x}, t-n)\}$, then we have a robust difference:

$$d(\mathbf{x}, t) = |\mathbf{I}(\mathbf{x}, t) \bigotimes h(t)|, \tag{5.7}$$

where $h(t)$ is the wavelet band pass filter, $d(\mathbf{x}, t)$ is the frame difference value at position $\mathbf{x}$ and time t, and $\bigotimes$ represents the convolution. The filtering result gives the frame difference over some number of frames. So, it will be more robust than direct frame-differencing. We can treat this direct two consecutive frame differencing as a Harr wavelet filtering in the temporal direction. The algorithm is simple and easy to implement. Davis *et al.* [14] claimed that this can detect very low contrast and very small objects.

5.2.3.3 Lie Group Wavelet Motion Detection

Lie group wavelets [36] and [39] can perform low pass filtering along the edges in the spatial direction and motion direction, and band pass filtering perpendicular to the edges. Here we review the Kong *et al.* algorithm [36]. This technique performs the filtering in every possible direction. The wavelet referential transformation is given by:

$$\begin{pmatrix} \vec{x}' \\ t' \\ 1 \end{pmatrix} = \begin{pmatrix} aR(\theta) & \vec{v} & \vec{b} \\ 0 & 1 & \tau \\ 0 & 0 & 1 \end{pmatrix} \begin{pmatrix} \vec{x} \\ t \\ 1 \end{pmatrix}, \tag{5.8}$$

where the parameters of interest here are the spatial translation $\vec{b} \in \mathbf{R}^2$, the temporal translation $\tau \in \mathbf{R}$, the velocity $\vec{v} \in \mathbf{R}^2$, the scale $a \in \mathbf{R}_+ \backslash \{0\}$, the orientation $\theta \in [0, 2\pi)$. For the group element $g = \{\vec{b}, \tau, \vec{v}, a, \theta\}$, the group in the spatio-temporal Hilbert space is:

$$[T_a \hat{\psi}](\vec{k}, \omega) = a^{-1/2} e^{i(\vec{k}\cdot\vec{b}+\omega\tau)} \hat{\psi}(aR(\theta)\vec{k}, \vec{v}\cdot\vec{k}+\omega), \tag{5.9}$$

where the hat ^ stands for Fourier transform, $\vec{k}$ and ω stand as the spatial and temporal frequencies, θ is a rotation angle. The wavelet ψ is a mother wavelet, it must satisfy the condition of admissibility calculated from square integrability. Mostly anisotropic Morlet wavelets can be used in this application with rotation and translation features because of their admissibility:

$$\begin{aligned} \hat{\Psi}(\vec{k}, \omega) &= \hat{\Psi}(\vec{K}) \\ &= |det(D)^{\frac{1}{2}}|(e^{-\frac{1}{2}(\vec{K}-\vec{K}_0)^T D(\vec{K}-\vec{K}_0)} \\ &\quad -e^{-\frac{1}{2}\vec{K}_0^T D\vec{K}_0} e^{-\frac{1}{2}\vec{K}^T D\vec{K}}), \end{aligned} \tag{5.10}$$

where $\vec{K} = (\vec{k}, \omega)^T \in \mathbf{R}^2 \times \mathbf{R}, \vec{K}_0 = (k_{0x}, k_{0y}, \omega_0)^T$, D is a positive definite diagonal matrix and controls the wavelet shape. T means transpose.

If we fix the scale a , τ and ω_0, the filtered image $\mathbf{I}$ can be a 6 dimensional image with dimension $(x, y, t, \alpha, v_x, v_y)$. So for one pixel (x_0, y_0, t_0), the edge orientation α^* and the velocity $\vec{v}^* = (v_x^*, v_y^*)$ can be estimated by:

$$(\vec{v}^*, \alpha^*) = \arg\max_{\vec{v},\alpha} \sum_{x,y,t\in\mathbf{N}} |I(x, y, t, \alpha, v_x, v_y)|^2, \tag{5.11}$$

where $\mathbf{N}$ is the neighborhood set of (x_0, y_0, t_0). From here we find that only the edge portion in the image can be detected. Then segmentation will be obtained by grouping the edges with similar velocities where the local energy is large. For those moving objects, the velocities of their edges are not zero. In conclusion, this method is motion adaptive. Because we need to filter the image sequence in all possible edge orientations and all possible velocities, it is computationally very expensive.

5.2.3.4 Adaptive Frame Differencing with Background Estimation

If the camera is fixed, it is possible that the background could be estimated by averaging the frames over the time. If we assume the camera SNR (Signal to Noise Ratio) is σ, the standard deviation of the difference of two consecutive frames will be $\sqrt{2}\sigma$. And the standard deviation of frame difference averaged of N frames will be $\frac{\sqrt{N}}{\sqrt{N-1}}\sigma$. So when $N \to \infty$, the standard deviation will be σ. Because the background intensity may change from time to time, such as the natural light during the day and night, adaptive background estimation becomes more important. That is:

$$\bar{I}(x, y, t) = \alpha \bar{I}(x, y, t-1) + (1-\alpha) I(x, y, t-1), \tag{5.12}$$

where $\bar{I}(x, y, t)$ is the adaptive background at time t, $I(x, y, t)$ is the image value at position (x, y) at time t. $\alpha \in [0, 1]$ is a constant which is determined by the motion of objects. To have a good estimation of background, the slower the motion, the larger the required value of α. Thus if the difference between current pixel value $I(x, y, t)$ and the adaptive background value $\bar{I}(x, y, t)$ is within a threshold, we can classify this pixel into a background pixel. Otherwise, it will be classified as a pixel on the moving objects.

Since we only record the averaged background information, this technique may not be able to deal with some random motions, such as tree or water motion with wind. To solve this problem, Grimson *et al.* [21] and Kanade *et al.* [33] proposed similar algorithms which estimate several copies of the background pixels. This means we need to estimate the distribution of its background for each pixel. If the distributions of background pixel values are assumed Gaussian, then every pixel has $\mathbf{D} = \{d_1, d_2, ..., d_n\}$, and d_i is $N(0, \sigma_i)$, where $i = 1, 2, ..., n$. Then at each time, we calculate probabilities based on these models. If the largest probability among the models is smaller than a threshold, that is, the sample is not possibly a background pixel, then it is associated with a moving object. This technique is easy to implement in real-time for its simplicity. The result is shown in Fig. 5.3. From the image we eliminate the tree motion, and the person is detected with dots. The problem with this method is that the object can not be very large and the motion of the object can not be very slow. Let us look at Missa sequence in Fig. 5.4. Most parts of the body are relegated to the background. That is not what we want.

As can be seen, the above methods only give the dots which are associated with the moving objects. Because of the noise in the background and the noise inside the objects, some post-processing step is needed to get the object out. Some post-processing algorithm should be studied carefully in these kinds of approaches.

5.2.3.5 Combined PDE Optimization Background Estimation

A different background estimation approach was proposed by Kornprobst *et al.* [37]. As a by-product, it gives the segmentation results. The main limitation of this method is the same as the previous methods with fixed cameras. The goal of this method is to estimate the background frame from the observed image sequence. Thus the sequence segmentation is straightforward. So it needs to operate on the entire sequence, rather than on two or a few frames. Let $N(x, y, t)$ be a given noisy image defined for $(x, y, t) \in \mathbf{R}^2 \times \mathbf{R}_+ \backslash 0$, B^* the recovery background image, $C^*(x, y, t)$ the moving object region. If pixel (x, y) belongs to a moving object at time t, $C(x, y, t) = 0$. Otherwise, $C(x, y, t) = 1$. Then we have:

$$\begin{aligned}\{B^*(x,y), C^*(x,y,t)\} = \quad & \arg\min_{B,C} \textstyle\int_t \int_y \int_x C^2(B-N)^2 dxdydt \\ & +\alpha_c \textstyle\int_t \int_y \int_x (C-1)^2 dxdydt \\ & +\alpha_b^r \textstyle\int_y \int_x \phi_1(|\bigtriangledown B|) dxdy \\ & +\alpha_c^r \textstyle\int_t \int_y \int_x \phi_2(|\bigtriangledown C|) dxdydt\end{aligned}, \quad (5.13)$$

where $\alpha_c, \alpha_b^r, \alpha_c^r$ are positive constants, ϕ_1 and ϕ_2 are functions still to be defined. If $\phi_i(x) = x^2$, $i = 1, 2$, this problem is transfered to the Tikhonov regularization. The problem with this function is that we can not preserve the motion edges. So a robust minimization procedure is to use a convex function ϕ such as:

$$\phi(x) = \sqrt{1 + x^2} - 1. \quad (5.14)$$

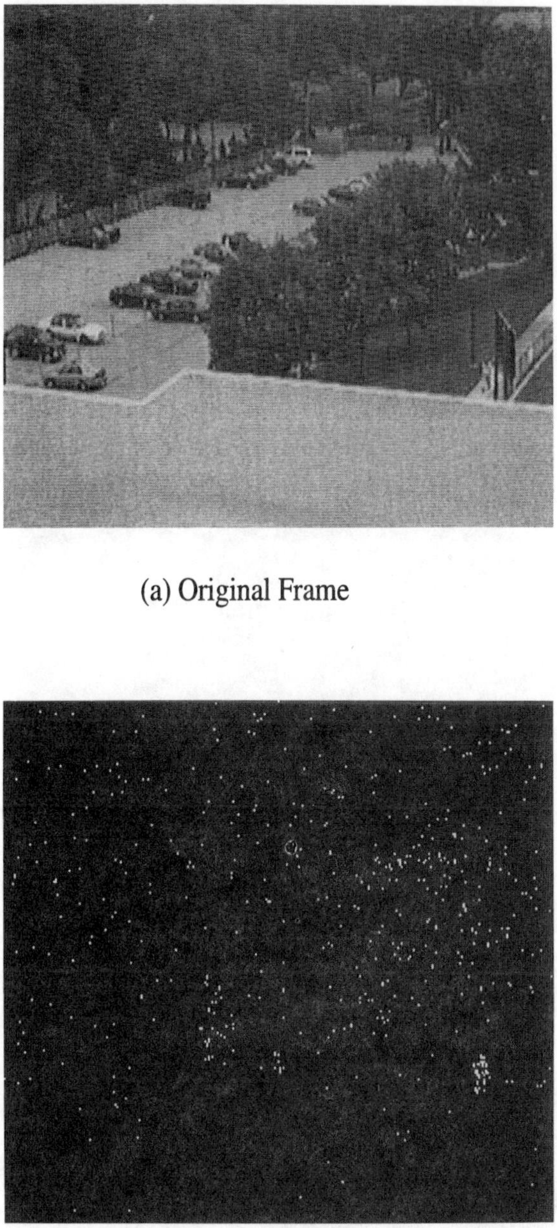

(a) Original Frame

(b) Outlier of Background

Figure 5.3: Adaptive Background Detection for Outdoor Sequence.

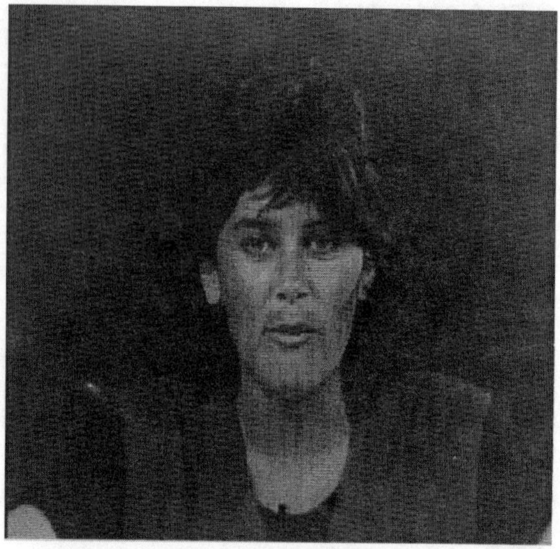

(a) Original Frame

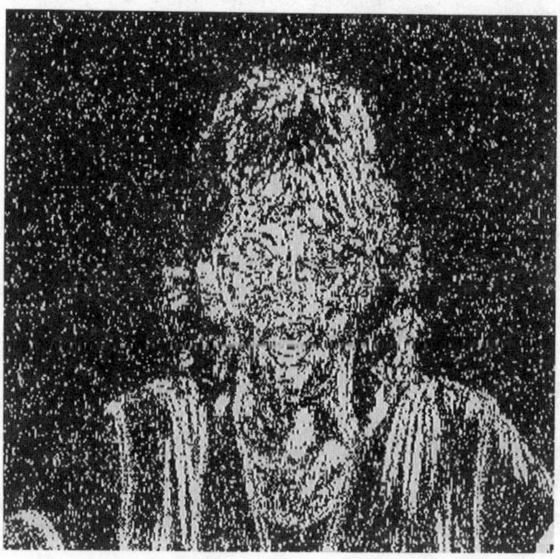

(b) Outlier of Background

Figure 5.4: Adaptive Background Detection for Missa Sequence.
(See color insert)

Geman and Reynolds [19] proposed a method to solve this minimization. Although it is robust, the computation is very expensive. Furthermore, it needs the whole sequence to get the segmentation and background.

5.2.4 Semi-Automatic Segmentation

The techniques we mentioned so far are all automated in that they need no operator intervention other than setting parameters for the algorithms. Recently, there has been some interest in semi-automated techniques [83], [22], [5], [24], where an operator would provide an initial segmentation manually on the first or first few frames of an image sequence. That is, we assign an initial curve which is close to the moving object which we want to segment. Sometimes there are several objects in the scene, but we are only interested in one of them. Sometimes the moving object is not a rigid object, within which there is no uniform motion. Thus, motion segmentation with dense field classification will fail. The other advantage for semi-automatic methods is in computation efficiency and accuracy if we assign an initial curve. This could also eliminate noise effect. Although we call this a semi-automatic technique, many edge detection and segmentation techniques can be incorporated into this method, which will make the moving object boundaries more accurate. The technical nature of the semi-automated techniques is generally different from that of the automated techniques: the former are concerned more with object tracking, while the latter, with object segmentation. This Chapter is concerned mainly with automated techniques.

5.2.5 Our Approach and Their Related Techniques

We developed a new approach to image sequence segmentation that is computationally efficient, does not require a dense motion field, is insensitive to noise and global or background motion, and produces whole objects. This approach contains three parts: global motion compensation, robust frame-differencing, and curve evolution. While the roles of the first two parts are self-evident, the third part, curve evolution, is used to extract *whole* regions or objects from the result of frame-differencing.

For the global motion compensation part, many algorithms can be found in the recent motion estimation literature. Hoetter [28] used a 3 parameter model to estimate the global motion with zoom and pan. Morimoto *et al.* [46]

proposed a fast algorithm which does feature-based multi-resolution motion estimation. Sawhney *et al.* [60] proposed a 3-D perspective model with 12 parameters to obtain global motion by robust M-estimation. Hansen *et al.* [25] used a pyramidal hardware (VFE-100) to estimate the affine motion by multiresolution method iteratively. All of the above algorithms need to estimate the motion vector for every pixel before the global motion is obtained. We adopt Zhang *et al.*'s [82] method which is computationally efficient. It only needs a sparse set of pixels which is evenly distributed in the image frame, which can significantly reduce the amount of computation. To get the accurate global motion, regression is used to reject the outlier of the pixels which are not related to the background. We will discuss this in Section 5.4.

The use of curve evolution for image sequence segmentation has also been investigated in [13] and [50]. Our approach uses a robust variation of frame-differencing and is computationally more efficient than [13], which applies (for each frame) the "color snake" [59] to a combined image intensity and motion field. The original color snake was proposed to detect the objects' contours. The edges of the color image can be extracted from the eigenvalues of local structure tensor. Our approach also differs from [50], which uses simple frame-differencing which is sensitive to noise and global motion.

5.3 A New Multiresolution Technique for Color Image Segmentation

As one of the image sequence segmentation approaches, intra-frame segmentation is now also very important for determining the exact motion boundaries [1]. With the combination of motion segmentation, which only detects moving objects, this method can improve the accuracy of motion boundary location.

In addition to image sequence segmentation applications, the color image segmentation itself is a very important technique. It has many applications, such as skin lesion analysis for cancer detection, object detection and recognition, hyperspectral image segmentation and other industrial and medical application, etc.

The main idea of color image segmentation is to separate the objects from background by color or to separate regions with different colors.

5.3.1 Previous Technique for Color Image Segmentation

There are many color image segmentation methods, such as histogram with threshold, clustering, region splitting and merging, etc. For the histogram method, the critical aspect is how to pick the threshold in the valleys. Lim *et al.* [41] proposed a fuzzy C-means clustering method which is popular since it is adaptive and unsupervised. These methods all consider the image pixels independent. That is to say, there is no relationship between a pixel and its neighbors. The problem of this will make the segmentation noisy and fragmented. To avoid this problem, Chang *et al.* [12] proposed a Bayesian segmentation algorithm with MRF which improved the segmentation. In this method, the spatial constraint is embedded in the MRF minimization. The algorithm considered the three components of color image independent. As we know, the color components are highly correlated. Zhang [80] proposed an EM algorithm image segmentation method which only deals with the gray scale images. Sapiro [59] proposed a color snake which can detect the region boundaries very well and less well in region segmentation.

Saeed *et al.* [56] proposed a multiresolution method for image segmentation, which is still in the traditional multiresolution framework. Although the algorithm will be faster than a single resolution algorithm because of good initial value from the lower resolution segmentation, it still needs to process the whole image in high resolution. To significantly accelerate the computation, new ideas should be brought in the multiresolution implementation.

5.3.2 Our New Multiresolution Technique for Color Image Segmentation

5.3.2.1 Motivation

As we discussed before, we want to look for a technique that can produce a smooth region segmentation. The new technique is unsupervised, and adaptive. Also, it can be significantly faster than single and traditional multiresolution processing. To have such kinds of characteristics, we need to apply the MRF and mean field theory to obtain smooth segmentation. With the EM algorithm, we can adaptively estimate the cluster centers, and also have an unsupervised classification of image pixels, segmentation. To dramatically accelerate the computation, we have developed a new "Narrow Band" multiresolution technique.

In our new technique for color image segmentation, we divide it into four parts. They are: 1) Transform RGB color image to L*u*v* or L*a*b* perceptual color space. 2) EM algorithm for parameter estimation. 3) MRF and mean field theory to produce accurate and smooth regions. 4) A new fast multiresolution technique, "Narrow Band".

5.3.2.2 Color Space Transform

Some algorithms first transform the color image into a gray scale image [17], then solve a gray scale image segmentation problem. This will lose some color information and it is not efficient. The transformation can extract the intensity, the PCT (Principle Component Transform) component as a gray image or convert the image from one color space to another color space. We can process the image in RGB, L*u*v*, L*a*b* and YUV, etc. In Luo *et al.*'s paper [42], they defined their own color space with a special transformation. The goal of the color space transformation is to find a good representation in which the distance between two colors is proportional to the human eye perception. That means the larger the distance in the new color space measurement, the larger the color difference the eyes sense. L*u*v* and L*a*b are two common perceptual color spaces [75] which are widely used in many color image processing algorithms [59], [12].

Next we discuss the transformation from RGB to L*u*v* and L*a*b*. CIE 1976 ($L^*a^*b^*$)-space and ($L^*u^*v^*$)-space are two uniform color spaces. Both are related to the conceptual color space. Here, the uniform means that the Euclidean distance in these spaces is proportional to the perceptual difference sensed by human eyes.

According to Wyszecki *et al.*'s book [75], both of their conversions will use the CIE(**X,Y,Z**) space. From (R,G,B)- space to (X,Y,Z)-space, we have:

$$\begin{pmatrix} X \\ Y \\ Z \end{pmatrix} = \begin{pmatrix} 0.60700 & 0.17400 & 0.20100 \\ 0.29900 & 0.58700 & 0.11400 \\ 0.00000 & 0.06600 & 1.11700 \end{pmatrix} \begin{pmatrix} R \\ G \\ B \end{pmatrix}, \tag{5.15}$$

where R, G and B are a value between 0 and 1. This is a linear transformation.

From (X, Y, Z)-space to $(L^*a^*b^*)$-space conversion, we have

$$\begin{aligned} L^* &= \begin{bmatrix} 116\left(\frac{Y}{Y_n}\right)^{1/3} - 16 & if \frac{Y}{Y_n} \geq 0.008856 \\ 903.3\frac{Y}{Y_n} & otherwise \end{bmatrix} \\ a^* &= 500\left[\left(\frac{X}{X_n}\right)^{1/3} - \left(\frac{Y}{Y_n}\right)^{1/3}\right] \\ b^* &= 200\left[\left(\frac{Y}{Y_n}\right)^{1/3} - \left(\frac{Z}{Z_n}\right)^{1/3}\right], \end{aligned} \tag{5.16}$$

where X_n=0.982, Y_n=1.000 , Z_n=1.183.

From (X, Y, Z)-space to $(L^*u^*v^*)$-space conversion, we have:

$$\begin{aligned} L^* &= \begin{bmatrix} 116\left(\frac{Y}{Y_n}\right)^{1/3} - 16 & if \frac{Y}{Y_n} \geq 0.008856 \\ 903.3\frac{Y}{Y_n} & otherwise \end{bmatrix} \\ u^* &= 13L^*(u' - u'_n) \\ v^* &= 13L^*(v' - v'_n), \end{aligned} \tag{5.17}$$

In the above equation, u', v' and u'_n, v'_n are calculated from:

$$\begin{aligned} u' &= \frac{4X}{X+15Y+3Z} \\ v' &= \frac{9Y}{X+15Y+3Z} \\ u'_n &= \frac{4X_n}{X_n+15Y_n+3Z_n} = 0.201116 \\ v'_n &= \frac{9Y_n}{X_n+15Y_n+3Z_n} = 0.460806, \end{aligned} \tag{5.18}$$

where X_n=0.982, Y_n=1.000, Z_n=1.183.

Both of the above transformations from (X, Y, Z) are nonlinear.

5.3.2.3 Color (Vector) Image Segmentation

Our new color image segmentation method is an extension of Zhang's work [80]. Zhang's work was originally for gray scale image segmentation. We extend this work to a color image or a vector image segmentation where the number of pixel value dimensions can be more than one. Generally, the number of dimensions is three for color images.

Let $\mathbf{y}$ be an observed image. $\mathbf{\Phi}$ is the parameters for an color image, which includes cluster center mean $\{\mu_j\}$, cluster center covariance matrix $\{\Sigma_j\}$, and cluster proportions $\{\pi_j\}$, $j = 1...K$. And $\mathbf{z}$ is the segmentation of $\mathbf{y}$. For example, segmentation for i^{th} pixel in the image is:

$$\mathbf{z}_i = \begin{bmatrix} 0 \\ 0 \\ \cdot \\ \cdot \\ \cdot \\ 1 \\ \cdot \\ \cdot \\ \cdot \\ 0 \end{bmatrix}, \tag{5.19}$$

where 1 is in the jth position of the array, thus this i^{th} pixel in the image belongs to the cluster j.

With the mean field theory, the formulation of segmentation will be changed to

$$\mathbf{z}_i = \begin{bmatrix} p_0 \\ p_1 \\ \cdot \\ \cdot \\ \cdot \\ p_j \\ \cdot \\ \cdot \\ \cdot \\ p_{K-1} \end{bmatrix} \tag{5.20}$$

and

$$\sum_{j=0}^{K-1} p_j = 1, 0 \leq p_j \leq 1, j = 0, ..., K-1, \tag{5.21}$$

where the segmentation is represented by the probabilities of each cluster center. We determine that the ith pixel belongs to cluster j if p_j is the largest among the K clusters.

After we have above notation, we now go over our image segmentation algorithm. For given $\mathbf{\Phi}$, or given the parameters of the clusters, we want to find the classification. This leads to the problem of Maximum A Posterior

(MAP) inference. The formulation is:

$$\begin{aligned}\hat{\mathbf{z}} &= \arg\max_{\mathbf{z}} \log p(\mathbf{z}|\mathbf{y}, \mathbf{\Phi}) \\ &= \arg\max_{\mathbf{z}}[\log p(\mathbf{y}|\mathbf{z}, \mathbf{\Phi}) + \log p(\mathbf{z}|\mathbf{\Phi})].\end{aligned} \tag{5.22}$$

For the mean field theory, we need to consider the conditional mean inference to get the MAP. Then, Eqn. (5.22) will be converted to:

$$\hat{\mathbf{z}} = < \mathbf{z}|\mathbf{y}, \mathbf{\Phi} > . \tag{5.23}$$

Based on the above formulations and cluster center parameters, we can easily classify the observed image $\mathbf{y}$ and obtain a segmentation.

Because in most cases the cluster centers are not available, or the cluster centers are different from image to image, we need to estimate the cluster centers based on the image itself. So, this leads to a parameter estimation problem. To find an estimation of $\mathbf{\Phi}$, we use the Maximum Likelihood method (ML), that is:

$$\hat{\mathbf{\Phi}}_{ML} = \arg\max_{\mathbf{\Phi}} \log p(\mathbf{y}|\mathbf{\Phi}). \tag{5.24}$$

The EM algorithm gives a connection between MAP and ML processings. The purpose of using the EM algorithm is to solve the ML inference problem, while it can get a by-product with conditional mean inference, the segmentation. The algorithm is carried out iteratively with the E-step and M-step. At the beginning, we need to initialize the parameters as $\hat{\mathbf{\Phi}}^{(0)}$. With the E-step, we compute:

$$Q(\mathbf{\Phi}|\hat{\mathbf{\Phi}}^{(p)}) = < \log p((\mathbf{y}, \mathbf{z}|\mathbf{\Phi})|\mathbf{y}, \hat{\mathbf{\Phi}}^{(p)}) > . \tag{5.25}$$

With the M-step, we update $\hat{\mathbf{\Phi}}$ by:

$$\hat{\mathbf{\Phi}}^{(p+1)} = \arg\max_{\mathbf{\Phi}} Q(\mathbf{\Phi}|\hat{\mathbf{\Phi}}^{(p)}). \tag{5.26}$$

In the above Eqn. (5.25), we have:

$$\begin{aligned}\log p((\mathbf{y}, \mathbf{z}|\mathbf{\Phi})|\mathbf{y}, \hat{\mathbf{\Phi}}^{(p)}) = \quad & \log p((\mathbf{y}|\mathbf{z}, \mathbf{\Phi})|\mathbf{y}, \hat{\mathbf{\Phi}}^{(p)}) \\ & + \log p((\mathbf{z}|\mathbf{\Phi})|\mathbf{y}, \hat{\mathbf{\Phi}}^{(p)}),\end{aligned} \tag{5.27}$$

where the first term is a multivariable Gaussian density, the second term is an MRF distribution which is associated with the smoothness constraint.

For the entire segmentation processing, here are the estimation formulas:

$$
\begin{aligned}
\hat{z}_{ik}^{(p)} &= E[z_{ik}|\mathbf{y}, \hat{\mathbf{\Phi}}^{(p)}] = \frac{\hat{\pi}_k^{(p)} f(\mathbf{y}_i|\mathbf{e}_k, \hat{\mathbf{\Phi}}^{(p)})}{\sum_{j=1}^{K} \hat{\pi}_k^{(p)} f(\mathbf{y}_i|\mathbf{e}_j, \hat{\mathbf{\Phi}}^{(p)})} \\
\hat{\mu}_k^{(p+1)} &= \frac{1}{\hat{N}_k^{(p)}} \sum_{i=1}^{n} \hat{z}_{ik}^{(p)} \mathbf{y}_i \\
\hat{\Sigma}_k^{(p+1)} &= \frac{1}{\hat{N}_k^{(p)}} \sum_{i=1}^{n} \hat{z}_{ik}^{(p)} (\mathbf{y}_i - \hat{\mu}_k^{(p+1)})(\mathbf{y}_i - \hat{\mu}_k^{(p+1)})^T \\
\hat{N}_k^{(p)} &= \sum_{i=1}^{n} \hat{z}_{ik}^{(p)}, \hat{\pi}_k^{(p)} = \frac{\hat{N}_k^{(p)}}{N},
\end{aligned}
\tag{5.28}
$$

5.3.2.4 Multiresolution

Because an EM algorithm is used, the computation load is very heavy. The solution for this is using a multiresolution method. The most traditional multiresolution technique is: Assuming that the low resolution segmentation is already obtained, we propagate the result (segmentation) to high level resolution as initial values. Then, we perform the calculation again. Because we use the "good" initial value for high resolution, the calculation will be much faster than in a single resolution.

To significantly accelerate the computation, we have developed a new multiresolution technique, "Narrow Band," in which the calculation is only performed in a strip around the boundary area, other than the whole image domain. Let us look at Fig. 5.5. (a) is the previous multi-resolution method, in which the calculation in the high resolution will be performed over the whole image, such as [40] and [56]. (b) is the new technique method, in which the calculation in high resolution will only be performed in the boundary area as shown. The pixels in other area are already classified. So the computation is dramatically down. Usually, the width of the narrow band is about 10 pixels. The complexity of this method can be reduced to $O(n)$ from $O(n^2)$ with the assumption of image size $n \times n$.

To obtain the low resolution level image faster, we only use the sub-sample technique, that is, just pick one value of the 4 pixels to represent the low resolution image value.

When we propagate the result from low resolution to high level resolution, we copy the cluster centers from low resolution. Also, we set the segmentation value of the high resolution pixels as that of the associated pixel in low resolution. Then, we process the EM algorithm again within the boundary area.

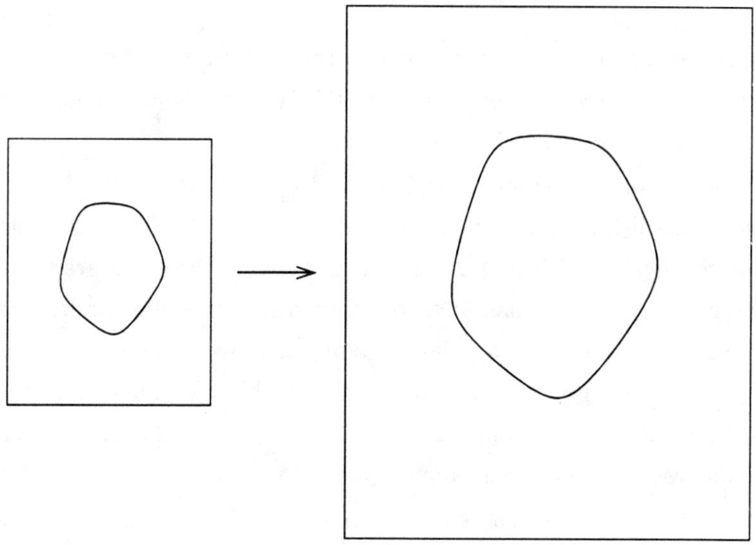

(a) Previous multiresolution technique

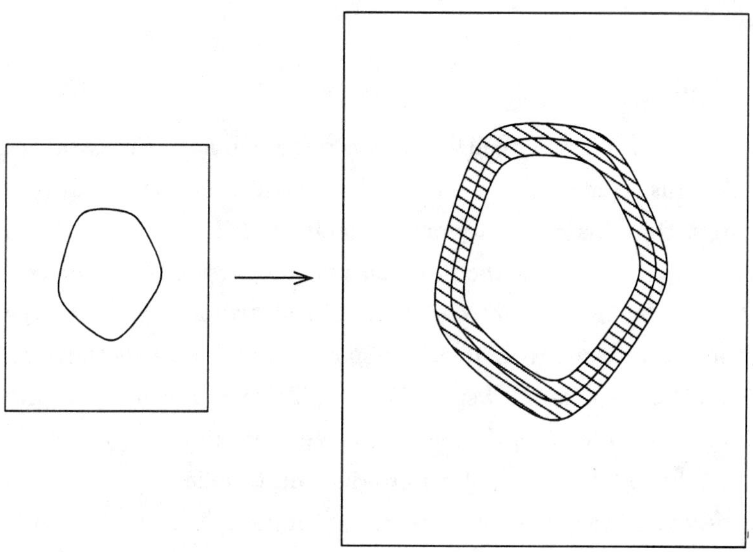

(b) New multiresolution technique

Figure 5.5: Multi-Resolution Schemes: a) Previous Method, b) Our Method.

5.3.3 Experimental Results

Our image segmentation has been tested in the medical application, skill lesion segmentation, and TV sequences. We use L*u*v* color space. The results for skin lesions are displayed in Fig. 5.6 and Fig. 5.7.

For the above skin lesion image, Fig. 5.6, with a size of 924x748, the processing time using the new multiresolution technique (4 levels, 2 clusters) is about 46 seconds in a PII 300 machine with Linux operating system. On the contrary, it will take more than 383 seconds with the traditional multiresolution method (4 levels). And in a single resolution, it will take more than 1941 seconds. From our experimental results, it is about 8 times faster for our method than the traditional multiresolution method, and 45 times faster than single multiresolution methods on average.

The results for TV sequences are shown on Fig. 5.8. We use 3 multi-levels, 7 clusters, image size of 360 × 288 pixels, and it took about 3 minutes CPU time in PII 300 machine. For this image, if we use (R,G,B) color space other than the perceptual $L^*U^*V^*$ color space, this will lead the segmentation to split the background into two regions.

5.3.4 Summary

We have developed a new multiresolution technique for color image segmentation, which is significantly faster than single and traditional multiresolution processing with the same quality of segmentation. It has dramatically lowered the computation load, while the processing is only carried out in the boundary area, "Narrow Band", in high resolution. The algorithm is based on the color (vector) image with multivariable Gaussian distribution model for individual pixels and MRF mean field for spatial model. This will give more accurate and smoother results. EM algorithm is used to estimate the cluster centers adaptively and robustly. It is straightforward that this technique can be extended to a hyperspectral image or texture image segmentation. The other extension can be an image sequence intra-frame segmentation. When we have the previous intra-frame segmentation, we can propagate it to the current frame, and process the boundary area where the pixels need to be refined for the segmentation.

The disadvantage of this algorithm is that we need to give the number of clusters. And the computation will increase dramatically while the number of

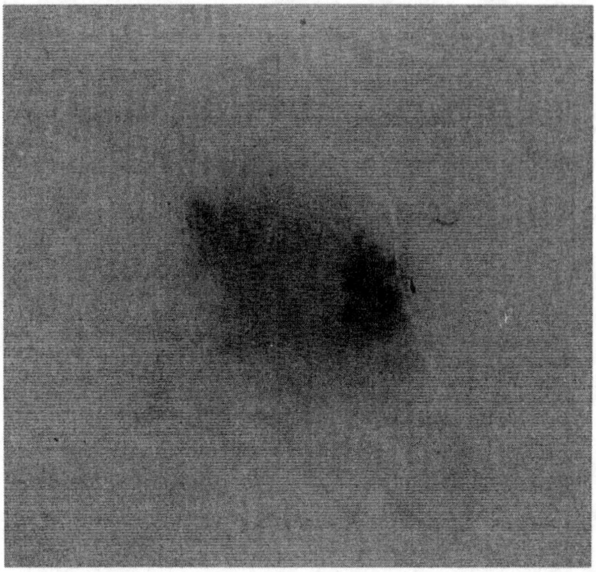

(a) Original Image (924x748)

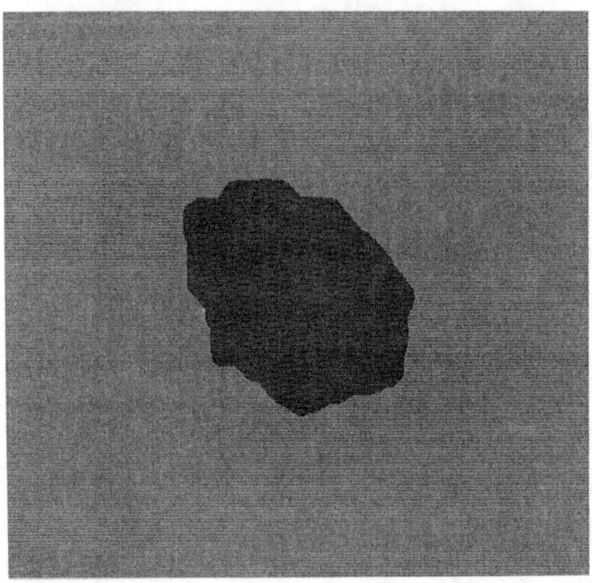

(b) Segmentation Result (2 clusters)

Figure 5.6: Image Segmentation for Skin Lesion 1.
(See color insert)

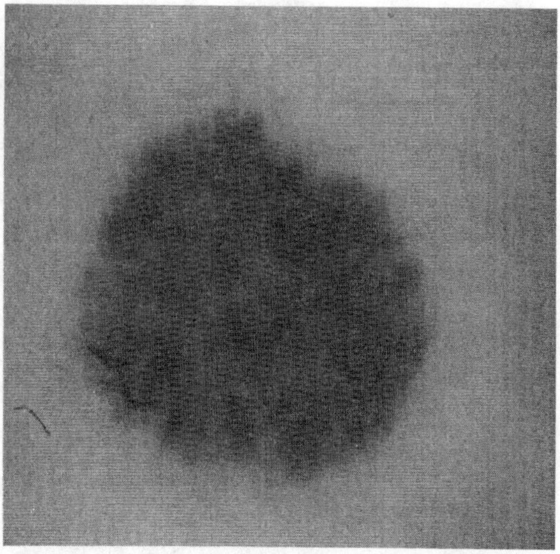

(a) Original Image

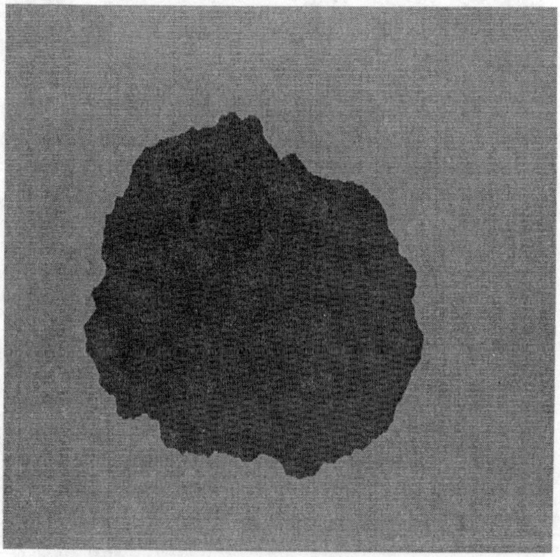

(b) Segmentation Result

Figure 5.7: Image Segmentation for Skin Lesion 2.
(See color insert)

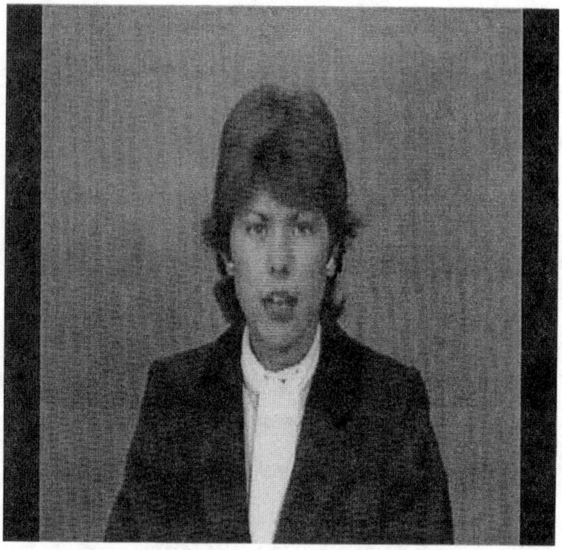

(a) One Frame of Claire Sequence

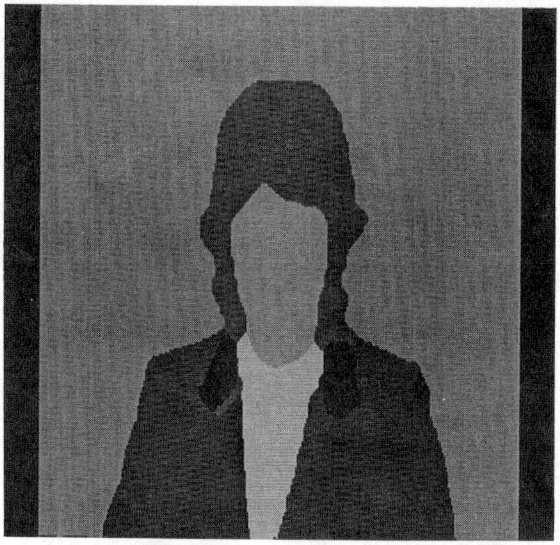

(b) Segmentation Result (7 clusters)

Figure 5.8: Image Segmentation for One Frame of Claire Sequence.
(See color insert)

clusters increases.

5.4 Our Approach for Image Sequence Segmentation

We will begin by introducing some notation. For the sake of simplicity, we view an image sequence as a function defined over continuous space and time. Specifically, let a pixel or a spatial location be denoted by a vector, $\mathbf{x} = [x_1, x_2]^t$, where $\mathbf{x} \in \mathbf{M}$, which is a bounded region in the 2D plane. Then, an image sequence can be represented as $f(\mathbf{x}, t)$, where t is the time. Our approach to image sequence segmentation contains three parts, namely, global motion compensation, robust frame-differencing and curve evolution.

5.4.1 Global Motion Compensation

We have introduced the motion estimation and global motion estimation in Section 5.2. Here we review Zhang *et al.*'s [82] method to estimate the global motion. This is a fast, robust and efficient method. The algorithm is composed of three parts: block matching for sparse set of points, global motion estimation by Taylor expansion and robust regression by probabilistic thresholds.

In this method, a 6-parameter affine motion model is used. This model was introduced in Section 5.2 with Eqn. (5.3). Although we can use Eqn. (5.5), perspective model from our experimental results, the final global compensation results are almost the same as that of perspective model, but the computation load for an affine model is less. So in this Chapter, we only use the affine motion model.

5.4.1.1 Block Matching for Sparse Set of Points

The first step of Zhang *et al.*'s method is to obtain a sparse set of displacement (p, q). The sparse set of pixels is evenly distributed on the sequence frames. With these initial motion displacements, an affine model is used to fit these motion displacements. A pixel may relate to a moving object if it fails the affine model. Generally, the number of sparse set is from 49 to 500 as [82] suggested. This method dramatically reduces the computational load for motion estimation.

A block matching method is used to estimate the motion displacement for the sparse set of pixels. This is a small difference from the general block-matching method. The algorithm used is to find the pixel and its small neighbor (such as (15×15)) matching a pixel in the next frame. For general block-matching algorithm, the image frame is divided into blocks, and the displacement of best matching will be the motion vector of this block. In this Chapter, we use full searching block-matching which will give a good estimation, but the computation will be a little higher. Some new techniques, such as the multiresolution blockmatching algorithm, can obtain high performance in speed. The search window size is 64×64.

5.4.1.2 Global Motion Estimation by the Taylor Expansion Equation

With the initial best matching displacement (p, q), a Taylor expansion-based affine motion estimation is introduced by Zhang *et al.* [82].

Using the Taylor expansion equation, the local compensation error function at a block position (i, j) can be expressed by:

$$\begin{aligned} E_{i,j}(u,v) = \ & \bar{E}_{i,j}(p_{i,j}, q_{i,j}) + (u - p_{i,j})\frac{\partial E_{i,j}}{\partial u} + (v - q_{i,j})\frac{\partial E_{i,j}}{\partial v} \\ & + \tfrac{1}{2}(u - p_{i,j})^2\frac{\partial^2 E_{i,j}}{\partial u^2} + \tfrac{1}{2}(v - q_{i,j})^2\frac{\partial^2 E_{i,j}}{\partial v^2} \\ & + (u - p_{i,j})(v - q_{i,j})\frac{\partial^2 E_{i,j}}{\partial u \partial v}. \end{aligned} \tag{5.29}$$

Let **S** be the 3×3 values of the motion compensation error surrounding the best matched displacement (p, q) as:

$$\begin{aligned} S = \ & (e(p-1, q-1), e(p-1, q), e(p-1, q+1), \\ & e(p, q-1), e(p, q), e(p, q+1), \\ & e(p+1, q-1), e(p+1, q), e(p+1, q+1))^t, \end{aligned} \tag{5.30}$$

where $e(x, y)$ denotes the value of the motion compensation error at position (x, y). Using differential operators, the partial derivative items in Eqn. (5.29) can be expressed as:

$$\begin{aligned} \bar{E}(p,q) &= \tfrac{1}{9}(-1, 2, -1, 2, 5, 2, -1, 2, -1)\mathbf{S} \\ \frac{\partial E(p,q)}{\partial u} &= \tfrac{1}{6}(-1, 0, 1, -1, 0, 1, -1, 0, -1)\mathbf{S} \\ \frac{\partial E(p,q)}{\partial v} &= \tfrac{1}{6}(-1, -1, -1, 0, 0, 0, 1, 1, 1)\mathbf{S} \\ \frac{\partial E^2(p,q)}{\partial u^2} &= \tfrac{1}{3}(1, -2, 1, 1, -2, 1, 1, -2, 1)\mathbf{S} \\ \frac{\partial E^2(p,q)}{\partial v^2} &= \tfrac{1}{3}(1, 1, 1, -2, -2, -2, 1, 1, 1)\mathbf{S} \\ \frac{\partial E^2(p,q)}{\partial u \partial v} &= \tfrac{1}{4}(1, 0, -1, 0, 0, 0, -1, 0, 1)\mathbf{S}, \end{aligned} \tag{5.31}$$

To facilitate discussion, we can rewrite Eqn. 5.3 in a matrix form as:

$$\begin{pmatrix} u \\ v \end{pmatrix} = \mathbf{P}(\mathbf{x}_{ij})\mathbf{a}, \tag{5.32}$$

where

$$\mathbf{P}(\mathbf{x}_{ij}) = \left\{ \begin{array}{cccccc} 1 & x_{ij} & y_{ij} & 0 & 0 & 0 \\ 0 & 0 & 0 & 1 & x_{ij} & y_{ij} \end{array} \right\} \tag{5.33}$$

$$\mathbf{a} = (a_0, a_1, a_2, a_3, a_4, a_5)^t. \tag{5.34}$$

If we substitute (u, v) in Eqn. (5.29) by Eqn. (5.32), the global motion estimation can be obtained by minimizing:

$$\sum_{i,j} E_{i,j}(\mathbf{P}(\mathbf{x}_{ij})\mathbf{a}), \tag{5.35}$$

where $\mathbf{x}_{ij}$ denotes the center position of the block (i, j). This leads to Euler's equation as:

$$\frac{\partial \sum_{i,j} E_{i,j}(\mathbf{P}(\mathbf{x}_{ij})\mathbf{a})}{\partial \mathbf{a}} = 0, \tag{5.36}$$

and therefore:

$$\mathbf{Aa} - \mathbf{b} = 0, \tag{5.37}$$

where:

$$\mathbf{A} = \sum_{i,j} \left\{ \begin{array}{cc} \frac{\partial^2 E_{i,j}}{\partial u^2}\mathbf{U}(\mathbf{x}_{ij}) & \frac{\partial^2 E_{i,j}}{\partial u \partial v}\mathbf{U}(\mathbf{x}_{ij}) \\ \frac{\partial^2 E_{i,j}}{\partial u \partial v}\mathbf{U}(\mathbf{x}_{ij}) & \frac{\partial^2 E_{i,j}}{\partial v^2}\mathbf{U}(\mathbf{x}_{ij}) \end{array} \right\} \tag{5.38}$$

$$\mathbf{U}(\mathbf{x_{ij}}) = \left\{ \begin{array}{ccc} 1 & x & y \\ x & x^2 & xy \\ y & xy & y^2 \end{array} \right\} \tag{5.39}$$

$$\mathbf{b} = \sum_{i,j} \mathbf{P}(\mathbf{x}_{ij})^t \begin{pmatrix} -\frac{\partial E_{i,j}}{\partial u} + \frac{\partial^2 Ei,j}{\partial u^2} p_{i,j} + \frac{\partial^2 E_{i,j}}{\partial u \partial v} q_{i,j} \\ -\frac{\partial E_{i,j}}{\partial v} + \frac{\partial^2 Ei,j}{\partial v^2} q_{i,j} + \frac{\partial^2 E_{i,j}}{\partial u \partial v} p_{i,j} \end{pmatrix}. \tag{5.40}$$

By solving the Eqn. (5.37), we can obtain the affine coefficients as:

$$\mathbf{a} = \mathbf{A}^{-1}\mathbf{b}. \tag{5.41}$$

Here is an example to test this algorithm. Let us look at Fig. 5.9, (a) and (b) are two consecutive frames. There is a vehicle in the sequence. (c) is the directly difference. And (d) is the compensated error. Comparing (c) and (d), we found the moving object easily without background noise.

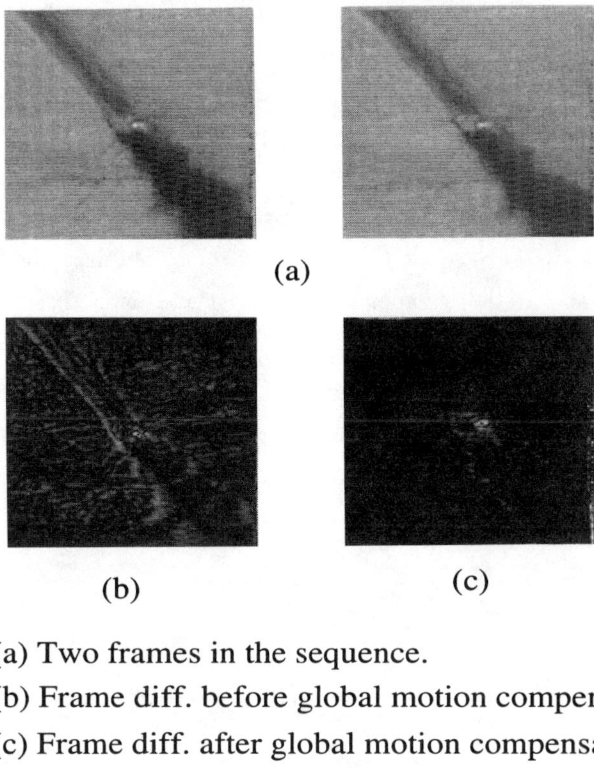

(a)

(b) (c)

(a) Two frames in the sequence.

(b) Frame diff. before global motion compensation.

(c) Frame diff. after global motion compensation.

Figure 5.9: Frame Difference Before and After Global Motion Compensation.

5.4.1.3 Robust Regression Using Probabilistic Thresholds

To eliminate the local motion or object motion influence, Zhang *et al.* [82] proposed a robust regression method, which is based on the statistical distribution of the compensation error and uses a pair of probability thresholds to classify inliers and outliers. The basic idea of this method is to assume that in each iteration, only a small portion of the compensation error, which is related to local motion or outliers, is much greater than the average compensation error. The classification is based on the assumption that the motion parameters are computed only using inliers. Technically, this is divided into 2 steps. One step is to determine the outlier when the error is larger than a threshold, a lower threshold. The other step is from the outlier points. We may find the misclassification in which the error is smaller than another threshold, an upper threshold. When this process is repeated a certain number of times, we shall be able to eliminate the local motion pixel influence and obtain a good global motion estimation and motion compensation. Upper and lower thresholds are calculated as:

$$\begin{aligned} T_{upper} &= \bar{E} + C_{upper}\sigma \\ T_{lower} &= \bar{E} + C_{lower}\sigma, \end{aligned} \tag{5.42}$$

where

$$\bar{E} = \frac{1}{K} \sum_{\mathbf{x}_{i,j} \in Inliers} E_{i,j}(\mathbf{P}(\mathbf{x}_{ij})\mathbf{a}) \tag{5.43}$$

$$\sigma = \sqrt{\frac{1}{K-1} \sum_{\mathbf{x}_{i,j} \in Inliers} (E_{i,j}(\mathbf{P}(\mathbf{x}_{ij})\mathbf{a}) - \bar{E})^2}, \tag{5.44}$$

where K is the number of inliers, $E_{i,j}$ is motion estimate error at position (i, j). P is defined in Eqn. (5.33), and $\mathbf{a}$ is defined in Eqn. (5.34). C_{upper} and C_{lower} are two constants.

5.4.2 Robust Frame Differencing

5.4.2.1 The Tensor Method

To estimate a local orientation in an image, one direct method is to compute the gradient. Let $g(x, y)$ be an image, its gradient is $(\frac{\partial g}{\partial x}, \frac{\partial g}{\partial y})$. We could use the magnitude of the gradient as an orientation-independent certainty measurement:

$$|\nabla g| = \left[\left(\frac{\partial g}{\partial x} \right)^2 + \left(\frac{\partial g}{\partial y}^2 \right) \right]^{1/2}, \tag{5.45}$$

and determine the direction of the orientation by:

$$\phi = \arctan\left(\frac{\partial g}{\partial x} / \frac{\partial g}{\partial y} \right). \tag{5.46}$$

The problem with this method is that the orientation is not reliable in practical images when there is some noise in the image. A new robust orientation estimation should be developed, which can solve this problem.

Tensor in Frequency Domain Bigun and Granlund [7], [31] developed a method which can determine the local orientation more reliably in the Fourier domain. We will review this technique as described in Jahne's book [31]. The procedure used is:

- With a window function, we select a small local neighborhood from an image.
- We perform the Fourier transform in a local windowed image.
- Local orientation is then determined by fitting a straight line to the spectral density distribution. This yields the angle of the local orientation from the slope of the line.

The main idea is to fit a straight line to the spectral density in the Fourier domain. We cannot solve this problem exactly since it is generally overdetermined, but we can obtain a solution by minimizing the measurement error. So, we have:

$$J = \int_{-\infty}^{\infty} d^2k d^2(\mathbf{k}, \bar{\mathbf{k}}) |\hat{g}(\mathbf{k})|^2 \rightarrow minimum, \tag{5.47}$$

where $\bar{\mathbf{k}}$ is the unit vector of which represents the orientation in the Fourier domain. $|\hat{g}(\mathbf{k})|^2$ is the spectral density. The distance function is abbreviated using $d(\mathbf{k}, \bar{\mathbf{k}})$.

From Fig. 5.10, the distance vector d can be:

$$\mathbf{d} = \mathbf{k} - (\mathbf{k}^T \mathbf{k})\bar{\mathbf{k}}. \tag{5.48}$$

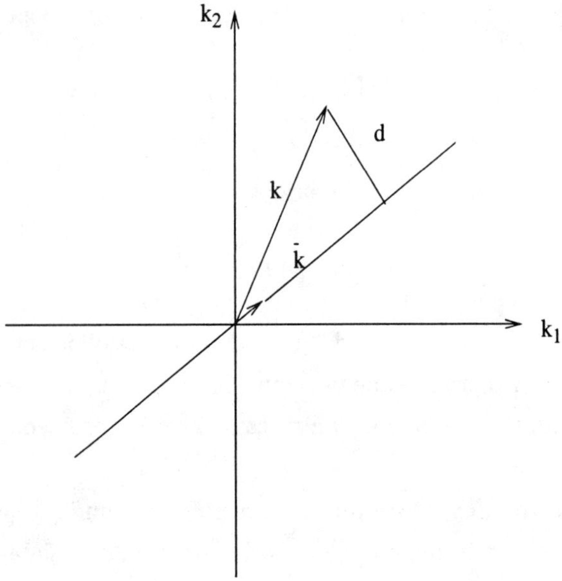

Figure 5.10: Distance $d(\mathbf{k}, \bar{\mathbf{k}})$ Calculation [31].

The square of the distance is then given by:

$$\begin{aligned} |\mathbf{d}|^2 &= [\mathbf{k} - (\mathbf{k}^T k)\bar{\mathbf{k}}]^T[\mathbf{k} - (\mathbf{k}^T k)\bar{\mathbf{k}}] \\ &= \mathbf{k}^T\mathbf{k} - (\mathbf{k}^T\bar{\mathbf{k}})^2 \\ &= \bar{\mathbf{k}}^T(\mathbf{I}(\mathbf{k}^T\mathbf{k}) - (\mathbf{k}\mathbf{k}^T)\bar{\mathbf{k}})^2. \end{aligned} \tag{5.49}$$

Substituting this expression into Eqn. (5.47), we obtain:

$$J = \bar{\mathbf{k}}^T\mathbf{J}\bar{\mathbf{k}}, \tag{5.50}$$

where $\mathbf{J}$ is called tensor with the diagonal elements:

$$J_{pp} = \sum_{q \neq p} \int_{-\infty}^{\infty} d^n k k_q^2 |\hat{g}(\mathbf{k})|^2, \tag{5.51}$$

and the off-diagonal elements:

$$J_{pq} = -\int_{-\infty}^{\infty} d^n k k_p k_q |\hat{g}(\mathbf{k})|^2, \tag{5.52}$$

where n is the number of the space dimensions.

In the two-dimensional case, that is n=2, we can write:

$$J(\bar{\mathbf{k}}) = \begin{bmatrix} \bar{k}_1 & \bar{k}_2 \end{bmatrix} \begin{bmatrix} J_{11} & J_{12} \\ J_{12} & J_{22} \end{bmatrix} \begin{bmatrix} \bar{k}_1 \\ \bar{k}_2 \end{bmatrix}. \tag{5.53}$$

From this equation, we can readily find $\bar{\mathbf{k}}$ so that J shows a minimum value. So, this is an eigen decomposition problem as:

$$J(\bar{\mathbf{k}}) = \begin{bmatrix} \bar{k}_1' & \bar{k}_2' \end{bmatrix} \begin{bmatrix} J_1 & 0 \\ 0 & J_2 \end{bmatrix} \begin{bmatrix} \bar{k}_1' \\ \bar{k}_2' \end{bmatrix} = J_1 \bar{k}_1'^2 + J_2 \bar{k}_2'^2. \tag{5.54}$$

If $J_1 < J_2$, then J is minimal in the $\bar{k}_1\prime$ direction.

Tensor in Spatial Domain Jahne's book [31] also gave information about tensor in spatial domain to estimate the local orientation. In the spatial domain, the diagonal elements are:

$$J_{pp} = \sum_{q \neq p} \int_{window} \left(\frac{\partial g}{\partial x_q} \right)^2 d^2x, \tag{5.55}$$

and the off-diagonal elements are:

$$J_{pq} = - \int_{window} \frac{\partial g}{\partial x_p} \frac{\partial g}{\partial x_q} d^2x. \tag{5.56}$$

The integration area corresponds to the window we use to select a local neighborhood. On a discrete image matrix, the integral can be entirely performed by convolution. Integration over a window limiting the local neighborhood means convolution with a smoothing mask B of the corresponding size. The partial derivatives are computed with the derivative operators D_x and D_y. Consequently, the elements of the tensor are essentially computed with nonlinear operators:

$$J_{pq} = B(D_p \cdot D_q). \tag{5.57}$$

It is important to note that the operators J_{pq} are nonlinear operators containing both linear convolution operations and nonlinear point operations in the spatial domain. In particular, this means that we must not interchange the multiplication of the partial derivative with the smoothing operations.

5.4.2.2 Tensor Method for Robust Frame Differencing

Due to image noise, frame difference at the non-moving part of the scene can often be much larger (in magnitude) than that in the moving parts, making it an unreliable indication of object motion, (see Fig. 5.11.(b)).

In this work, we use a robust frame difference from the 3D (spatial-temporal) structure tensor [30], [23]. Like the Lie group wavelets, this technique involves spatial and temporal filtering and is highly noise resistant. Unlike the Lie group wavelets, however, it achieves motion-adaptiveness locally without having to filter along all possible motion directions and edge directions.

The 3D structure tensor technique was originally proposed for optical flow computation (motion estimation) and has been shown to perform significantly better than previous techniques [30], [23]. For an image sequence $f(\mathbf{x}, t)$, the 3D structure tensor is a 3×3 matrix, defined as:

$$\mathbf{R}(\mathbf{x}, t) = \int h(\mathbf{x} - \mathbf{x}', t - t')\nabla f(\mathbf{x}, t)\nabla f(\mathbf{x}, t)^T \, d\mathbf{x} \, dt, \tag{5.58}$$

where $h(\mathbf{x}, t)$ is a spatial-temporal Gaussian function and ∇ is the gradient operator. Intuitively, the 3D structure tensor can be viewed as a correlation matrix for the gradient vectors in Eqn. (6.3) in a principle component analysis. Indeed, under relatively mild conditions, the eigen vector associated with the smallest eigenvalue of $\mathbf{R}(\mathbf{x}, t)$ is associated with the direction of motion for the pixel at $(\mathbf{x}, t)$. This eigenvalue, denoted by $\lambda_3(\mathbf{x}, t)$, the smallest eigenvalue, can be viewed as the average power of the frame difference along the motion direction. We found that compared to the power of the simple frame difference, $\lambda_3(\mathbf{x}, t)$ is much more robust to noise. Hence, it is taken as a robust version of the frame difference and used for image sequence segmentation.

To calculate the eigenvalues, a Jacobi transformation method [54] is used because of the symmetric matrix of structure tensor and its low dimensions.

To test the local tensor field, we have a synthetic image sequence whose first frame is shown in Fig. 5.12.(a). There are two rectangle "objects" in the sequence. The upper one has a velocity of 2 pixel/frame going down. The other one does not have motion. (b) is the largest eigenvalue field. (c) is the second largest eigenvalue field, and (d) is the smallest eigenvalue field. Table 5.4.2.2 is the average value of eigenvalues of different areas of the above sequence, which include Moving Edges 1, Moving Edges 2, Moving Objects Still Edges, Still Objects and Still Background. Moving Edges 1 are the edges associated with the edges perpendicular to the motion direction. Moving Edges 2 are the edges along with the motion direction. We found that in the smallest eigenvalue field, the non-moving pixels' value is not larger than 0.238 which reflects the noise level. And all moving pixels either in the edges or inside the object are larger than 0.5. In the moving object area, the average of this value is more than 0.50 which is as large as 3 times of that on the background. The largest eigenvalue

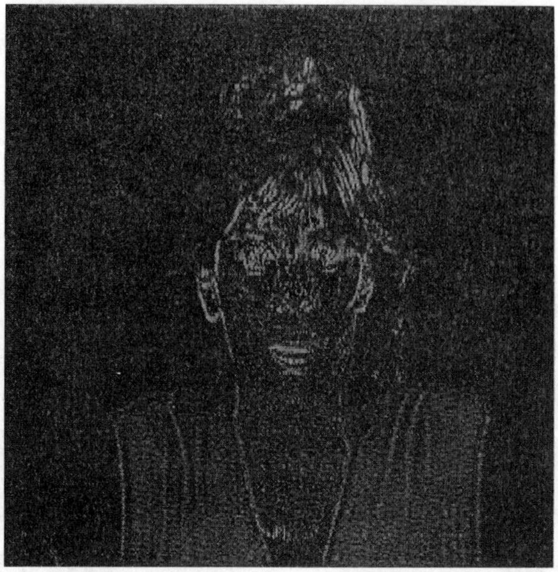

(a) Simple frame difference.

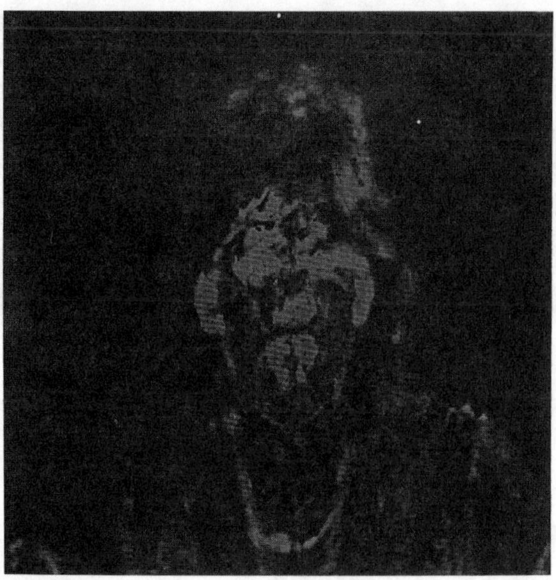

(b) Tensor based frame difference.

Figure 5.11: Simple Frame Difference and Tensor Based Frame Difference.

(a) First Frame of Image Sequence

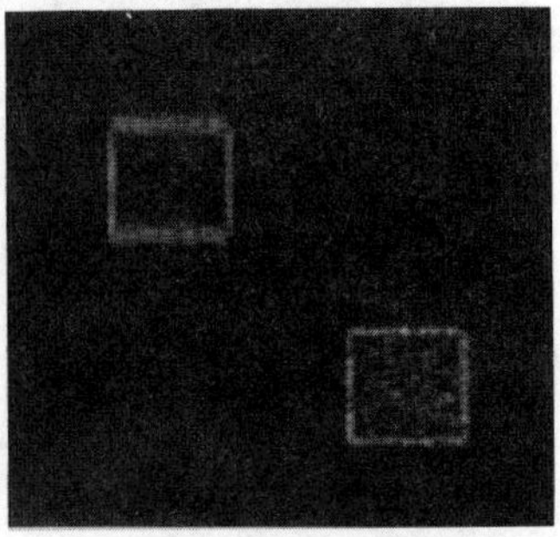

(b) Largest Eigenvalue Field

(c) Second Largest Eigenvalue Field

(d) Smallest Eigenvalue Field

Figure 5.12: Local Structure Tensor Fields.

Area	λ_1	λ_2	λ_3
Moving Edges 1	37.0	1.95	0.739
Moving Edges 2	40.9	1.60	0.50
Moving Objects	5.08	2.62	0.88
Still Edges	47.7	3.97	0.221
Still Objects	10.7	5.10	0.238
Still Background	0.38	0.23	0.15

Table 5.1: The Eigenvalues of Different Areas.

field is associated with the edges of the objects in the spatial direction. And the second largest eigenvalue field is mostly related to the corners of the objects.

For color image sequences, we use Di Zenzo's method [78] to calculate the multivariable image tensor field. Originally it was used in the 2-D image. We extended it to the spatio-temporal image sequence to generate this 3D structure tensor. If we have the color image (l, u, v), then:

$$\begin{aligned}
J_{xx} &= \left(\tfrac{\partial l}{\partial x}\right)^2 + \left(\tfrac{\partial u}{\partial x}\right)^2 + \left(\tfrac{\partial v}{\partial x}\right)^2 \\
J_{xy} &= \left(\tfrac{\partial l}{\partial x}\right)\left(\frac{\partial l}{\partial y}\right) + \left(\tfrac{\partial u}{\partial x}\right)\left(\frac{\partial u}{\partial y}\right) + \left(\tfrac{\partial v}{\partial x}\right)\left(\frac{\partial v}{\partial y}\right) \\
J_{xt} &= \left(\tfrac{\partial l}{\partial x}\right)\left(\tfrac{\partial l}{\partial t}\right) + \left(\tfrac{\partial u}{\partial x}\right)\left(\tfrac{\partial u}{\partial t}\right) + \left(\tfrac{\partial v}{\partial x}\right)\left(\tfrac{\partial v}{\partial t}\right) \\
J_{yy} &= \left(\frac{\partial l}{\partial y}\right)^2 + \left(\frac{\partial u}{\partial y}\right)^2 + \left(\frac{\partial v}{\partial y}\right)^2 \\
J_{yt} &= \left(\frac{\partial l}{\partial y}\right)\left(\tfrac{\partial l}{\partial t}\right) + \left(\frac{\partial u}{\partial y}\right)\left(\tfrac{\partial u}{\partial t}\right) + \left(\frac{\partial v}{\partial y}\right)\left(\tfrac{\partial v}{\partial t}\right) \\
J_{tt} &= \left(\tfrac{\partial l}{\partial t}\right)^2 + \left(\tfrac{\partial u}{\partial t}\right)^2 + \left(\tfrac{\partial v}{\partial t}\right)^2 .
\end{aligned} \tag{5.59}$$

5.4.3 Curve Evolution

5.4.3.1 Basic Theory of Curve Evolution

The original curve evolution was proposed by Kass *et al.* [34]. Let $C(q) : [0, 1] \to \mathbf{R}^2$ be a planar curve and let $I : [0, a] \times [0, b] \to \mathbf{R}^+$be a given image in which we want to detect the objects boundaries. The curve C with an energy E is given by:

$$E(C) = \alpha \int_0^1 |C'(q)|^2 dq + \beta \int_0^1 |C''(q)|^2 dq - \lambda \int_0^1 | \bigtriangledown I(C(q))| dq, \tag{5.60}$$

where α, β, and λ are real positive constants. $\bigtriangledown$ is the gradient operator. This deforms a curve based on the internal and external forces. The internal force, the first two terms in Eqn. (5.60), associated with the first and second derivative of the curve, governs the curve change with continuity. In other words, they control the smoothness of the contours to be detected. The external force, the third term in Eqn. (5.60), is responsible for attracting the contour towards the object in the image. Given a set of constants α, β, and λ, we can solve the snake problem by minimizing E to get the curve C.

In Fleming *et al.*'s [16] work, they used a statistical model to measure the external force to replace the third term of Eqn. (5.60). The results are promising in the dermatoscopic imagery for detecting the globule blobs. The problem in this kind of method is that it can not deal with the topological change, such as curve splitting and merging. That is, when two snakes evolve, if they have a common boundary or edge, they can not merge together. Or if there are two objects inside an initial snake, it is not possible to be two snakes after the curve evolution.

5.4.3.2 Level Set Curve Evolution

We follow Caselles *et al.*'s direction [10]. They proposed a geodesic active contour approach which is based on the relationship between active contours and the computation of geodesics or minimal distance curves. This approach for object segmentation allows connecting classical "snakes" based on energy minimization and geometric active contours based on the theory of curve evolution. To obtain this, they set the $\beta = 0$, and change the third term of the Eqn. (5.60). Then, the general energy function is given by:

$$E(C) = \alpha \int_0^1 |C'(q)|^2 dq + \lambda \int_0^1 |g(\nabla I(C(q))|)^2 dq, \tag{5.61}$$

where g is a strictly decreasing function in $[0, +\infty)$, and $g(r) \to 0$ as $r \to \infty$, the graph of g as shown in Fig. 5.13.

Since $|C'(q)|dq = ds$, minimizing Eqn. (5.61) is equivalent to minimizing the following:

$$\begin{aligned} E(C) &= \int_0^1 g(|\nabla I(C(q))|)|C'(q)|dq \\ &= \int_0^{L(C)} g(|\nabla I(C(q))|)ds, \end{aligned} \tag{5.62}$$

Furthermore, the equation can be solved by curve evolution equation:

$$\frac{\partial C(t)}{\partial t} = g(|\nabla I|)\kappa\vec{N} - (\nabla g \cdot \vec{N})\vec{N} \ , \tag{5.63}$$

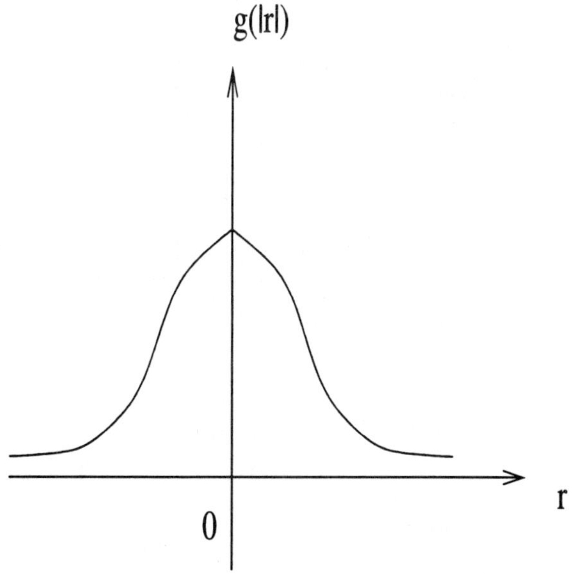

Figure 5.13: Shape of $g(|r|)$.

where κ is the Euclidean curvature of the curve, $\vec{N}$ is the unit inward normal vector.

In the simplest case, curve evolution solves the following problem: evolving an initial curve over time according to a partial differential equation such that eventually, the curve attracts to the outer boundary of an object (see Fig. 5.14). Specifically, suppose $\mathbf{C} = \mathbf{C}(s) = [x(s), y(s)]$, $s \in [0,1]$, is a closed contour on the plane. Curve evolution amounts to evolving $\mathbf{C}$ over time by a differential equation:

$$\mathbf{C}_t = \beta\vec{N}, \tag{5.64}$$

where subscript t denotes the partial derivative with respect to time t, $\vec{N}$ is a normal vector on the curve, and β is a speed (notice both β and $\vec{N}$ are functions of (x, y, t)). Eqn. (5.63) can be converted to the above equation by letting $\beta = g(|\bigtriangledown I|)\kappa - \bigtriangledown g \cdot \vec{N}$.

Recently, the level-set method [62] has become a standard technique for implementing curve evolution. Osher *et al.* [49] converted the curve evolution problem to a surface evolution problem. Among other advantages, it automatically handles topological changes (for multiple object detection, one initial curve can split into multiple curves during evolution). The level-set technique

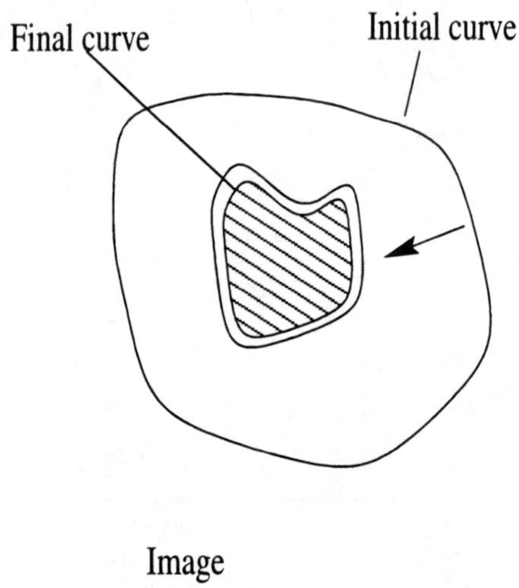

Figure 5.14: Curve Evolution.

implements curve evolution by embedding **C** in a surface $u(x, y; t)$ which evolves in time according to:

$$u_t + \beta|\nabla u| = 0, \tag{5.65}$$

where β is the same a in Eqn. (6.4). While the details of Eqns. (6.4) and (6.5) can be found in [10], [59] and [62]. The most important aspect to our application in image sequence segmentation is the selection of β, the speed function.

A popular speed function used for extracting objects from a single image $I(x, y)$ is (see [10]).

$$\beta = g(||\nabla I||)(c + \kappa) - (\nabla g \cdot \vec{N}), \tag{5.66}$$

where ∇I is the image gradient, $g(v)$ is a monotonically decreasing function that approaches zero when v is large, c is a constant, κ is the curvature of the curve. The first term in this speed function becomes zero (i.e., stops the curve from evolving) when the curve hits object boundaries while the second term stops to fill gaps in object boundaries.

This method was originally applied to the image segmentation. We want to demonstrate it with one example of its topological characteristics. According to Sapiro's paper [59], we implemented the color snake algorithm. Here is the result by this color snake algorithm. There are 3 balls in the original image, Fig. 5.15.(a). After 20 iterations, we come to an intermediate result of the evolution. The three balls are within one curve, which is demonstrated in Fig. 5.15.(b). The final result is shown in Fig. 5.15.(c), which is after 100 iterations. Finally, the one curve is split into several curves.

5.4.3.3 Curve Evolution for Image Sequence Segmentation

To apply curve evolution to image sequence segmentation, we replace the norm of the image gradient $||\nabla I||$ by the robust frame difference λ_3 in the speed function of Eqn. (6.7). That is:

$$\beta = g(||\lambda_3||)(c + \kappa) - (\nabla g \cdot \vec{N}), \tag{5.67}$$

where λ_3 is the smallest eigenvalue of local tensor field.

5.4.3.4 Implementation Details

To implement the resultant curve evolution, we have used a narrow-band algorithm [52], which is a faster level set method.

We initially set the surface $u(x, y, 0)$ as the distance between the pixels to the initial curve $C(0)$. We will set the surface of pixels to a positive sign if they are inside the initial curve. Otherwise, a negative sign will be set. Fig. 5.16 gives more visual information about this setup.

The entire process is:

1. Initialize the surface, based on the initial curve.

2. Create a narrow-band set around the zero level set.

3. Update the surface $u(x, y, t)$ with Eqn. (5.67) within the narrow-band set for a given amount of iterations.

4. Detect the zero level set or result curve.

5. If the curve is still moving, or the number of iterations is smaller than a given value, reinitialize the surface and go to step 2.

6. Output the final curve.

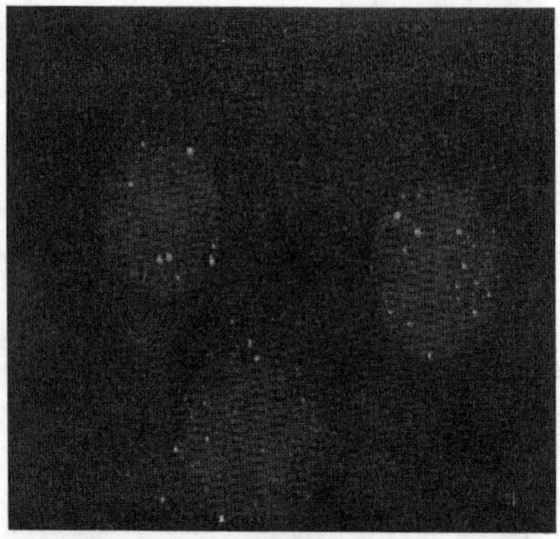

(a) Original Image

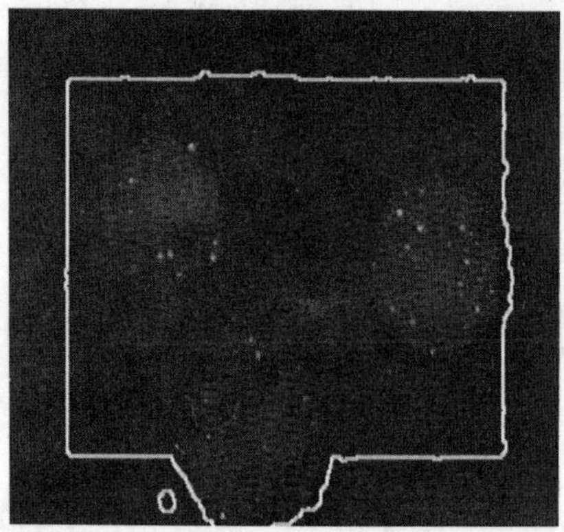

(b) Evolution Result after 20 Iterations

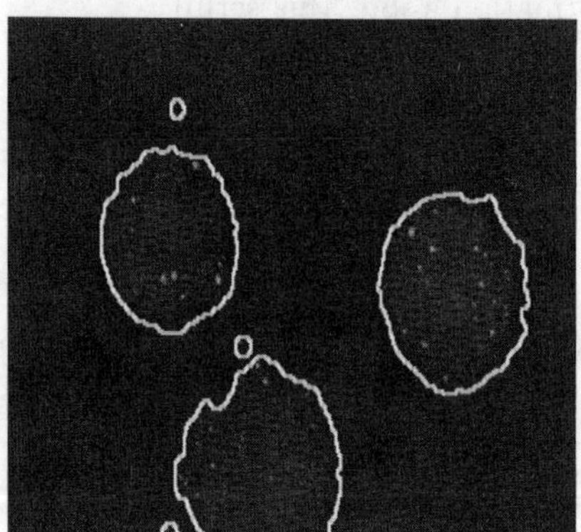

(c) Evolution Resolution after 100 Iterations

Figure 5.15: Color Snake with the Splitting of Curves.
(See color insert)

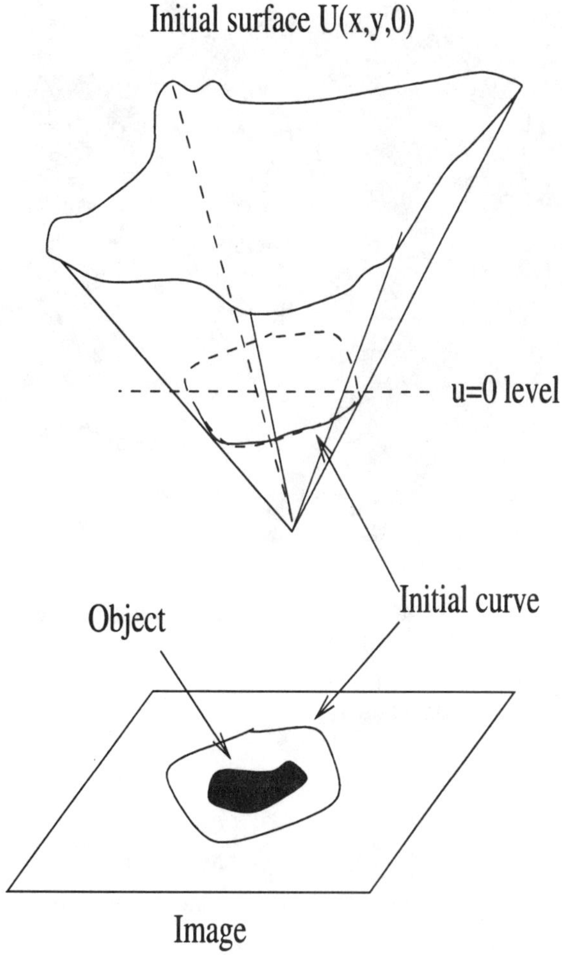

Figure 5.16: Surface Initialization Based on Initial Curve.

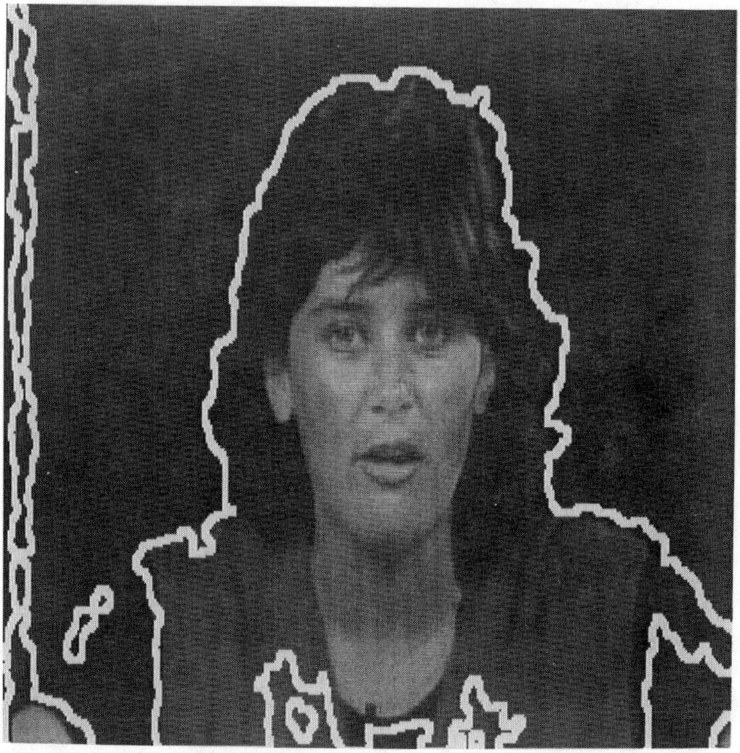

Figure 5.17: Segmentation of Miss America Sequence.

5.4.4 Experimental Results

To demonstrate the efficiency of our algorithm, we have tested our approach on a number of TV and surveillance image sequences. Some typical results are shown in Figs. 5.17-5.19. Fig. 5.17 shows a segmented frame of the Miss America sequence. This sequence is very noisy and the object motion is relatively small. Simple frame difference failed to produce any clear indication of object motion (see Fig. 5.11.(a)). Using the tensor-based frame differencing (see Fig. 5.11.(b)), however, good segmentation results can be obtained.

Fig. 5.18 shows a segmented frame from an infra-red video surveillance sequence obtained from a moving camera. Due to global motion and low object-background contrast, this sequence is difficult to segment. Our approach, however, produced good results.

Finally, Fig. 5.19 shows a segmented frame from a surveillance sequence.

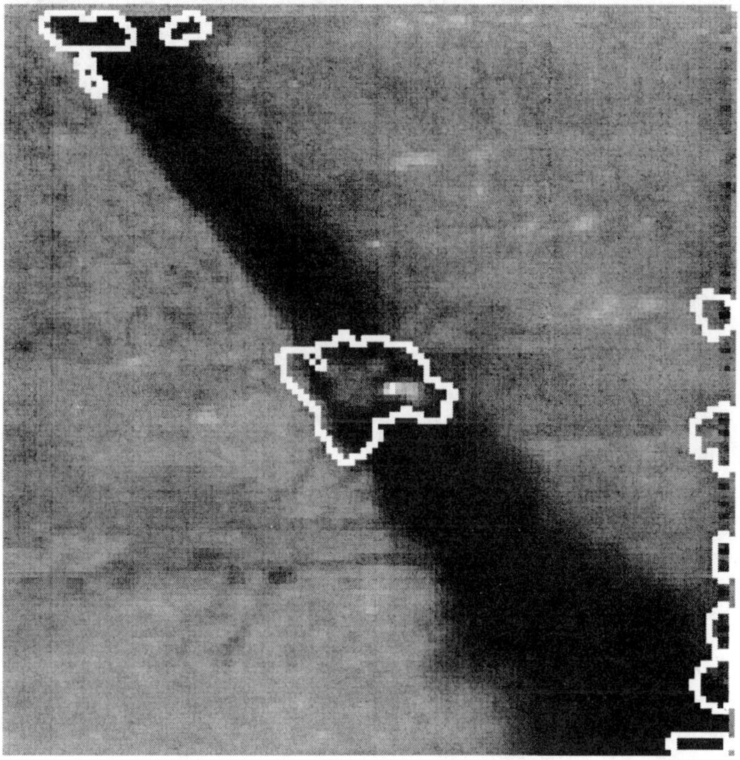

Figure 5.18: Segmentation of Infra-red Sequence.

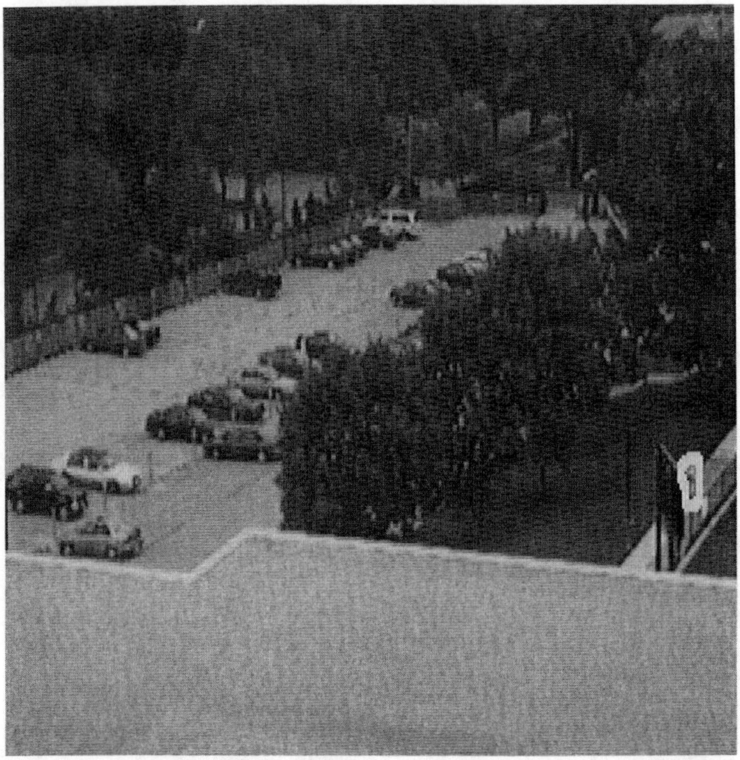

Figure 5.19: Segmentation of Outdoor Sequence (moving person on lower right, indicated by white outline).

The interesting feature here is that there are two types of motion in the scene: the random motion of the trees (caused by wind) and the motion of the walking person and cars. The tensor based frame-differencing is capable of suppressing the trees' random motion such that it does not show up in the final segmentation.

5.4.5 Summary

In this Chapter, we have presented our image sequence segmentation algorithm and experimental results. The algorithm is composed of three parts: global motion compensation, robust differencing and curve evolution. We give the details of these techniques. The global motion compensation includes a sparse set of block-matching, Taylor expansion, and regression. This is a fast and accurate global motion estimator. The robust differencing gives motion detection more reliably for the local structural tensors. Level set curve evolution is used to segment out the moving object with the tensor motion detector. We have tested the efficiency with many sequences.

5.5 Conclusions and Directions for Future Work

In this Chapter, we have described a new multiresolution color image segmentation method and a novel approach to image sequence segmentation. The new multiresolution color image segmentation is an unsupervised algorithm, with MRF and mean field theory. This gives accurate and smooth segmentation results. Some results of color image segmentation are demonstrated. Our new multiresolution implementation, "Narrow Band", significantly accelerates the compensation.

Our new image sequence segmentation contains three parts: global motion compensation, a robust frame differencing scheme based on the 3D structure tensor field, and level set based curve evolution to produce whole objects. This is insensitive to noise and global motion, produces whole objects, and is relatively fast. The efficacy of the approach was demonstrated on a number of relatively difficult image sequences, such as TV and infrared-surveillance sequences.

For future work, we would like to further increase the processing speed by looking into fast marching techniques (for the curve evolution part) [62] or other fast implementation. A more detailed study will be carried out for the local structure tensor field. Also, we would like to use some hardware to accelerate the computation. Practical applications may be studied, such as target tracking, school children monitoring, and video compression.

Bibliography

[1] Alatan, A. A., Onural, L., Wollborn, M., Mech, R., Tuncel, E. and Sikora, T., Image sequence analysis for emerging interactive multimedia services - the European cost 211 framework, IEEE Trans. on Circuits and Systems for Video Technology, Vol. 8, No.7, pp. 802-813, Nov. 1998.

[2] Anandan, P., Bergen, J.R., Hanna, K.J. and Hingorani, R., Hierarchical model-based motion estimation, Motion Analysis and Image Sequence Processing, Sezan, M. I. and Lagendijk, R. L. eds., Kluwer, 1993.

[3] Bartolini, F., Cappellini, V. and Giani, C., Motion estimation and tracking for urban traffic monitoring, IEEE International Conference on Image Processing, ICIP'96, Vol. 3, pp. 787-790, 1996.

[4] Bergen, L. and Meyer, F., Motion segmentation and depth ordering based on morphological segmentation, European Conference on Computer Vision, ECCV'98, Vol. 2, pp. 531-547, 1998.

[5] Betalmio, M., Sapiro, G. and Randall, G., Morphing active contours: a geometric approach to topology-independent image segmentation and tracking, IEEE International Conference on Image Processing, ICIP'98, pp. 318-322, Vol. 3, 1998.

[6] Bierling, M. and Thoma, R., Motion compensating field interpolation using a hierarchically structured displacement estimator, Signal Processing, Vol. 11, No. 4, pp. 387-404, Dec. 1986.

[7] Bigun, J. and Granlund, G. H., Optimal orientation detection of linear symmetry, Proceedings - First International Conference on Computer Vision, pp. 433-438, 1987.

[8] Black, M. J., Sapiro, G., Marimont, D. and Heeger, D., Robust anisotropic diffusion, IEEE Transactions on Image Processing, Special issue on Partial

Differential Equations and Geometry Driven Diffusion in Image Processing and Analysis, Vol. 7, No. 3, pp. 421-432, March 1998.

[9] Burt, P. J., Bergen, J. R., Hingorani, R., Kolczynski, R., Lee, W. A., Leung, A., Lubin, J. and Shvaytser, H., Object tracking with a moving camera, Workshop on Visual Motion, Washington, DC, USA, pp. 2-12, Mar. 28-31, 1989.

[10] Caselles, V., Kimmel, R. and Sapiro G., Geodesic active contours, International Joural of Computer Vision, Vol. 22, No. 1, pp. 61-79, Feb.-Mar. 1997.

[11] Chan, M. H., Yu, Y. B. and Constantinides, A. G., Variable size block matching motion compensation with applications to video coding, Proceedings of IEEE, Part I: Communications, Speech and Vision, Vol. 137, No. 4, pp. 205-212, Aug. 1990.

[12] Chang, M. M., Sezan, M. I. and Tekalp, A. M., Adaptive Bayesian estimation of color images, Journal of Electronic Imaging, Vol. 3, No. 4, pp. 404-414, October 1994.

[13] Ciampini, R., Blanc-Feraud, L. Barlaud, M. and Salerno, E., Motion-based segmentation by means of active contours, IEEE International Conference on Image Processing, ICIP'98, Vol. 2, pp. 667-670, 1998.

[14] Davies, D., Palmer, P. L. and Mirmehdi, M., Detection and tracking of very small low-contrast objects, Submitted to the 9th BMVC (British Machine Vision Conference), 1998.

[15] De Smet, P. and De Vleeschauwer, D., Motion-based segmentation using a thresholded merging strategy on watershed segments, IEEE International Conference on Image Processing, ICIP'97, Vol. 2, pp. 490-493, 1997.

[16] Fleming, M. G., Steger, C., Zhang, J., Gao, J., Cognetta, A. B., Pollak, I. and Dyer, C. R., Techniques for a structural analysis of dermatoscopic imagery, Computerized Medical Imaging and Graphics, Vol. 22, No. 5, pp. 375-389, 1998.

[17] Gao, J., Zhang, J., Fleming, M. G., Pollak, I. and Cognetta, A., Segmentation of dermatoscopic images by stabilized inverse diffusion equations,

IEEE International Conference on Image Processing, ICIP'98, Vol. 3, pp. 823-827, Oct. 4-7, 1998.

[18] Geman, S. and Hwang, C.-R., Diffusions for global optimization, SIAM Journal of Control and Optimization, Vol. 24, No. 5, pp. 1031-1043, September 1986.

[19] Geman, D. and Reynolds, G. Constrained restoration and the recovery of discontinuities, IEEE Transactions on Pattern Analysis and Machine Intelligence, Vol. 14, No. 3, pp. 367-383, March 1992.

[20] Ghanbari, M., The cross-search algorithm for motion estimation, IEEE Transactions on Communications, Vol. 38, No. 7, pp. 950-953, 1990.

[21] Grimson, E., Stauffer, C., Romano, R., Lee, L., Viola, P. and Faugeras, O., Forest of sensors: using adaptive tracking to classify and monitor activities in a site, Proceedings of 1998 DARPA Image Understanding Workshop, Vol. 1, pp. 33-41, 1998.

[22] Gu, C. and Lee, M.-C., Semantic video object segmentation and tracking using mathematical morphology and perspective motion mode, IEEE Int. Conf. Image Processing, ICIP'97, Vol. 2, pp. 514–517, Oct. 1997.

[23] Haag, M. and Nagel, H. H., Beginning a transition from a local to a more global point of view in model-based vehicle tracking, European Conference on Computer Vision, ECCV'98, Vol. 1, pp. 812-827, 1998.

[24] Hall, J., Greenhill, D. and Jones, G. A., Segmenting film sequences using active surfaces, IEEE International Conference on Image Processing, ICIP'97, Vol. 1, pp. 751-754, 1997.

[25] Hansen, M., Anandan, P., Dana, K., Van der Wal, G. and Burt, P., Real-time scene stabilization and mosaic construction, IEEE Workshop on Application of Computer Vision, pp. 54-62, 1994.

[26] Han, S. C. and Woods, J. W., Object-based subband/wavelet video compression, Wavelet Image and Video Compression, Topiwala, Pankaj, ed., Kluwer Academic Press, Boston, 1998.

[27] Hildreth, E. C., Computations underlying the measurement of visual motion, Artif. Intel., Vol. 23, pp. 309-354, 1984.

[28] Hoetter, M., Differential estimation of the global motion parameters zoom and pan, Signal Processing, Vol. 16, pp. 249-265, 1989.

[29] Horn, B. K. P. and Schunck, B. G., Determining optical flow, Artif. Intell., Vol. 17, pp. 185-203, 1981.

[30] Jahne, B., Haubecker, H., Scharr, H., Spies, H., Schmundt, D. and Schurr, U., Study of dynamical processes with tensor-based spatiotemporal image processing techniques, European Conference on Computer Vision, ECCV'98, Vol. 2, pp. 322-336, 1998.

[31] Jahne, B., Digital Image Processing: Concepts, Algorithms, and Scientific Appliations, Third Edition, Springer-Verlag, Berlin, New York, 1995.

[32] Jain, J. R. and Jain, A. K., Displacement measurement and its application in interframe image coding, IEEE Trans. Commun., Vol. 29, pp. 1799-1808, 1981.

[33] Kanade, T., Collins, R., Lipton, A., Burt, P. and Wixson, L., Advances in cooperative multi-sensor video surveillance, Proceedings of DARPA Image Understanding Workshop, Vol. 1, pp. 3-24, 1998.

[34] Kass, M., Witkin, A. and Terzopoulos, D., Snakes: Active contour models, International Journal of Computer Vision, Vol. 1, No. 4, pp. 321-331, 1988.

[35] Kimmel,R., Curve Evolution on Surfaces, Ph.D Thesis, Technion, Israel, 1995.

[36] Kong, M., Leduc, J.-P., Ghosh, B. K. and Wickerhauser, V. M., Spatio-temporal continuous wavelet transforms for motion-based segmentation in real image sequences, IEEE International Conference on Image Processing, ICIP'98, Vol. 2, pp. 662-666, 1998.

[37] Kornprobst, P., Deriche, R. and Aubert, G., Image sequence restoration: a PDE based coupled method for image restoration and motion segmentation, European Conference on Computer Vision, Freiburg (Allemagne), Vol. 2, pp. 548-562, 1998.

[38] Torres, L. and Kunt, M., Video Coding: The Second Generation Approach, Kluwer Academic Pub., Boston, 1996.

[39] Leduc, J.-P., Mujica, F., Murenzi, R. and Smith, M., Spatio-temporal wavelet transforms for motion tracking, IEEE International Conference on Acoustics, Speech, and Signal Processing, ICASSP-97, Vol. 4, pp. 3013-3016, 1997.

[40] Li, C.-T. and Wilson, R., Image segmentation based on a multiresolution Bayesian framework, IEEE International Conference on Image Processing, ICIP'98, PP. 761-765, 1998.

[41] Lim, Y. W. and Lee, S. U., On the color image segmentation algorithm based on the thresholding and the fuzzy C-means techniques, Pattern Recognition, Vol. 23, No. 9, pp. 935-952, 1990.

[42] Luo, J., Gray, R. T. and Lee, H.-C., Towards physics-based segmentation of photographic color images, IEEE International Conference on Image Processing, ICIP'97, Vol. 3, pp. 58-61, 1997.

[43] Marques, F., Pardas, M. and Salembier, P., Coding-oriented segmentation of video sequences, Video Coding: The Second Generation Approach, by Torres, L. and Kunt, M. (Editor), Kluwer Academic Pub., Boston, March 1996.

[44] Meier, T. and Ngan, K. N., Video object plane segmentation using a morphological motion filter and Hausdorff object tracking, IEEE International Conference on Image Processing, ICIP'98, Vol. 2 , pp. 652-656, 1998.

[45] Memin, E. and Perez, P., Dense estimation and object-based segmentation of the optical flow with robust techniques, IEEE Transactions on Image Processing, Vol. 7, No. 5 , pp. 703-719, May 1998.

[46] Morimoto, C. and Chellappa, R., Evaluation of image stabilization algorithms, Proc. IEEE Int. Conf. on Acoustics, Speech and Signal Processing, ICASSP'98, Vol. 5, pp. 2789-2792, 1998.

[47] Moscheni, F., Bhattacharjee, S. and Kunt, M., Robust spatiotemporal segmentation based on region merging, IEEE Trans. on PAMI, Vol. 20, pp. 897-915, Sept. 1998.

[48] Nagel, H.-H. and Enkelmann, W., An investigation of smoothness constraints for the estimation of displacement vector fields from image se-

quences, IEEE Trans. Pattern Analysis and Machine Intelligence, Vol. 8, pp. 565-593, Sept. 1986.

[49] Osher, S. J. and Sethian, J. A., Fronts propagation with curvature dependent speed: Algorithms based on Hamilton-Jacobi formulations, Journal of Computational Physics, Vol. 79, pp. 12-49, 1988.

[50] Paragios, N. and Deriche, R., PDE-based level-set approach for detection and tracking of moving objects, Proceedings of the 6th International Conference on Computer Vision, ICCV'98, pp. 1139-1145, 1998.

[51] Perona, P. and Malik, J., Scale-space and edge detection using anisotropic diffusion, IEEE Trans. PAMI, Vol. 12, pp. 629-639, 1990.

[52] Plankers, R., A level set approach to shape recognition, EPFL Technical Report, Swiss Federal Institute of Technology, 1997.

[53] Pollak, I. , Willsky, A. and Krim, H., Image Segmentation and Edge Enhancement with Stabilized Inverse Diffusion Equations, LIDS report, MIT, Boston, 1997.

[54] Press, W. H., Teukolsky, S. A., Vetterling, W. T. and Flannery, B. P., Numerical recipes in C: the art of scientific computing, 2nd edition, Cambridge University Press, New York, 1993.

[55] Robbins, J. D. and Netravali, A. N., Recursive motion compensation: A review, Image Sequence Processing and Dynamic Scene Analysis, Huang, T. S., ed., pp. 76-103, Berlin, Germany: Springer-Verlag, 1983.

[56] Saeed, M., Karl, W. C., Nguyen, T. Q. and Rabiee, H. R., A new multiresolution algorithm for image segmentation, IEEE International Conference on Acoustics, Speech and Signal Processing, ICASSP'98, Vol. 5, pp. 2753-2756, 1998.

[57] Salembier, P. and Pardas, M., Hierarchical morphological segmentation for image sequence coding, IEEE Transactions on Image Processing, Vol. 3, No. 5, pp. 639-651, Sept. 1994.

[58] Salembier, P., Brigger, P., Casas, J. R. and Pardas, M., Morphological operators for image and video compression, IEEE Transactions on Image Processing, Vol. 5, No. 6, pp. 881-898, June 1996.

[59] Sapiro, G., Color snakes, Computer Vision and Image Understanding, Vol. 68, No. 2, pp. 247-253, 1997.

[60] Sawhney, H. S. and Ayer, S., Compact representations of videos through dominant and multiple motion estimation, IEEE Trans. on PAMI, Vol. 18, No. 8, pp. 814-830, 1996.

[61] Schutz, M. and Ebrahimi, T. E., Matching error based criterion of region merging for joint motion estimation and segmentation techniques, International Conference on Image Processing, ICIP'96, Vol. 2, pp. 509-512, 1996.

[62] Sethian, J. A., Level Set Methods and Fast Marching Methods: evolving interfaces in computational geometry, fluid mechanics, computer vision, and materials science, 2nd edition, Cambridge University Press, New York, 1999.

[63] Shi, J., Belongie, S., Leung, T. and Malik, J., Image and video segmentation: the normalized cut framework, IEEE International Conference on Image Processing, ICIP '98, Vol. 1, pp. 943-947, 1998.

[64] Siggelkow, S., Grigat, R.-R. and Ibenthal, A., Segmentation of image sequences for object oriented coding, IEEE International Conference on Image Processing, ICIP'96, Vol. 2, pp. 477-480, 1996.

[65] Smith, S. M., Real-time motion segmentation and object tracking, Technical Report TR95SMS2b, University of Surrey, Guildford, Surrey, UK, 1995.

[66] Smith, S. M., Reviews of optic flow, motion segmentation, edge finding and corner finding, Technical Report TR97SMS1, University of Surrey, Guildford, Surrey, UK, 1997.

[67] Stiller, C., Object based motion computation, IEEE International Conference on Image Processing, ICIP'96, Vol. 1, pp. 913-916, 1996.

[68] Sullivan, G., Multi-hypothesis motion compensation for low bit-rate video coding, Proc. IEEE Int. Conf. ASSP, Minneapolis, MN, Vol. 5, pp. 437-440, 1993.

[69] Tekalp, A. M.,Digital Video Processing, Upper Saddle River, NJ, Prentice-Hall, 1995.

[70] Ullman, S., High-level vision: object recognition and visual cognition, Cambridge, Mass., MIT Press, 1996.

[71] Wang, J. Y. A. and Adelson, E., Representing moving images with layers, IEEE Trans. on Image Proc., Vol. 3, pp. 625-638, Sept. 1994.

[72] Wang, J. Y. A. and Adelson, E. H., Spatio-temporal segmentation of video data, Proc. SPIE, Vol. 2182, pp. 120-131, 1994.

[73] Waxman, A. M., Kamgar-Parsi, B. and Subbarao, M., Closed-form solutions to image flow equations for 3-D structure and motion, Int. J. Comp. Vision, Vol. 1, pp. 239-258, 1987.

[74] Wolberg, G., Digital Image Warping, Los Alamitos, CA, IEEE Comp. Soc. Press, 1990.

[75] Wyszecki, G. and Stiles, W. S., Color Science: Concepts and Methods, Quantitative Data and Formulae, Wiley-Interscience Pub., New York, 1982.

[76] Yang, X. and Ramchandran, K., A low-complexity region-based video compression framework using morphology, 1996 IEEE International Conference on Image Processing, ICIP'96, Vol. 2, pp. 485-488, 1996.

[77] Yemez, Y., Sankur, B., and Anarim, E., Region growing motion segmentation and estimation in object-oriented video coding, IEEE International Conference on Image Processing, ICIP'96, Vol, 2, pp. 521-524, 1996.

[78] Di Zenzo, S., A note on the gradient of a multi-image, Computer Vision, Graphics, and Image Processing, Vol. 33, pp. 116-125, 1986.

[79] Zhang, Z., On the epipolar geometry between two images with lens distortion, Proc. Int'l Conf. Pattern Recognition, Vol. 1, pp. 407-411, Aug. 1996.

[80] Zhang, J., The mean field theory in EM procedures for Markov Random Fields, IEEE Trans. Signal Processing, Vol. 40, pp. 2570-2583, 1992.

[81] Zhang, J. and Hanauer, G. G., Application of mean field theory to image motion estimation, IEEE Transactions of Image Processing, Vol. 4, No. 1, pp. 19-33, Jan. 1995.

[82] Zhang, K. and Kittler, J., Global motion estimation and robust regression for video coding, IEEE International Conference on Acoustics, Speech and Signal Processing, Vol. 5, pp. 2589-2592, 1998.

[83] Zhong, D. and Chang, S.-F., AMOS: An active system for MPEG-4 video object segmentation, IEEE International Conference on Image Processing, ICIP'98, Vol. 2, pp. 647-651, 1998.

Chapter 6

Motion Imagery Segmentation Via PDE

Jun Zhang[1] *and Weisong Liu*[2]

6.1 Introduction

Separating moving objects from the background in a video clip is known as the image sequence segmentation problem. In recent years, it has attracted considerable interest due to its applications in a wide range of areas. These include object-based video compression (e.g., MPEG4), video surveillance and monitoring, automatic target detection and tracking, and the analysis of medical and other scientific image sequences.

Most previous work in image sequence segmentation can be classified into three approaches: 1) intra-frame segmentation, 2) motion field clustering/ segmentation, and 3) frame differencing. In the first approach (e.g., see [1]), each frame in an image sequence is segmented independently (i.e., intra-frame) into regions of homogeneous intensity or texture, using traditional *image segmentation* techniques. Then regions in consecutive frames are matched and tracked. This would work well if intra-frame segmentation produced a small number of regions closely related to real-world objects. However, since image segmentation using intensity or texture remains a difficult problem, this approach often encounters difficulties, as many image segmentation techniques produce over-segmentation.

In the second approach, a dense motion field is used for segmentation. For example, pixels with similar motion vectors are grouped into regions (e.g., see [2]-[3]). Alternatively, small regions generated from intra-frame segmentation

[1]University of Wisconsin-Milwaukee, Milwaukee, WI, USA
[2]University of Wisconsin-Milwaukee, Milwaukee, WI, USA

can also be grouped based on the similarity of their motion vectors (e.g., see [5]). This approach produces good results when a reliable motion field can be obtained from motion estimation. However, most motion estimation techniques can not guarantee this, especially on real-world image sequences.

In the third approach, image segmentation is achieved *partially* through frame-differencing (see e.g., [6]-[8]). The idea here is to take the difference between two consecutive frames (or a frame and a "background"): if a pixel position has a large frame difference, it is linked to a moving object. This approach, although extremely computation efficient, generally does not produce whole objects (various post processing is needed for that). Furthermore, it is very sensitive to noise and fails completely if there is global motion.

In recent work [9], we have developed an approach to image sequence segmentation that is computationally efficient, does not require a dense motion field, is insensitive to noise and global/background motion, and produces whole objects. It contains three parts: global motion compensation, robust frame-differencing, and curve evolution, where the curve evolution is used to extract *whole* regions or objects. While this approach produced good results on a variety of image sequences, it was implemented as an off-line algorithm [9]. To make this approach more useful in practice, especially for real-time applications, we have subsequently investigated its real-time implementation, which is the subject of this paper.

Using curve evolution for image sequence segmentation has also been investigated in [10] and [11]. Our approach uses a robust variation of frame-differencing and is computationally more efficient than [10], which for each frame applied the "color snake" [12] to a combined image intensity and motion field. It also differs from [11], which uses simple frame-differencing and is sensitive to noise and global motion.

The rest of the paper is organized as follows. Section II provides a brief review of our curve evolution approach to image sequence segmentation and Section III describes its real-time implementation. Section IV presents some typical experimental results.

6.2 Approach

For the sake of simplicity, we view an image sequence as a function defined over continuous space and time. Specifically, let $\mathbf{x} = [x_1, x_2]^T$ denote a spatial location and let $\mathbf{x} \in \mathbf{M}$, a bounded rectangular region in the 2D plane. Then, an image sequence can be represented as $f(\mathbf{x}, t)$, where t denotes time. If the image sequence is colored rather than black and white, we take $f(\mathbf{x}, t)$ to be the Y (intensity) component of its YIQ representation[3]. Our approach to image sequence segmentation contains three parts, namely, global motion compensation, robust frame-differencing, and curve evolution.

A. Global Motion Compensation

Since our approach uses robust frame differencing, when there is global motion, such as that caused by camera motion, global motion compensation needs to be used first. Generally[4], this amounts to finding a motion vector field $\mathbf{u} = \mathbf{u}(\mathbf{x})$ such that

$$f(\mathbf{x} - \mathbf{u}\Delta t, t + \Delta t) \simeq f(\mathbf{x}, t), \tag{6.1}$$

where $f(\mathbf{x}, t)$ and $f(\mathbf{x}, t + \Delta t)$ are, respectively, two consecutive frames in the image sequence (in this sense $\mathbf{u}$ is also dependent on t).

A wide variety of global motion can be realistically modeled by the affine model [6]

$$\mathbf{u}(\mathbf{x}) = \mathbf{A}\mathbf{x} + \mathbf{b} \tag{6.2}$$

where $\mathbf{A}$ is a 2 by 2 matrix and $\mathbf{b}$ is a 2 by 1 column vector. The problem of global motion compensation, then, is to estimate $\mathbf{A}$ and $\mathbf{b}$ from $f(\mathbf{x}, t)$ and $f(\mathbf{x}, t + \Delta t)$. A number of numerical techniques have been proposed to do this [6] and in our previous work [9], we have adopted a technique proposed by Zhang and Kittler [13]. This technique has two advantages: fast and relatively robust to local motion. It was implemented in the off-line version of our image sequence segmentation algorithm in [9]. However, it has not been implemented our current real-time version since, as described in Section III, the camera in our current system is stationary (no global motion).

B. Robust Frame Differencing

---

[3]A more sophisticated technique for dealing with color image sequences that also involves more computational effort is described in [9]

[4]That is, assume the illumination is relatively constant and the effect of occlusions can be ignored.

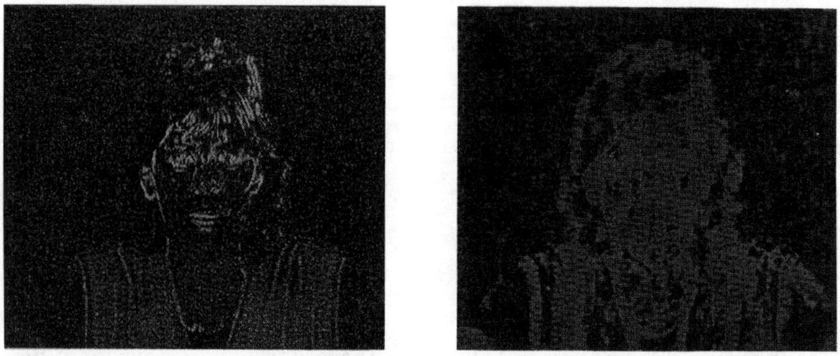

(a) (b)

Figure 6.1: Comparison of Simple Frame Difference and Tensor Based Frame Difference. (a) Simple frame difference. (b) Tensor based frame difference.

Due to image noise and low object-background contrast, the frame difference at non-moving parts of the scene can often be quite large in magnitude, sometimes even larger than that at the moving parts, making it an unreliable indicator of object motion. To deal with this problem, we have derived a robust frame difference measure in [9] based on the 3D (spatial-temporal) structure tensor of [14]. For an image sequence $f(\mathbf{x}, t)$, the 3D structure tensor is a 3×3 matrix defined as

$$\mathbf{R}(\mathbf{x}, t) = \int h(\mathbf{x} - \mathbf{x}', t - t') \nabla f(\mathbf{x}', t') \nabla f(\mathbf{x}', t')^T \, d\mathbf{x}' \, dt' \tag{6.3}$$

where $h(\mathbf{x}, t)$ is a spatial-temporal lowpass filter and ∇ is the gradient operator[5]. Intuitively, the 3D structure tensor can be viewed as a correlation matrix for the gradient vectors of (6.3) in a principle component analysis. Indeed, under relatively mild conditions, the eigenvector associated with the smallest eigenvalue of $\mathbf{R}(\mathbf{x}, t)$ is associated with the direction of motion for the pixel at $(\mathbf{x}, t)$ [14]. We proposed that this smallest eigen value, denoted by $\lambda_3(\mathbf{x}, t)$, can be viewed as the average power of a smoothed frame difference along the motion direction and we observed in experiments that, compared to the simple frame difference, $\lambda_3(\mathbf{x}, t)$ is much more robust to noise and low object-background contrast. Hence, it is taken as a robust version of the frame difference and used for image sequence segmentation. As an illustration, Fig. 6.1 shows the simple

[5] In numerical simulations, we implemented the gradient operation by smoothing the image or image sequence first by a Gaussian.

frame difference (see Fig. 6.1a) and $\lambda_3(\mathbf{x},t)$ (see Fig. 6.1b) computed for the Miss America sequence. Notice that $\lambda_3(\mathbf{x},t)$ is large near the left part of her hair and overall, provides better object boundary integrity. Indeed, our previous study [9] indicates when objects move at relatively normal speeds (e.g., a person walking or a car moving), $\lambda_3(\mathbf{x},t)$ provides a more robust motion indicator.

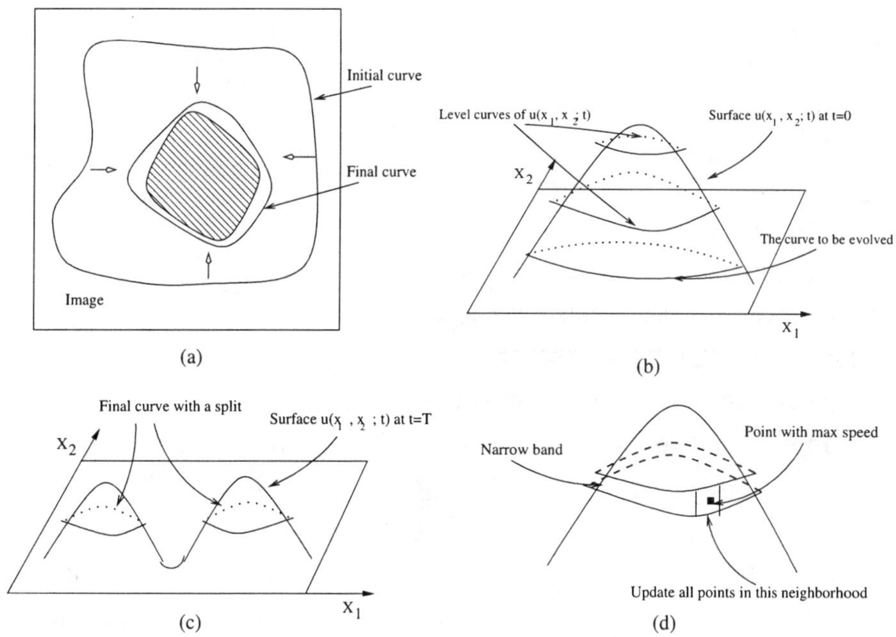

Figure 6.2: Level Set Curve Evolution. (a) Curve evolution. (b) Embed the curve in a surface. (c) Curve evolution result. (d) Illustration of Hermes algorithm.

C. Curve Evolution

In recent years, there has been much interest in the subject of curve evolution and its various applications [15]. In our work, curve evolution is used to single out whole objects from the output of the robust frame differencing. In this section we briefly review relevant aspects of this technique and describe how it is used in our approach to image sequence segmentation. For more comprehensive treatments of the theory and applications of curve evolution, see e.g., [15].

Imagine an image containing one or more objects. In the simplest case, curve evolution solves the following problem: how to evolve a closed curve on the image plane over time[6] such that eventually, the curve attracts to the outer boundary of the object or objects (see Fig. 6.2a). Specifically, suppose $\mathbf{C} = \mathbf{C}(s) = [x_1(s), x_2(s)]^T$, $s \in [0, 1]$, is a closed curve on the image plane. Curve evolution amounts to evolving $\mathbf{C}$ over time by a (vector) differential equation,

$$\mathbf{C}_t = \beta \vec{\mathbf{N}}, \tag{6.4}$$

where subscript t denotes the partial derivative with respect to time t, $\vec{\mathbf{N}}$ is a normal vector on the curve and β is a speed function. Notice that both β and $\vec{\mathbf{N}}$ are functions of x_1, x_2, t.

The direct discrete implementation of the curve evolution of eqn. (6.4) is cumbersome. For example, the number of points in a discretized curve could change over time as the curve evolves. Furthermore, when there are more than one object, the curve needs to split. Problems like these lead to complicated book-keeping and the requirement of ad hoc special case handling procedures [15]. Recently, a new technique, known as the level-set method [15], has overcome most of the difficulties in the implementation of curve evolution algorithms. Among its many advantages, the level-set method automatically handles topological changes (e.g., the split and merge of curves during evolution) and makes book-keeping very simple. It implements curve evolution by embedding $\mathbf{C}$ in a surface $u(x_1, x_2; t)$ (see Fig. 6.2b). Specifically, at $t = 0$, the curve is the level-set given by $\{(x_1, x_2) | u(x_1, x_2; 0) = 0\}$. As the surface evolves over time, so does the embedded curve. When the evolution of $u(x_1, x_2; t)$ stops at $t = T$, the evolved curve can be obtained from the level-set $\{(x_1, x_2) | u(x_1, x_2; T) = 0\}$ (see Fig. 6.2c). The evolution equation for the surface $u(x_1, x_2; t)$ can be derived from the curve evolution equation of (6.4) and, as shown in [15], this is

$$u_t = \beta |\nabla u|, \tag{6.5}$$

[6] Here, the word time mean iterations and is different from the time as in space-time.

where β is the same as in (6.4), computed on the "level-curves" of u (see also Fig. 6.2b).

Several fast implementations of the level-set method have been proposed (e.g., see [15], [11]). In this work, we have used the narrow-band technique of [15]. In each iteration during the evolution of the surface $u(x_1, x_2; t)$, this technique only updates a small neighborhood of points surrounding the largest curvature point on the curve $C(\mathbf{x}, t)$ (see Fig. 6.2d). The advantage of this technique is that it is faster and also allows relatively arbitrary speed functions. To conclude the brief review of curve evolution and level-set method, we describe the initialization process. As the initial curve, we use the largest possible curve, i.e., the boundary of the image. As this curve evolves it generally moves inward and stops at object boundaries. Since the curve evolution is implemented using the level-set method, an initial surface containing the initial curve, i.e., $u(x_1, x_2, 0)$, also needs to be given. Here we have used the "distance function" of [15]. Specifically, $u(x_1, x_2, 0)$ is given by

$u(x_1, x_2, 0) =$ The minimum distance between (x_1, x_2) and the boarder of the image. (6.6)

Given the basic equations, fast algorithms, and initialization procedure for the curve evolution and level-set method, the most important thing to our image sequence segmentation application now is the selection of β, the speed function. A popular choice used for extracting objects from a single image $I(x_1, x_2)$ is (see [16])

$$\beta = g(|\nabla I|)(c + \kappa) - \nabla g(|\nabla I|) \cdot \vec{\mathbf{N}} \tag{6.7}$$

where $|\nabla I|$ is the norm of the gradient of the image, $g(v)$ is a monotonically decreasing function that approaches zero when $|v|$ is large, for example, we took

$$g(v) = e^{-\alpha |v|} \tag{6.8}$$

with $\alpha > 0$, c is a constant, κ is the curvature of the evolving curve, and $\vec{\mathbf{N}}$, as in eqn. (6.4), is the normal vector of the curve. The first term in this speed function becomes zero and stops the curve from evolving when the curve hits object boundaries. The second term increases the attraction of the curve towards object boundaries [16]. As noted previously, in the level-set implementation the curvature κ and normal vector $\vec{\mathbf{N}}$ are computed on the level curves of the embedding surface $u(x_1, x_2; t)$.

To apply curve evolution to image sequence segmentation, we replace the norm of the image gradient $|\nabla I|$ by the robust frame difference measure $\lambda_3(\mathbf{x}, t)$ in the speed function of (6.7). In this way, image sequence segmentation can be accomplished by the three steps of global motion compensation (if there is global motion), $\lambda_3(\mathbf{x}, t)$ computation, and level-set based curve evolution.

6.3 Implementation

The real-time implementation of the curve evolution approach for image segmentation, described in Section II, was investigated along two directions. The first is to find computationally efficient ways to implement the 3D structure tensor and curve evolution. The second is to find a proper hardware and software platform.

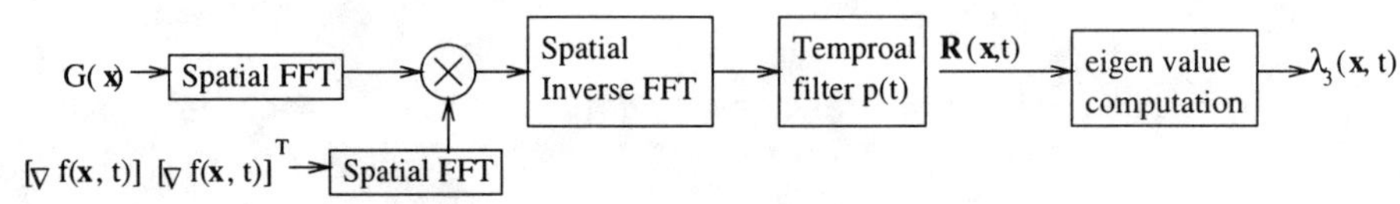

Figure 6.3: Spatial Temporal Filtering in 3D Structure Tensor and $\lambda_3(\mathbf{x}, t)$ Computations.

A. 3D Structure Tensor and Curve Evolution

We first look at how the 3D structure tensor and its associated robust frame difference can be implemented. From eqn. (6.3), the 3D tensor $\mathbf{R}(\mathbf{x}, t)$ is defined by a spatial-temporal lowpass filtering operation (convolution). Hence, its implementation lies in the implementation of the lowpass filter $h(\mathbf{x}, t)$. Normally, a spatial-temporal Gaussian filter is used. However, since the Gaussian filter is non-causal in time, it cannot be implemented in "real-time." To solve this problem, we select a separable filter

$$h(\mathbf{x}, t) = G(\mathbf{x})p(t) \tag{6.9}$$

where $G(\mathbf{x})$ is a spatially (non-causal) Gaussian filter and $p(t)$ is a time causal lowpass filter. In discrete implementation, $G(\mathbf{x})$ filters each frame (more precisely, $[\nabla f(\mathbf{x}, t)][\nabla f(\mathbf{x}, t)]^T$ for each fixed t) and is realized by using spatial

FFT (see Fig. 6.3). Similarly, the discrete implementation of $p(t)$ is as a simple time recursive lowpass filter (see Fig. 6.3), given by

$$y_o(\mathbf{x}, t) = a y_o(\mathbf{x}, t-1) + (1-a) y_i(\mathbf{x}, t) \tag{6.10}$$

where $0 < a < 1$ and i and o denote, respectively, the input and output of filter $p(t)$.

Having implemented the 3D tensor computation, we then used the Jacobi algorithm [18], a fast algorithm for computing eigenvalues, to obtain $\lambda_3(\mathbf{x}, t)$, the robust frame difference measure (see Section II.B).

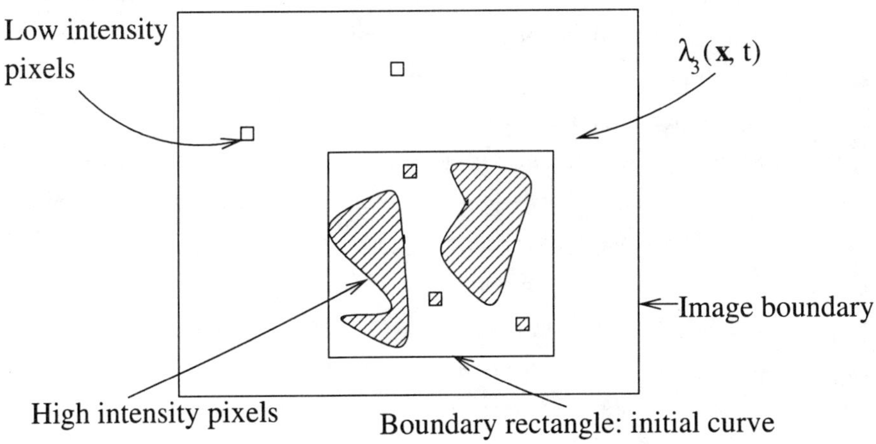

Figure 6.4: Initial Curve in Curve Evolution.

As described in Section II.C, we implemented curve evolution by using the fast algorithm of [11]. In addition, we also devised a fast initialization scheme to provide additional acceleration. Specifically, for each t, i.e., each frame, the robust frame difference $\lambda_3(\mathbf{x}, t)$ can be viewed as an image. We classify each "pixel" in this image into one of two classes: low intensity (background/noise) and high intensity (potential moving objects). We then find the maximum bounding rectangle for high intensity pixels and use it as the initial curve for the curve evolution, see Fig. 6.4. Since the objects in many applications are relatively small compared to the size of the entire image and since $\lambda_3(\mathbf{x}, t)$ usually does a good job in separating background/noise and object pixels, this bounding rectangle is much smaller than the boundary of the image (see Fig. 6.4). Hence, curve evolution using this as the initial curve can be much faster than using the image boundary as the initial curve. Indeed, for the typical test sequences used in our experiments (see Section IV), this initialization makes our curve evolution 4 times faster.

B. Hardware/Software Platform

The platform for our real-time implementation is a standard PC (Pentium 400) running a Windows 98 operating system (other Windows operating systems, e.g., 95, 2000 or NT can also be used). For video input, we used a 3Com Home Connect USB Web Camera, connected to the PC through a USB. This camera is a standard Windows video capture device which means it can be recognized, and subsequently be controlled, by standard drivers in Windows. Our choice of the PC, Windows operating system, and the 3Com camera, while somewhat standard, makes our software development easier and makes our software highly portable and easy to maintain. For example, the use of a PC rather than specialized hardware generally makes software development easier and faster. Indeed, as many of today's PC's are very fast, developing real-time image processing applications running on a PC has becoming a trend. Similarly, the use of the USB connection eliminates the need for a frame grabber. This not only makes programming simpler but also reduces system cost[7]. Finally, the fact that the 3Com camera is a standard Windows video capture device allows us to make our image sequence segmentation program highly portable and easy to maintain. This is described in more detail below.

Under the Windows 98 operating system, there are two ways to implement video I/O operations, such as video capture. The first is to write functions (in C, for example) to control the camera directly. The second, which requires that the camera be a Windows standard video capture device, is to "leave them to the Windows operating system." The second approach has two advantages. First, it eliminates the need for writing our own video I/O functions – we need only to write the video processing functions (i.e., those for curve evolution based video segmentation). Second, when a different camera is used, we do not need to make any changes to our programs as long as the camera is a Windows standard video capture device. In the same way, our programs can be ported to another Windows-based PC easily as long as it has a camera that is a standard

[7]To be sure, a frame grabbers is generally needed when an applications requires very high image resolutions and frame rates, which is not the case here.

Windows video capture device.

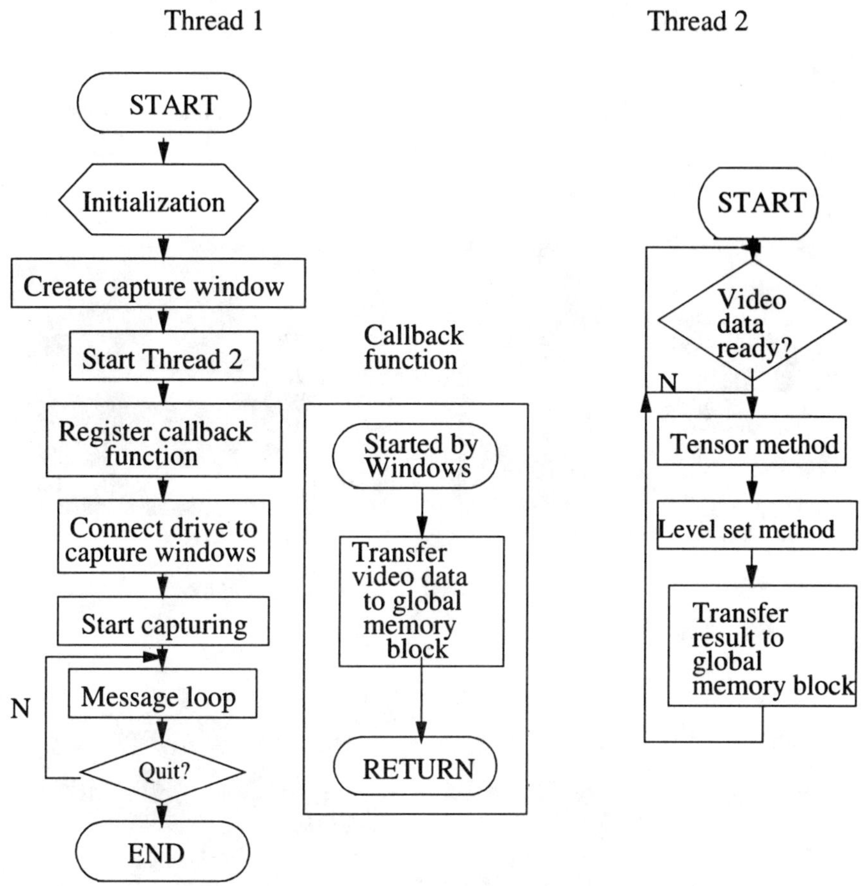

Figure 6.5: The Flowchart of the Multithread Implementation.

Due to these advantages, we have adopted the second approach for implementing video I/O operations. In this approach, we first "ask" the Windows to start capturing video by sending it a "message". When a frame is captured and ready for processing, which is an "event" (i.e., "frame ready"), the Windows automatically calls a "callback" function to respond to this "event." To process the captured current frame, we embed our curve evolution based image segmentation program (C functions) in the callback function. In practice, however, this approach has a problem – before we finish processing the captured current frame, no more new frames will be captured. That is, the Windows will only resume video capture after the callback function is returned. This would cause the system to "miss" some of the frames, thereby reducing its temporal resolution. To solve this problem, we used the multi-thread technique, with two threads. As shown in Fig. 6.5, the first thread uses the Windows to capture video frames with the captured frames sent to a memory block by the callback function[8]. Similarly, the second thread is the video processing thread, it segments the captured frames in the memory block.

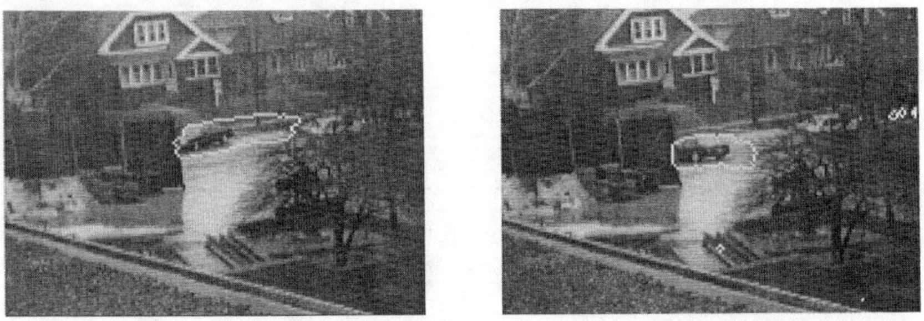

Figure 6.6: Segmentation Results for the Outdoor Sequence.
(See color insert)

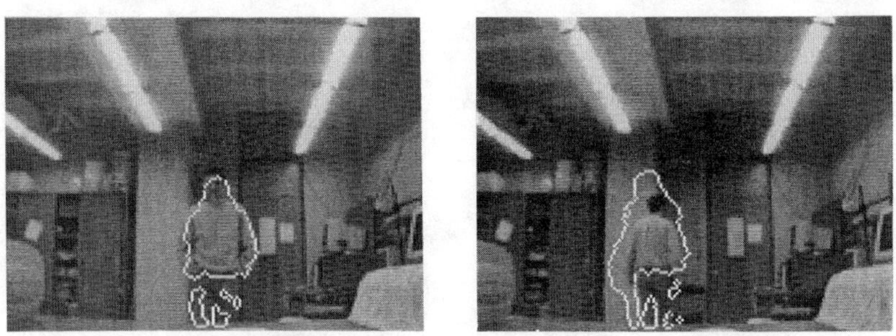

Figure 6.7: Segmentation Results for the Indoor Sequence.
(See color insert)

6.4 Experimental Results

We have performed real-time image sequence segmentation experiments using the system described in Section III. Some typical results are shown in Figs. 6.6 and 6.7 where the segmented moving objects are indicated by their boundaries.

[8]The callback function no longer performs image sequence segmentation operations

Fig. 6.6 is an image sequence obtained by pointing our camera to the street and the moving object is a car. Fig. 6.7 is an image sequence obtained from the inside our lab and the moving object is a walking person. Although our inexpensive camera produces a lot of noise, our system produced good segmentation results at 5 frames per second with a frame resolution of 160×120. We believe higher frame rate and higher resolution segmentation results can be obtained if we change our 400 MHz PC to a 1GHz PC. The latter is quite common today and not expensive.

Bibliography

[1] Marques, F., Pardas, M. and Salembier, P., Coding-oriented segmentation of video sequences, Video Coding: The Second Generation Approach, Torres, L. and Kunt, M. (Editor), Kluwer Academic Pub, March 1996.

[2] Burt, P.J., et al, Object tracking with a moving camera, MOTION89, pp. 2-12, 1989.

[3] Wang, J. Y.A. and Adelson, E. H., Spatio-temporal segmentation of video data(SPIE), Proc. Society of Photo-Optical Instrumentation Engineers, Vol. 2182, pp. 120-131, 1994.

[4] Haag, M. and Nagel, H.-H., Beginning a transition from a local to a more global point of view in model-based vehicle tracking, European Conference on Computer Vision(ECCV) '98, pp. 812-827, 1998.

[5] Moscheni, F., Bhattacharjee, S. and Kunt, M., Robust spatiotemporal segmentation based on region merging, IEEE Trans. on PAMI, Vol. 20, pp. 897-915, Sept. 1998.

[6] Tekalp, A. M., Digital Video Processing, Prentice-Hall, 1995.

[7] Grimson, E., Stauffer, C., Romano, R., Lee, L., Viola, P. and O. Faugeras. Forest of sensors: using adaptive tracking to classify and monitor activities in a site, Proceedings of 1998 DARPA Image Understanding Workshop, Vol. 1, pp. 33-41, 1998.

[8] Kanade, T., Collins, R., Lipton, A., Burt, P. and L. Wixson, Advances in cooperative multi-sensor video surveillance, Proceedings of 1998 DARPA Image Understanding Workshop, Vol. 1, pp. 3-24.

[9] Zhang, J., Gao, J. and Liu, W., Image sequence segmentation using 3D structure tensor and curve evolution, to appear in IEEE Trans. Circuits and Systems for Video Technology.

[10] Ciampini, R., et al., Motion-based segmentation by means of active contours, Proc. International Conference on Image Processing(ICIP) '98, Vol. 2, pp. 667-670, 1998.

[11] Paragios, N. and Deriche, R., PDE-based level-set approach for detection and tracking of moving objects, Proc. International Conference on Computer Vision(ICCV) '98, pp. 1139-1145, 1998.

[12] Sapiro, G., Color snakes, Computer Vision and Image Understanding, Vol. 68, No. 2, pp. 247-253, 1997.

[13] Zhang, K. and Kittler, J., Global motion estimation and robust regression for video coding, Proc. International Conference on Image Processing(ICIP) '98, Vol. 3, pp. 994-947, Oct 4-7, 1998.

[14] Jhne, B., Hauecker, H., Spies, H., Schmundt, D., Schurr, U., Study of dynamical processes with tensor-based spatiotemporal image processing techniques, European Conference on Computer Vision (ECCV) '98, pp. 322-335.

[15] Sethian, J. A., Level Set Methods and Fast Marching Methods, Cambridge University Press, 1999.

[16] Caselles, V., Kimmel, R. and Sapiro, G., Geodesic active contours, International Journal of Computer Vision, Vol. 22, No. 1, pp. 61-79, Feb-Mar 1997.

[17] Liu, W., Real-time image sequence segmentation using curve evolution, MS Thesis, UWM, to be completed by Dec. 2001.

[18] Numerical Recipe.

Chapter 7

Medical Image Segmentation Using Level Sets

Jasjit S. Suri[1], *Sameer Singh*[2] *and Swamy Laxminarayan*[3]

7.1 Introduction

The role of fast shape recovery has always been a critical component in 2-D and 3-D medical imagery since it assists largely in medical therapy such as image guided surgery applications. The applications of shape recovery have been increasing since scanning methods became faster, more accurate and less artifacted. Shape recovery of medical organs is more difficult compared to other computer vision and imaging fields. This is primarily due to the large shape variability, structure complexity, several kinds of artifacts and restrictive body scanning methods (scanning ability limited to acquiring images in three orthogonal and oblique directions only). The recovery of the White Matter (WM) and Gray Matter (GM) boundaries in the human brain slices is a challenge due to its highly convoluted structure. In spite of the above complications, we have started to explore faster and more accurate software tools for shape recovery in 2-D and 3-D applications.

Brain segmentation in 2-D has lately shown to be of tremendous interest and a number of techniques have been developed (see the classification tree as shown in fig. 7.1). The major success has been in the deformation techniques. Deformations has played a critical role in shape representation and this Chapter uses level sets as a tool to capture deforming shapes in medical imagery. In fact, the research on deformation started in the late 1980's when the paper

[1]Marconi Medical Systems, Inc., Cleveland, OH, USA
[2]University of Exeter, Exeter, UK
[3]New Jersey Institute of Technology, Newark, NJ, USA

PDE & Level Sets: Algorithmic Approaches to Static & Motion Imagery
Edited by Jasjit Suri and Swamy Laxminarayan, Kluwer Academic/Plenum Publishers, 2002

called "snakes" (first class of deformable models or classical deformable models) was published by Terzopoulous and co-workers (see Kass *et al.* [2]). Since then, there has been an extensive burst of publications in the area of parametric deformable models and their improvements. For details on the majority of the parametric deformable model papers, see the recently published paper by Suri [3] and the references therein. The discussions of these references are outside the scope in this Chapter. The second class of deformable models is level sets. These deformable models were introduced by Osher and Sethian [4] which started from Sethian's Ph.D. thesis [5]. The fundamental difference between these two classes is: Parametric deformable methods are local methods based on energy-minimizing spline guided by external and image forces which pulls the spline towards features such as lines and edges in the image. On the other hand, level set methods are based on active contour energy minimization which solves the computation of geodesics or minimal distance curves. The level set methods are governed by the curvature dependent speeds of moving curves or fronts. Those familiar in the field of parametric deformable models will appreciate the major advantages and superiority of level sets compared to classical deformable models. We will, however, briefly cover these in this Chapter also.

The application of level sets in medical imaging was attempted by Sethian and his coworkers (see Malladi *et al.* [6]). Other authors who used the level sets were: Kichenassamy *et al.* [7], Yezzi *et al.* [8] and Siddiqui *et al.* [9]. The work done above uses plain gradient-based techniques as the speed functions. These methods are very noise sensitive and are non-robust, especially in a multi-spectral and multi-class brain volume scans. These methods fail to take advantage of the regional based statistics in the level set framework for curve propagation for WM/GM boundary estimation. Thus there was leaking or bleeding of the boundaries. Recently, Suri [10] tried to incorporate the fuzzy statistics into the level set framework to prevent leaking of the boundaries.

This Chapter presents a fast region-based level set system (so-called geometric snakes[4] based on regions) for extraction of white matter, gray matter and cerebrospinal fluid boundaries from the two dimensional magnetic resonance images of the human brain. This method uses a new technique of introducing the fuzzy classifier in the level set framework besides keeping the traditional

[4]called as geometric active contour

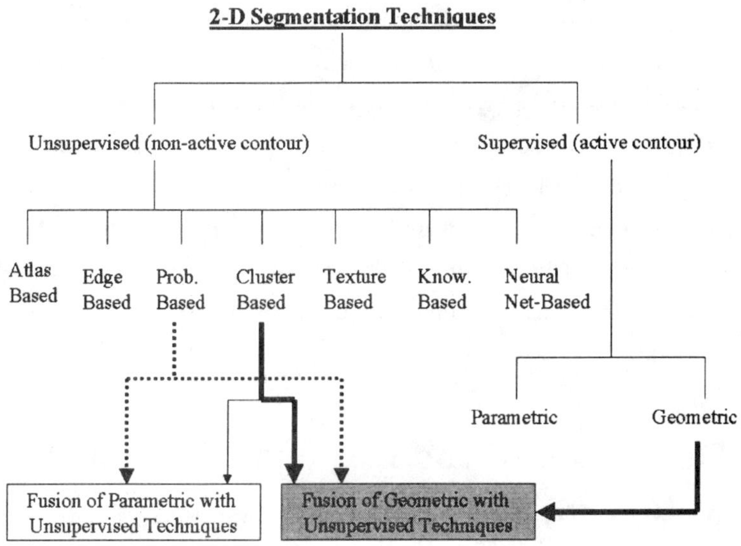

Figure 7.1: Classification tree for the 2-D brain segmentation techniques. The 2-D methods are primarily divided into two parts: unsupervised and supervised. They are also called in terms of deformation models as: (**1**) non-active and (**2**) active contour methods. As seen in the figure, the unsupervised methods are futher classified into seven categories: (**1**) atlas-based, (**2**) edge-based, (**3**) probability-based, (**4**) cluster-based, (**5**) texture-based, (**6**) knowledge-based and (**7**) neural network based. The supervised techniques are divided into two major classes: parametric and geometric. With the advancement in Computer Vision, Graphics and Image Processing techniques, we have started to see the fusion of unsupervised and supervised techniques. The shaded box shows the fusion of geometric and fuzzy clustering, the one used in this Chapter.

speed terms of curvature, shape and gradient. Please note that the shorter version of this Chapter will appear in the proceedings of the International Conference in Advances in Pattern Recognition [11].

The layout of this Chapter is as follows: Section 7.2 presents the derivation of geometric snakes from parametric models. The numerical implementation of integrating the speed functions in the level set framework is discussed in section 7.3. The methodology and the segmentation system are presented in section 7.4. The results on synthetic and real data are presented in section 7.5. The same section also discusses numerical stability issues related to this technique, sensitivity of level set parameters, accuracy and speed issues. The superiority of geometric snakes when fused with fuzzy clustering in level set framework is discussed in section 7.6. Comparison between the region-based level sets and the previous techniques are discussed in section 7.7. Finally, the Chapter concludes in section 7.8 with future directions.

7.2 Derivation of the Regional Geometric Active Contour Model from the Classical Parametric Deformable Model

Parametric Snake Model: In this section, we derive the level set equation by embedding the region statistics into the parametric classical energy model. This method is in the spirit of Xu's *et al.* [12] attempt. We will discuss part of that derivation here. To start with, the standard dynamic classical energy model as given by Kass *et al.* [2] was:

$$\gamma \frac{\partial \mathbf{X}}{\partial t} = \underbrace{\frac{\partial}{\partial s}(\alpha \frac{\partial \mathbf{X}}{\partial s}) - \frac{\partial^2}{\partial s^2}(\beta \frac{\partial^2 \mathbf{X}}{\partial s^2})}_{internal-energy} + \underbrace{F_{ext}(\mathbf{X})}_{external-energy} , \tag{7.1}$$

where $\mathbf{X}$ was the parametric contour[5] with parameter s and γ was the damping coefficient. As seen in equation 7.1, the classical energy model constitutes an energy-minimizing spline guided by external and image forces that pulled the spline towards features such as lines and edges in the image. The energy-minimizing spline was named "snakes" because the spline softly and quietly

[5]For some details on classical energy models, readers can refer to Chapter ??, for complete implementation of these equations, see Kass *et al.* [2].

moved while minimizing the energy term. The internal energy was composed of two terms: the first term was the first order derivative of the parametric curve which acted like a membrane and the second term was the second derivative of the parametric curve which acted as a thin plate (so-called the pressure force). These terms were controlled by the elastic constants α and β. The second part of the classical energy model constituted the external force given by $F_{ext}(\mathbf{X})$. This external energy term depended upon image forces which was a function of image gradient. Parametric snakes had flexibility to dynamically control the movements, but there were inherent drawbacks when they were applied to highly convoluted structures, sharp bends and corners, or on images with a large amount of noise. We therefore try to preserve the classical properties of the parametric contours but also bring the geometric properties which could capture the topology of the convoluted WM and GM. Next, we show the derivation of the geometric snake from the above model in the level set framework.

Derivation of the Geometric Snake: Since the second derivative term in Eq. 7.1 did not affect significantly the performance of the active geometric snakes (see Caselles *et al.* [13]), we dropped that term and replaced it with a new pressure force term given as: $F_p(\mathbf{X})$. This pressure force is an outward force which is a function of the unit normal, $\mathcal{N}$ of the deforming curve. Thus defining the pressure force as: $F_p(\mathbf{X}) = w_p(\mathbf{X})\mathcal{N}(\mathbf{X})$, where $w_p(\mathbf{X})$ is the weighting factor, the new parametric active contour could be written by replacing $\beta\frac{\partial^2\mathbf{X}}{\partial s^2}$ by $w_p(\mathbf{X})\mathcal{N}(\mathbf{X})$, we get:

$$\gamma\frac{\partial\mathbf{X}}{\partial t} = \frac{\partial}{\partial s}(\alpha\frac{\partial\mathbf{X}}{\partial s}) - w_p(\mathbf{X})\mathcal{N}(\mathbf{X}) + F_{ext}(\mathbf{X})\,. \tag{7.2}$$

Bringing Eq. 7.2 in terms of the curvature of the deformable curve by defining $\frac{\partial}{\partial s}(\frac{\partial\mathbf{X}}{\partial s})$ to be the curvature κ, and readjusting the terms by defining the constant $\epsilon = \frac{\alpha}{\gamma}$, $V_p = \frac{w_p(X)}{\gamma}\mathcal{N}(\mathbf{X})$ and $V_{ext} = \frac{F_{ext}}{\gamma}$, Eq. 7.2 can be rewritten as:

$$\frac{\partial\mathbf{X}}{\partial t} = (\epsilon\kappa + V_p + V_{ext}\,.\mathcal{N})\mathcal{N}\,. \tag{7.3}$$

The above Eq. is analogous to Sethian's [4] Eq. of curve evolution, given as: $\frac{\partial\phi}{\partial t} = V(\kappa)\mathcal{N}$, where $\mathcal{N} = -\frac{\nabla\phi}{|\nabla\phi|}$. Note, ϕ was the level set function and $V(\kappa)$ was the curvature dependent speed with which the front (or zero-level-curve) propagates. The expression $\frac{\partial\phi}{\partial t} = V(\kappa)\mathcal{N}$ described the time evolution of the level set function (ϕ) in such a way that the zero-level-curve of this evolving function was always identified with the propagating interface. We will interchangably use the term "level set function" with the term "flow field" or simply "field" during the course of this Chapter. Comparing Eq. 7.3 and $\frac{\partial \phi}{\partial t} = V(\kappa)\mathcal{N}$, and using the geometric property of the curve's normal $\mathcal{N}$ and considering only the normal components of internal and external forces,

$$\frac{\partial}{\partial s}(\alpha \frac{\partial \mathbf{X}}{\partial s}).\mathcal{N} = (\alpha\kappa)\,, \tag{7.4}$$

we obtain the level set function (ϕ) in the form of the partial differential equation (PDE) as:

$$\frac{\partial \phi}{\partial t} = (\epsilon\,\kappa + V_p)\,|\nabla\phi| - V_{ext}.\nabla\phi\,. \tag{7.5}$$

Note, V_p can be considered as a regional force term and and can be mathematically expressed as a combination of inside-outside regional area of the propagating curve. This can be defined as $\frac{w_R}{\gamma R}$, where R is the region indicator term that lies between 0 and 1, γ is the weighting constant and w_R is the term which controls the speed of the deformation process. An example of such a region indicator could come from a membership function of the fuzzy classifier (see Bezdek *et al.* [16]). Thus, we see that regional information is one of the factors which controls the speed of the geometric snake or propagating curve in the level set framework. A framework in which a snake propagates by capturing the topology of the WM/GM, navigated by the regional, curvature, edge and gradient forces is called geometric snakes. Also note that Eq. 7.5 has three terms: $\epsilon\,\kappa$, V_p and V_{ext}. These three terms are the speed functions which control the propagation of the curve. These three speed functions are known as curvature, regional and gradient speed functions, as they contribute towards the three kinds of forces responsible for navigating the curve propagation. In the next section, we show the numerical implementation used for solving the partial differential equation (PDE) (Eq. 7.5) to estimate the "flow field".

7.3 Numerical Implementation of the Three Speed Functions in the Level Set Framework for Geometric Snake Propagation

In this section, we mathematically present the speed control functions in terms of the level set function ϕ and integrating them to estimate ϕ over time. Let $I(x,y)$ represent the pixel intensity at image location (x,y), while $V_{reg}(x,y)$, $V_{grad}(x,y)$ and $V_{cur}(x,y)$ represent the regional, gradient and curvature speed terms at pixel location (x,y). Then, using the finite difference methods as discussed by Rouy *et al.* [14] and Sethian [15], the regional level set PDE Eq. 7.5 in time can be given as:

$$\phi^{n+1}_{x,y} = \phi^{n}_{x,y} - \triangle t \; \{ \; V_{reg}(x,y) + V_{grad}(x,y) - V_{cur}(x,y) \; \}\,, \qquad (7.6)$$

where $\phi^{n}_{x,y}$ and $\phi^{n+1}_{x,y}$ were the level set functions at pixel location (x,y) at times n and $n+1$, $\triangle t$ was the time difference. The important aspect to note here is that the curve is moving in the level set field and the level set field is controlled by these three speed terms. In other words, these speeds are forces acting on the propagating contour. In the next three sub-sections, we discuss the speed terms mathematically in terms of the level set framework.

7.3.1 Regional Speed Term Expressed in Terms of the Level Set Function (ϕ)

The regional speed term at a pixel location (x,y) is mathematically given as: $V_{reg}(x,y) = max\,(V_p(x,y),0)\ \nabla^+ + min\,(V_p(x,y),0)\ \nabla^-$, where $V_p(x,y)$, ∇^+ and ∇^- were given as: $V_p(x,y) = \frac{w_R}{\gamma\, R_{ind}(x,y)}$, $R_{ind} = 1 - 2\,u(x,y)$, $\nabla^+ = [\nabla^+_x + \nabla^+_y]^{\frac{1}{2}}$, and $\nabla^- = [\nabla^-_x + \nabla^-_y]^{\frac{1}{2}}$. ∇^+_x and ∇^-_x were mathematically given as:

$$\begin{cases} \nabla^+_x = [max\,(D^{-x}(x,y),0))^2 + min\,(D^{+x}(x,y),0))^2], \\ \nabla^-_y = [max\,(D^{-y}(x,y),0))^2 + min\,(D^{+y}(x,y),0))^2], \end{cases} \qquad (7.7)$$

Note, $u(x,y)$ was the fuzzy membership function for a particular tissue class which had a value between 0 to 1 for a given input image I. R_{ind} was the region indicator function that falls in the range between -1 to +1. The fuzzy membership computation and pixel classification were done using fuzzy clustering to compute the fuzzy membership values for each pixel location (x, y). The number of classes taken were four corresponding to WM, GM, CSF and background. Note, ∇_x^+ and ∇_y^+ are the forward level set gradients in the x and y directions. Similarly, ∇_x^- and ∇_y^- are the backward level set gradients in the x and y directions. Also note, ∇_x^+, ∇_y^+, ∇_x^- and ∇_y^- are expressed in terms of $D^{-x}(x, y)$, $D^{+x}(x, y)$, $D^{-y}(x, y)$, $D^{+y}(x, y)$ which are the forward and backward difference operators defined in terms of the level set function ϕ given in Eq. 7.9. We thus see that the regional speed term is expressed in terms of "flow field" and "flow field" is controlled by a regional force V_p, which in turn is controlled by a region indicator, which depends on the fuzzy membership function $u(x, y)$. Thus the pixel classifier is embedded in the level set framework to navigate the propagation of geometric snake to capture the brain topology, which is the novelty of this Chapter. We will see its implementation details ahead.

7.3.2 Gradient Speed Term Expressed in Terms of the Level Set Function (ϕ)

Here we compute the edge strength of the brain boundaries. The x and y components of the gradient speed terms were computed as: $V_{grad}(x, y) = V_{gradx}(x, y) + V_{grady}(x, y)$, where

$$\begin{cases} V_{gradx}(x, y) = max(p^n(x, y), 0)\ D^{-x}(x, y) + min(q^n(x, y), 0)\ D^{+x}(x, y), \\ V_{grady}(x, y) = max(q^n(x, y), 0)\ D^{-y}(x, y) + min(q^n(x, y), 0)\ D^{+y}(x, y), \end{cases} \tag{7.8}$$

$p^n(x, y)$ and $q^n(x, y)$ were defined as the x and y components of the gradient strength at a pixel location (x, y). These were given as: $p^n(x, y) = \nabla_x(w_e\ \nabla(G_\sigma * I))$ and $q^n(x, y) = \nabla_y(w_e\ \nabla(G_\sigma * I))$. Note, w_e was the weight of the edge and was a fixed constant. Also note that G_σ is the Gaussian operator with a known standard deviation σ and I is the original gray scale image and $(G_\sigma * I)$ was the simple Gaussian smoothing. Here, ∇_x and ∇_y were the x and y components of the edge gradient image, which was estimated by computing the gradient of the smoothed image. Again, note that the edge speed term is dependent upon the forward and backward difference operators which were defined in terms of the level set function ϕ given in Eq. 7.9.

$$\begin{cases} D^{-x}(x,y) = \frac{(\phi(x,y)-\phi(x-1,y))}{\Delta x} \ \& \ D^{+x}(x,y) = \frac{(\phi(x+1,y)-\phi(x,y))}{\Delta x} \\ D^{-y}(x,y) = \frac{(\phi(x,y)-\phi(x,y-1))}{\Delta y} \ \& \ D^{+y}(x,y) = \frac{(\phi(x,y+1)-\phi(x,y))}{\Delta y} \end{cases}, \tag{7.9}$$

where $\phi(x,y)$, $\phi(x-1,y)$, $\phi(x+1,y)$, $\phi(x,y-1)$, $\phi(x,y+1)$ were the level set functions at pixel locations (x,y), $(x-1,y)$, $(x+1,y)$, $(x,y-1)$, $(x,y+1)$, the four neighbours of (x,y). Note, Δx and Δy are the step sizes in x and y directions.

7.3.3 Curvature Speed Term Expressed in Terms of the Level Set Function (ϕ)

This is mathematically expressed in terms of the signed distance transform of the contour as:

$$V_{cur}(x,y) = \epsilon\, \kappa^n(x,y)[\,(D^{0x}(x,y))^2 + ((\,D^{0y}(x,y))^2\,]^{\frac{1}{2}}\,, \tag{7.10}$$

where ϵ was a fixed constant. $\kappa^n(x,y)$ was the curvature at a pixel location (x,y) at n^{th} iteration, given as: $\kappa^n(x,y) = \frac{\phi_{xx}^2\,\phi_y^2 - \phi_x^2\,\phi_y^2\,\phi_{xy}^2 + \phi_{yy}^2\,\phi_x^2}{(\phi_x^2+\phi_y^2)^{\frac{3}{2}}}$, and $D^{0x}(x,y)$ and $D^{0y}(x,y)$ were defined as: $D^{0x}(x,y) = \frac{(\phi(x+1,y)-\phi(x-1,y))}{2\,\Delta x}$ and $D^{0y}(x,y) = \frac{(\phi(x,y+1)-\phi(x,y-1))}{2\,\Delta y}$. Note that ϕ_x^2, ϕ_y^2 are the square of the first order finite difference of level set in x and y directions. Similarly, ϕ_{xx}^2 and ϕ_{yy}^2 are the square of the second order finite difference of level set in x and y directions. Also note that ϕ_{xy}^2 is the first order finite difference in x followed by y directions (details on finite difference can be seen in any book at undergraduate level). To numerically solve Eq. 7.6, all we needed were the gradient speed values $[p(x,y), q(x,y)]$, curvature speed $\kappa(x,y)$ and the membership function $u(x,y)$ at pixel locations (x,y). These speeds are integrated to compute the new "flow field" (level set function, ϕ). The integrated speed term helps in the computation of the new "flow field" for the next iteration $n+1$, given the "flow field" of the previous iteration n. So far, we discussed the "flow field" computation at every pixel location (x,y), but to speed up these computations, we compute the triplet speeds only in a "narrow band" using the "fast marching method", so-called optimization, which is discussed next.

7.4 Fast Brain Segmentation System Based on Regional Level Sets

Having discussed the derivation of geometric snakes in section 7.2 and its numerical implementation in section 7.3, we can use this model to segment the brain's WM, GM and CSF boundaries. This section presents the system or a procedure to estimate these boundaries, given a gray scale MR brain scan. Due to large brain volumes (typically of the size of 256 cubed data), it is necessary to devise a method where one can optimize the segmentation process. We thus use the methodology as adapted by Sethian and his coworkers, so-called "narrow banding", since it is simple and effective.

The layout of this section is as follows: We first present the steps/procedure or a system and its components to estimate the WM/GM boundaries in sub-section 7.4.1. Since the system uses the triplets of speed control functions and the regional speed control is the crux of the system, we will then focus on the estimation of the membership function which gets integrated into the regional speed function. We will discuss the regional speed computation using "Fuzzy C mean" (FCM) in sub-section 7.4.2. In sub-section 7.4.3, we discuss how to solve the fundamental Eikonal equation. Given the raw contour, the Signed Distance Transform (SDT) computation was implemented using the "fast marching method" in sub-section 7.4.4. Sub-section 7.4.4 presents the solution to the Eikonal equation when the speed is unity. A note on heap sorting is discussed in sub-section 7.4.5. Finally, we conclude this section by discussing the segmentation engine in sub-section 7.4.6, so-called initialization and re-initialization loops.

7.4.1 Overall System and Its Components

The "WM/GM boundary estimation system" for estimating the WM/GM boundaries is being presented using two diagrams: Fig. 7.2 shows the overall system which calls the "segmentation engine" shown in fig. 7.3. The inputs to the overall system were: the user-defined closed contour and the input gray scale image. The input to the segmentation engine (see the center ellipse in fig. 7.2) included the level set constants, the optimization module, the so-called "narrow band" method, speed terms and the signed distance transform of the raw input curve. The speed terms (regional and gradient) were computed first for the whole image just once, while the curvature speed terms were computed in the "narrow band". The segmentation engine was run over the initial field image (so-called SDT image) which was computed for the whole image or for the "narrow band". The major components of the main system are:

1. *Fuzzy membership value computation/Pixel classification*:
   A number of techniques exists for classifying the pixels of the MR image. Some of the most efficient techniques are the Fuzzy C Mean (see Bezdek *et al.* [16]), k-NN, neural networks, (see Hall *et al.* [17]), and Bayesian pixel classification (see the patent by Sheehan, Haralick, Lee and Suri [?]). We used the FCM method for our system due to its simplicity and effectiveness.

2. *Integration of different speed components and solving the level set function (ϕ)*:
   This includes the integration of regional, gradient and curvature-based speed terms, discussed in section 7.3.

3. *Optimization module ("fast marching method" in "narrow band")*:
   This involves application of the curve evolution and the level set to estimate the new "flow field" distribution in the "narrow band" using the "fast marching method".

4. *Isocontour extraction*:
   The last stage of this system required estimation of the WM/GM boundaries given the final level set function. This was accomplished using an isocontour algorithm at sub-pixel resolution (for details on these methods see, Berger *et al.* [19], Sethian *et al.* [20], Tababai *et al.* [?], Huertas *et al.* [?], and Gao *et al.* [?]).

7.4.2 Fuzzy Membership Computation / Pixel Classification

In this step, we classified each pixel. Usually, the classification algorithm expects one to know how many classes (roughly) the image would have. The number of classes in the image would be the same as the number of tissue types. A pixel could belong to more than one class; thus and therefore we used

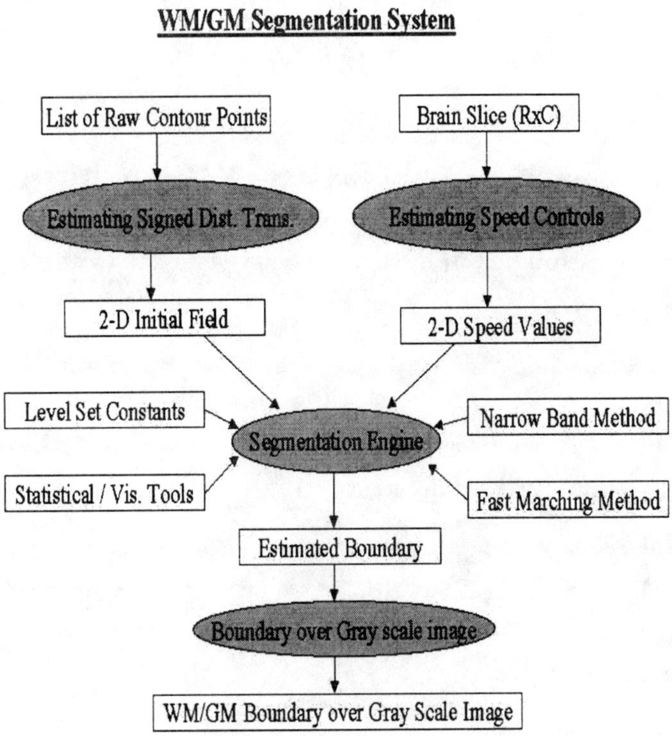

Figure 7.2: Overall system which calls the "segmentation engine". The user enters the raw contour and the initial field is estimated around that contour. A gray scale image is used to compute the gradient and regional speed functions. The segmentation engine receives the level set constants, gradient and regional speed values and the initial field to compute the final field in the narrow band using the "fast marching method" (four inputs to the central ellipse). The isocontour is extracted in the final field, which yields the WM/GM boundaries in the brain slice.

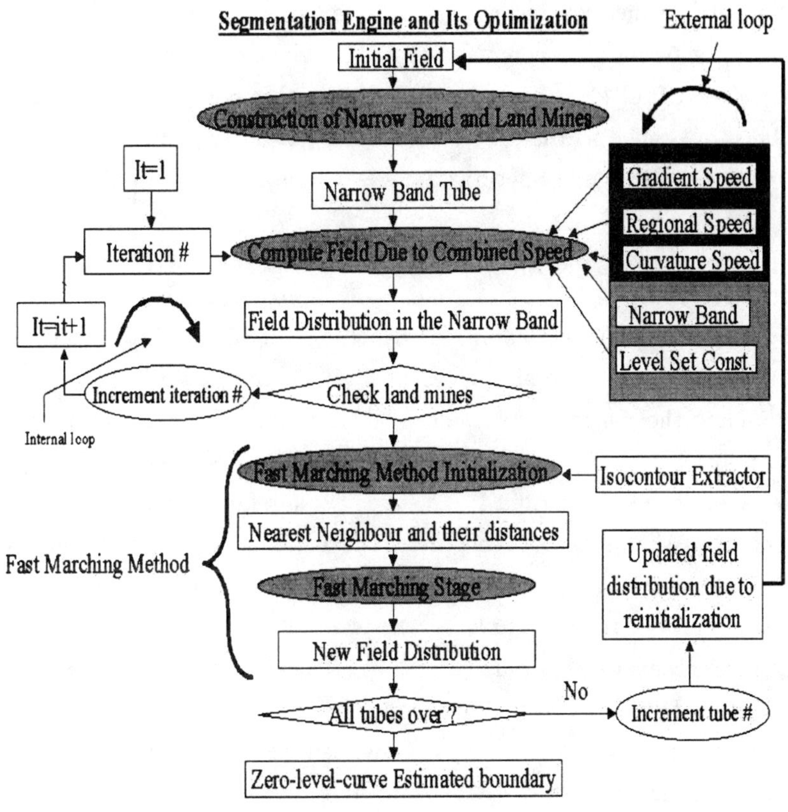

Figure 7.3: Brain "segmentation engine" and implementation details for running the region-based level set method in the narrow band using the "fast marching method". Given the initial field, we constructed the narrow tube of fixed thickness around the raw contour. The new field was computed using triplets of speed. The process exits if land mines were hit, or else the internal loop continued. The reinitialization process is activated and the next round of tubing starts, until all tubes were over.

the fuzzy membership function to associate with each pixel in the image. There are several algorithms used to compute membership functions and one of the most efficient ones is Fuzzy C Mean (FCM) based on the clustering technique. Because of its ease of implementation for spectral data, it is preferred over other pixel classification techniques. Mathematically, we expressed the FCM algorithm below but for complete details, readers are advised to see Bezdek *et al.* [16] and Hall *et al.* [17]. The FCM algorithm computed the measure of membership termed as the *fuzzy membership function.* Suppose the observed pixel intensities in a multi-spectral image at a pixel location j was given as:

$$\mathbf{y}_j = [y_{j1}\, y_{j2}\, ..., y_{jN}]^T, \tag{7.11}$$

where j takes the pixel location and N is the total number of pixels in the data set (note, not to get confused with the $\mathcal{N}$ used in derivation in section 7.2). In FCM, the algorithm iterates between computing the *fuzzy membership function* and the centroid of each class. This membership function is the pixel location for each class (tissue type) and the value of the membership function lies between the range of 0 and 1. This membership function actually represents the degree of similarity between the pixel vector at a pixel location and the centroid of the class (tissue type); for example, if the membership function has a value close to 1, then the pixel at the pixel location is close to the centroid of the pixel vector for that particular class. The algorithm can be presented in the following four steps. If $u_{jk}^{(p)}$ is the membership value at location j for class k at iteration p, then $\Sigma_{k=1}^{3} u_{jk} = 1$. As defined before, $\mathbf{y}_j$ is the observed pixel vector at location j and $\mathbf{v}_k^{(p)}$ is the centroid of class k at iteration p, thus, the FCM steps for computing the fuzzy membership values are:

1. Choose the number of classes (K) and the error threshold ϵ_{th} and set the initial guess for the centroids $\mathbf{v}_k^{(0)}$ where the iteration number p=0.

2. Compute the fuzzy membership function, given by the equation:

$$u_{jk}^{(p)} = \frac{||\mathbf{y}_j - \mathbf{v}_k^{(p)}||^{-2}}{\Sigma_{l=1}^{K} ||\mathbf{y}_j - \mathbf{v}^{(p)}||^{-2}} \tag{7.12}$$

   where $j = 1, ..., M$ and $k = 1, ..., K$.

3. Compute the new centroids, using the equation:

$$\mathbf{v}^{(p+1)} = \frac{\Sigma_{j=1}^{N} (u_{jk}^{(p)})^2\, \mathbf{y}_j}{\Sigma_{j=1}^{N} (u_{jk}^{(p)})^2}. \tag{7.13}$$

4. Convergence was checked by computing the error between the previous and current centroids ($||\mathbf{v}^{(p+1)} - \mathbf{v}^{(p)}||$). If the algorithm had converged, an exit would be required; otherwise, one would increment p and go to step 2 for computing the fuzzy membership function again. The output of the FCM algorithm was K sets of fuzzy membership functions. We were interested in the membership value at each pixel for each class. Thus, if there were K classes, then we threw out K number of images and K number of matrices for the membership functions to be used in computing the final speed terms. Since the algorithm computed the region properties of the image, we considered this factor to be a region-based speed control term which was plugged into Eq. 7.6.

7.4.3 Eikonal Equation and its Mathematical Solution

In this sub-section, we present the mathematical solution for solving the level set function with unity speed[6]. Such a method is needed to compute the signed distance transform when the raw contour crosses the background pixel grid. Let us consider a case of a "front" moving with a velocity $V = V(x, y)$, such that V is greater than zero. Using Sethian's level set equation, we can consider a monotonically advancing front represented in the form:

$$\phi_t = V(x, y)\ ||\nabla\,\phi||, \tag{7.14}$$

where ϕ_t is the rate of change of the level set and $\nabla\,\phi$ is the gradient of the ϕ. Let $T(x, y)$ be the time at which the front crosses the grid point (x, y). In this time, the surface $T(x, y)$ satisfies the equation:

$$||\nabla T||\ .\ V = 1. \tag{7.15}$$

Details on Eikonal equation can be seen by Osher and Sethian [4]. By approximation, the solution to the Eikonal equation would be given as:

$$\begin{aligned} max\ [\ max(D^{-x}\,T, 0), -min(D^{+x}\,T, 0)\ ]^2 + \\ max\ [\ max(D^{-y}\,T, 0), -min(D^{+y}\,T, 0)\ ]^2 = \frac{1}{V^2{}_{xy}}, \end{aligned} \tag{7.16}$$

[6]If one can perform the computation of curve evolution at unity speed, then the implementation can be done for any speed.

where ${V^2}_{xy}$ was the square of the speed at location (x, y) and $D^{-x}T$, $D^{+x}T$, $D^{-y}T$, $D^{+y}T$ are the backward and forward differences in time, given as:

$$\begin{cases} D^{+x}T = \frac{T(x,y+1)-T(x,y)}{2} \\ D^{-x}T = \frac{T(x,y)-T(x,y-1)}{2} \\ D^{+y}T = \frac{T(x+1,y)-T(x,y)}{2} \\ D^{-y}T = \frac{T(x,y)-T(x-1,y)}{2} \end{cases} \tag{7.17}$$

There are efficient schemes for solving Eikonal Eq. 7.15. For details, see Sethian *et al.* [15], Cao *et al.* [?] and Chen *et al.* [?]. We implemented Eq. 7.16 using Sethian's "fast marching" algorithm referred to in patent [26], discussed in the next sub-section.

7.4.4 Fast Marching Method for Solving the Eikonal Equation

The "fast marching method" (FMM) was used to solve the Eikonal equation, or a level set evolution with a given speed whose sign does not change. Its main usage was to compute the signed distance transform from a given curve (say, one with speed = 1). This signed distance function was the level set function that was used in the "narrow band" algorithm. FMM can also be used for a simple active contour model if the contour only moves either inward (pressure force in terms of parametric snakes) or outward (balloon force in terms of parametric snakes). The FMM algorithm consisted of three major steps: (1) initialization stage, (2) tagging stage and (3) marching stage (see fig. 7.3). We will briefly discuss these three stages.

1. *Initialization Stage*:

   Let us assume that the curve cuts the grid points exactly, which means that it passed through the intersection of the horizontal and vertical grid lines. If the curve did not pass through the grid points, then we found where the curve intersected the grid lines using the simple method recently developed by Adalsteinsson *et al.*'s [?] for curve-grid intersection (see figure 7.9). We implemented a robust method, which was a modified version of Adalsteinsson *et al.* [?]. In this method, we checked four neighbors (E, W, N, S) of a given central pixel and found 16 combinations where the given contour could intersect the grid. Since the central pixel could be inside or outside, there were 16 positive combinations and 16 negative combinations. At the end of this process, we noted the distances of all the grid points which were closest to the given curve.

2. *Tagging Stage*:
   Here, we created three sets of grid points: *Accepted set*, *Trial set* and *Far set.* The *Accepted set* included those points which lay on the given curve. All these points obviously had a distance of zero. We tagged them as ACCEPTED. If the curve did not pass through the grid points, then those points were the points of the initialization stage and we also tagged them as ACCEPTED. The *Trial set* included all points that were nearest neighbors to a point in the *Accepted set.* We tagged them as TRIAL. We then computed their distance values by solving the Eikonal Equation (Eq. 7.16). These points and their distances were put on the heap. The *Far set* were the grid points which were neither tagged as ACCEPTED nor TRIAL. We tagged them as FAR. They did not affect the distance computation of trial grid points. These grid points were not put onto the heap.

3. *Marching Stage*:

   (a) We first popped out a grid point (say P) from the top of the heap. It should have the smallest distance value among all the grid points in the heap. We tagged this point as ACCEPTED so that its value would not change anymore. We used the heap sort methodology for bubbling the least distance value on the heap.

   (b) We found the four nearest neighbors of the popped point P. This is what was done for these four points: if its tag was ACCEPTED, we did nothing; otherwise, we re-computed its distance by solving Eikonal Eq. 7.16. If it was FAR, it was relabled as TRIAL and was put on the heap. If it is already labeled as TRIAL, its value was updated in the heap. This prevented the same point from appearing twice in the heap.

   (c) Return to step (a) until there were no more points in the heap, i.e. all points had been tagged as ACCEPTED.

Note that the above method was an exhaustive search like the greedy algorithm discussed by Suri *et al.* [?]. The superiority of this method is evidenced by the fact that we visited every grid point no more than four times. The grid or pixel location (x, y) was picked up by designing the back pointer method as used by Sethian *et al.* [26].

7.4.5 A Note on the Heap Sorting Algorithm

We used the heap sorting algorithm to select the smallest value (see Sedwick *et al.* [30]). Briefly, a heap can be viewed as a tree or a corresponding ordered array. A binary heap had the property that the value at a given "child" position int(i) is always larger than or equal to the value at its "parent" position (int (i/2)). The minimum travel time in the heap is stored at the top of the heap. Arranging the tentative travel time array onto a heap effectively identified and selected the minimum travel time in the array. The minimum travel time on the heap identified a corresponding minimum travel time grid point. Values could be added or removed from the heap. Adding or removing a value to/from the heap included re-arranging the array so that it satisfied the heap condition ("heapifying the array"). Heapifying an array was achieved by recursively exchanging the positions of any parent-child pair violating the heap property until the heap property was satisfied across the heap. Adding or removing a value from a heap generally has a computation cost of order $O(\mathbf{log}\ n)$, where n is the number of heap elements.

7.4.6 Segmentation Engine: Running the Level Set Method in the Narrow Band

Having discussed the components of the brain segmentation system, we now present the steps for running the segmentation engine (see fig. 7.3). Below are the steps followed for computing the level set function ϕ in the "narrow band", given the speed functions (see fig. 7.3 and for details on narrow banding see, Malladi *et al.* [28]).

1. *Narrow Band and Land Mine Construction*:
   Here, we constructed a "narrow band" around the given curve where the absolute distance value was less than half the width of the "narrow band". These grid points are put onto the list. Now some points in the "narrow band" were tagged as land mines. They are the grid points whose absolute distance value was less than $\frac{W}{2}$ and greater than $(\frac{W}{2} - \Delta_l)$, where W was

the band-width and $\triangle_l$ was the width of the land mine points. Note that the formation of the "narrow band" was equivalent to saying that the first external iteration or a new tube had been formed.

2. *Internal Iteration for computing the flow field (ϕ):*
   This step evolved the active contour inside the "narrow band" until the land mine sign changed. For all the iterations, the level set function was updated by solving the level set Eq. 7.6. We then checked whether the land mine sign[7] of its ϕ had changed. If so, the system was re-initialized, otherwise the loop was continued (see fig. 7.3).

3. *Re-Initialization (ZLC[8] and SDT computation):*
   This step consisted of two parts: (i) Determination of the zero-level curve given the flow field ϕ. (ii) Given the zero-level curve, estimation of the signed distance transform was done. Part (i) is also called isocontour extraction since we estimated the front in the flow field which had a value of zero. We used the modified version of the Adalsteinsson *et al.* [?] algorithm for estimating the ZLC, however we needed the signs of the flow field to do that. In part (ii), we ran the "fast marching method" to estimate the signed distance transform (i.e., we re-ran sub-sections 7.4.4 and 7.4.3). The signed-distance-function was computed for all the points in the computational domain. At the end of step 3, the algorithm returned to step 1 and the next external iteration was started.

At the end of the process, a new zero-level curve was estimated which represented the final WM/GM boundary. Note, this technique used all the global information integrated into the system. We will discuss in detail the major advantages and superiority of this technique in section 7.6.

---

[7] if the sign of the ϕ was positive and changed to negative, then the sign changed occured. Similarly, if the sign of the ϕ was negative and changed to positive, then the sign change had occured.

[8] zero-level-curve

7.5 MR Segmentation Results on Synthetic and Real Data

7.5.1 Input Data Set and Input Level Set Parameters

This sub-section presents the segmentation results obtained by running the region-based level set technique in the "narrow band" using the "fast marching method". We performed our experiments over several normal volunteers. MR data was collected over five normal volunteers (in each of the three orthogonal planes), thereby acquiring 15 brain volumes, each having around 256 slices. Typical imaging parameters[9] were: T_E=12.1 msec, BW (band width)=15.6 kHz, T_R=500 msec, FOV=22.0 cm, PS=0.812, flip angle=90 degrees and slice thickness=5.0 mm using the Picker MR scanner. This data was converted into an isotropic volume using internal Picker software and then the MR brain slices were ready for processing. We ran our system over the sagittal, coronal and transverse slices of the MR data set, but here, complete one cycle of results are only shown over one sample MR brain scan.

Level Set Parameters: The following sets of parameters were chosen for all the experiments on real data. The factors which controlled the speed and error for the regional speed were: w_R=0.5 and ϵ_{th}=0.5. We took several combinations of the "narrow band" width (W) and land mine widths (Δ_l). For W, we increased it from 10 to 25 in increments of 5. For (Δ_l), we varied it from 2 to 10 in increments of 2. The level set constants α and γ and ϵ were fixed to 0.5, 1 and 1, respectively, for all of the experiments.

7.5.2 Results: Synthetic and Real

The inputs to the system (see figures 7.2, 7.3) were the gray scale image and the hand-drawn contour points. The speed model was first activated by computing three types of speed: curvature, gradient and region-based. The level set function was solved in the "narrow band" employing the "fast marching method" using these speed functions.

Results on Synthetic Data and its Validation:

Figure 7.10 shows the results of running the "fast marching" algorithm to compute the signed distance function in the "narrow band". Four kinds of synthetic

---

[9]For definitions of these MR parameters, see Chapter ??

shapes (from low convoluted shapes to high convoluted shapes) were taken into account to show the effect of signed distance transform on the convolution of shapes. The signed distance function performed well at the sharp curvature points. Also shown is the zero-level-curve or the input contour. This serves as a measure of our validation of the "fast marching method" and 2-D field estimation, which is one of the most critical stages.

7.5.2.1 Synthetic results for Toroid

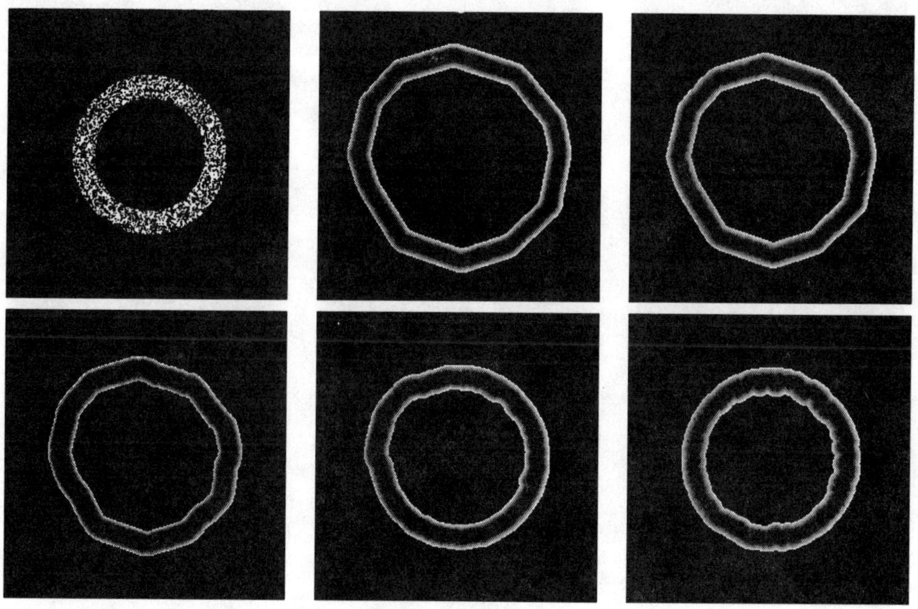

Figure 7.4: Synthetic results for demonstration of the shrinking field. **Top Left**: input image generated by perturbing the binary shape with Gaussian perturbation. **Top Middle** to **Bottom Right**: sequence of shrinking dynamic field. Note, the behavior of the changing dynamic field. Note, that the final field converges to the shape of the original toroid.

Results on Real MR Data and its Evaluation:
Figure 7.11 shows the results of pixel classification using the fuzzy C mean (FCM) algorithm. Shown are the membership function results when the class number was 0, 1, 2 and 3. Figure 7.12 shows the results of running the "fast marching method" in the "narrow band" to compute the signed distance trans-

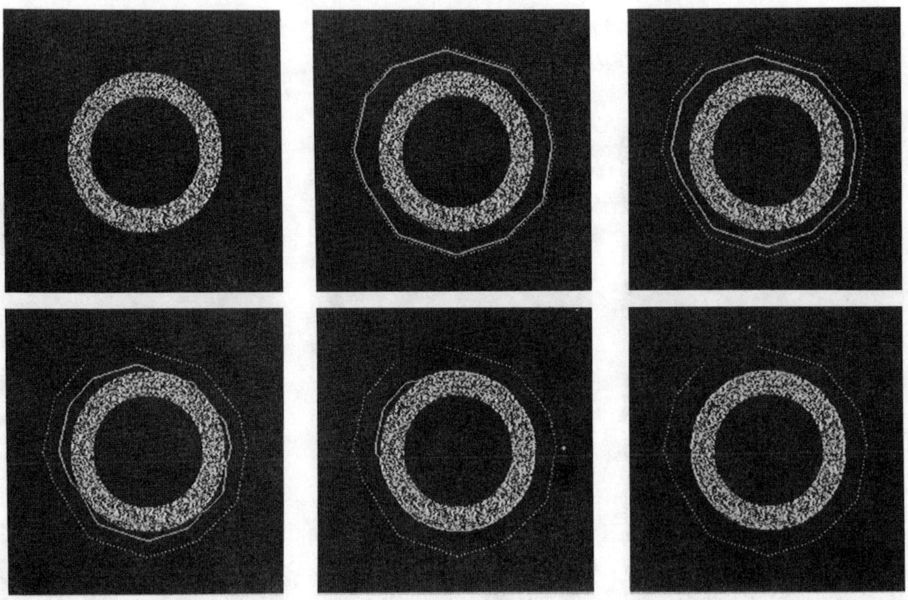

Figure 7.5: Synthetic results for the demonstration of the shrinking raw contour with respect to the original raw contour. **Top Left**: input image generated by perturbing the binary shape with Gaussian perturbation. The remainder of the images show the raw contour becoming attracted to the toroid. Note, there are two contours in each of these images. The dotted contour is the original contour and the thick continuous curve is the level set curve tracked towards the toroid.

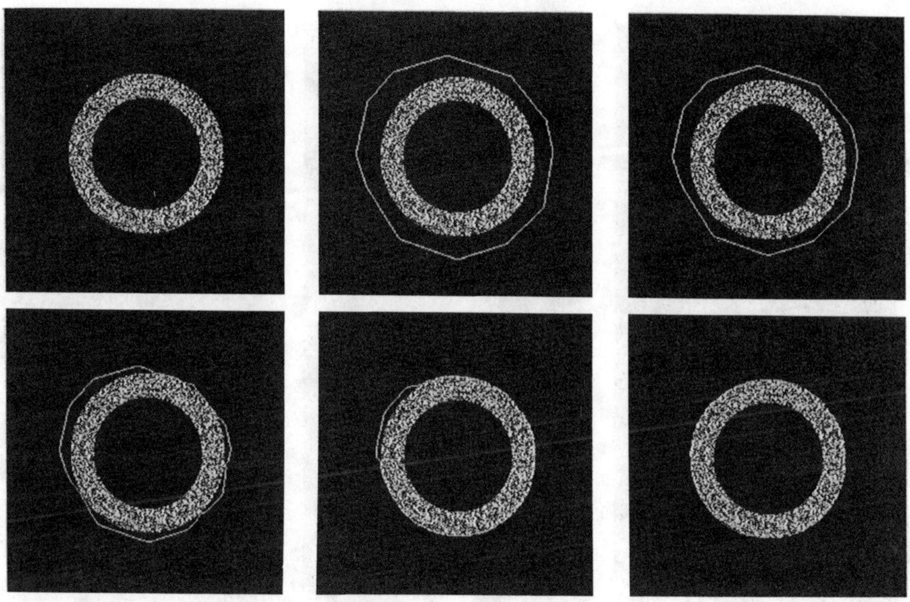

Figure 7.6: Synthetic results for the demonstration of the shrinking raw contour. **Top Left**: input image generated by perturbing the the binary shape with Gaussian perturbation. The rest of the images shows the raw contour getting attracted to the toroid.

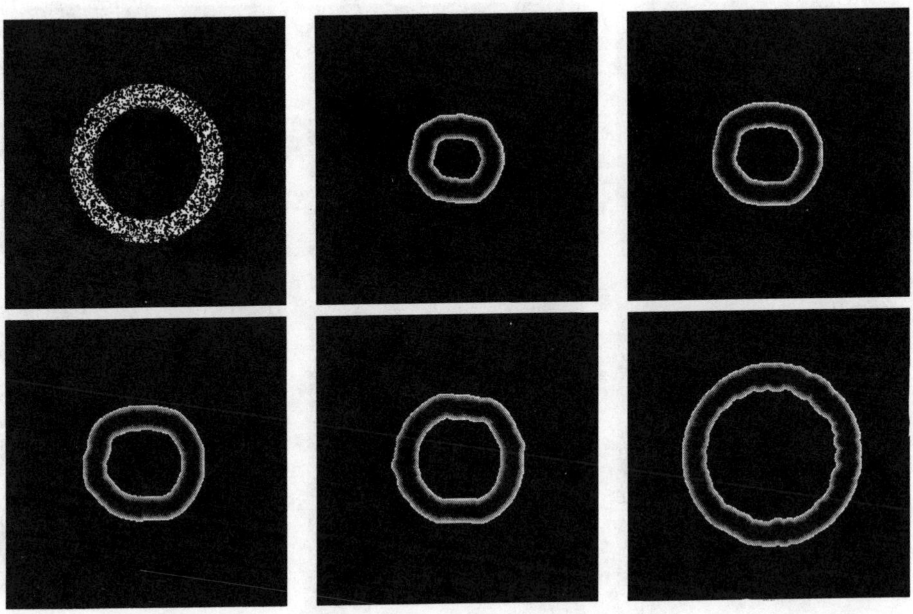

Figure 7.7: Synthetic results for the demonstration of the expanding field. **Top Left**: input image generated by perturbing the binary shape with Gaussian perturbation. The remainder of the images show the raw contour being attracted towards the outer edge of the toroid.

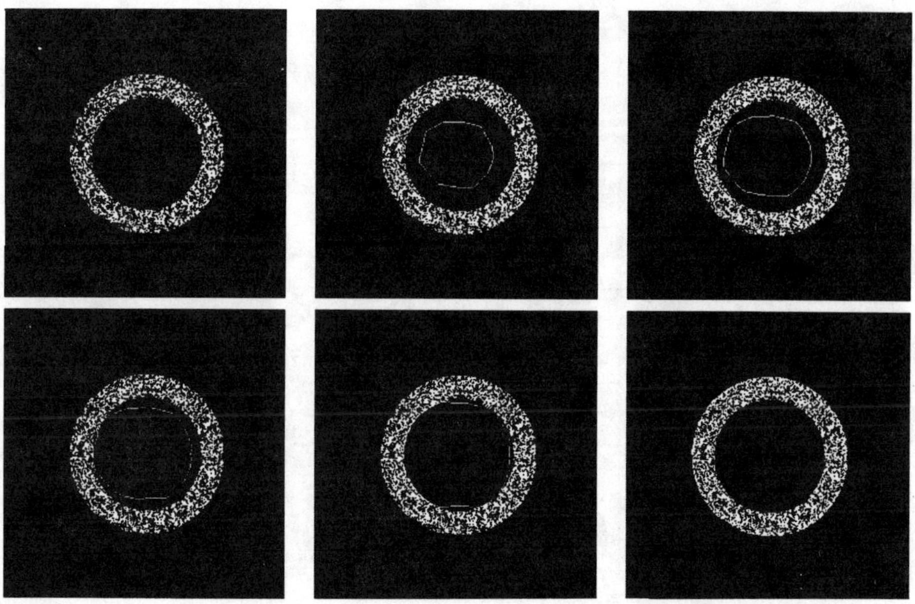

Figure 7.8: Synthetic results for the demonstration of the expanding contour. **Top Left**: input image generated by perturbing the binary shape with Gaussian perturbation. The remainder of the images show the raw contour being attracted to the toroid.

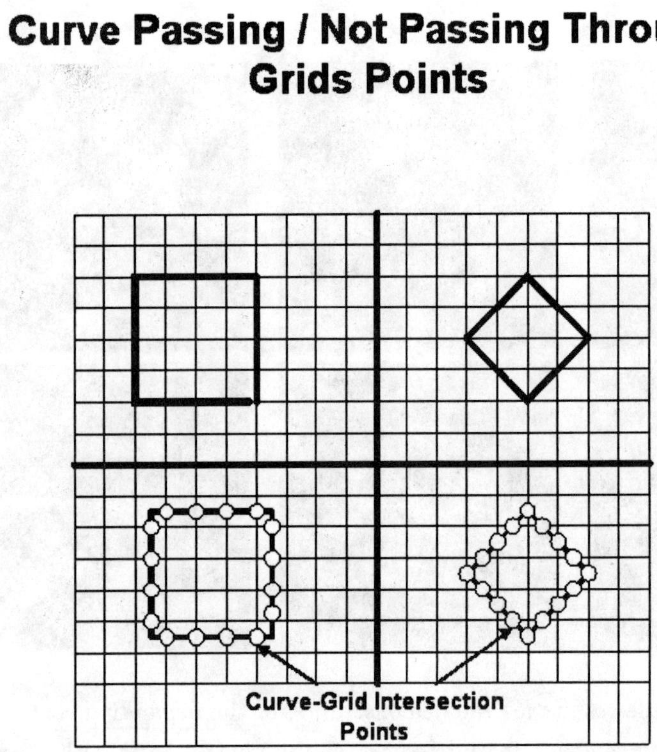

Figure 7.9: The figure shows the intersection of curve with the background grid. Note that for implementation of level sets, one needs the points where the curve interesects the background grid. This is shown in circles.

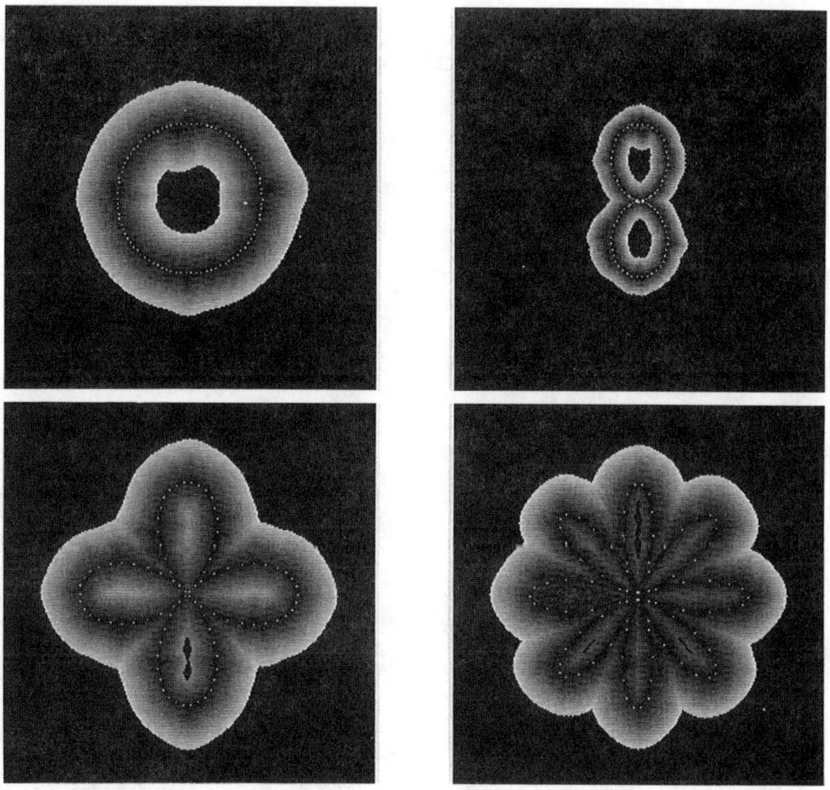

Figure 7.10: Results of running the "fast marching algorithm" in the "narrow band" on the synthetic circle, a flower with two petals, a flower with four petals and a flower with eight petal images. The synthetic shapes are sampled with white dots and the initial field (SDT) is estimated for the inner and outer regions (so-called, narrow band). The figure shows the field estimation to an accuracy of almost one hundred percent.

form during the re-initialization stage of the segmentation process. Also shown are the associated Zero-Level-Curves (ZLC's). Figure 7.13 shows how the region evolved during the course of the external iterative process. Figure 7.14 shows how the raw contour grew during the level set function generation process. Currently, we have made a visual inspection for the segmented boundary and overlay over the gray scale boundary to see the difference. We also compared our results from regional level set framework with plain clustering-based technique. We are however working on a better technique where an experienced technologist can trace the WM/GM boundaries in the brain scans (slice-by-slice) and compare the error between the human traced boundaries versus the boundaries estimated by the computer when the regional level set algorithm was run. We intend to use the polyline distance method as developed by Suri *et al.* [?], which has been well established and demonstrated over contours of the left ventricle of the heart and its segmentation.

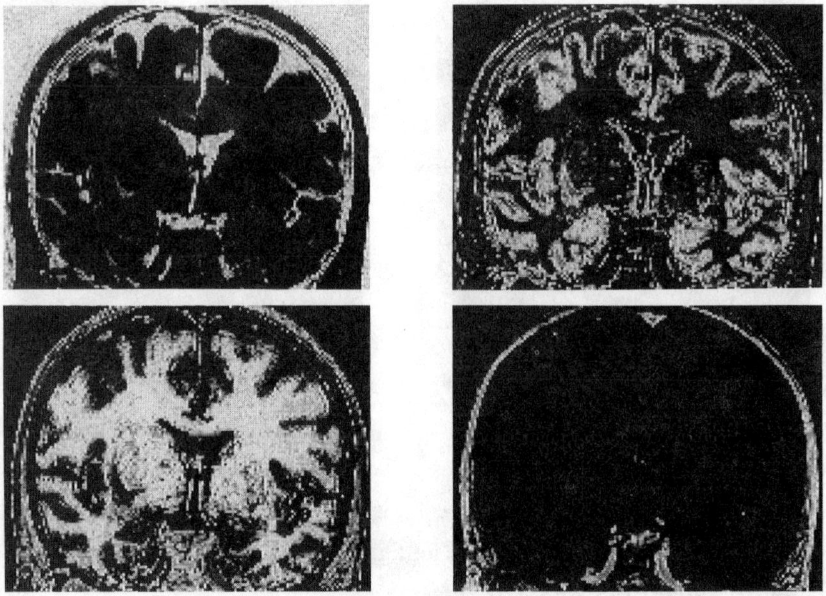

Figure 7.11: Results of the pixel classification algorithm with the number of classes equal to four on a sample MR brain scan. **Top Left**: class 0, **Top Right**: class 1, **Bottom Left**: class 2, **Bottom Right**: class 3.

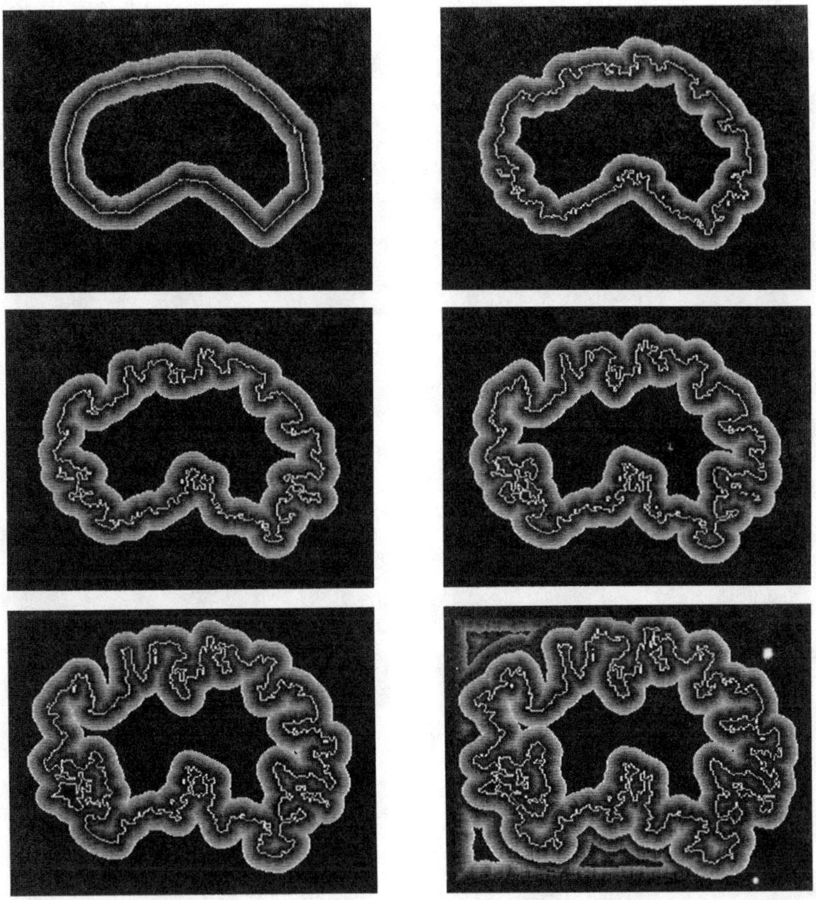

Figure 7.12: Results of the superimposition of the "zero-level-curve" and its level set (field) function using the "fast marching method" in the narrow band. The figure show the six tubes in the order from left to right and top to bottom. The important aspect to note is that as we go along the deformation process, the system captured the white matter topology. This topology characteristic was being provided by the fuzzy C mean algorithm in the level set framework.

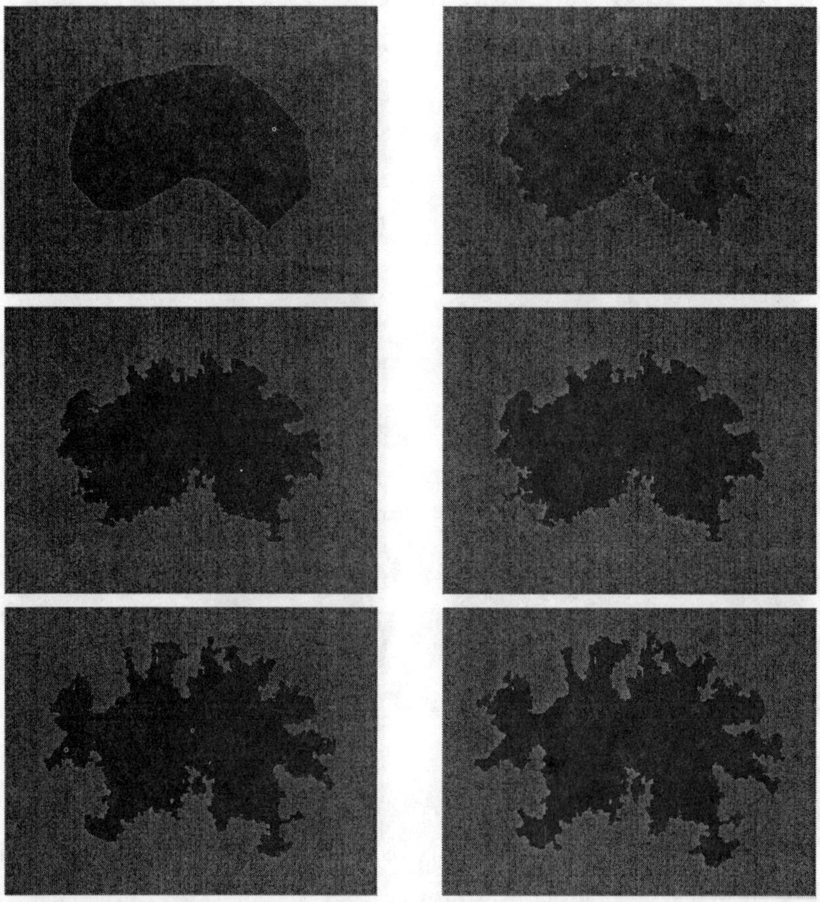

Figure 7.13: Results showing how the white matter evolves using the regional level set method. The order is from left to right and top to bottom. Note, the power of the pixel classification process in the level set framework to capture the topology of the white matter in the MR brain scan.

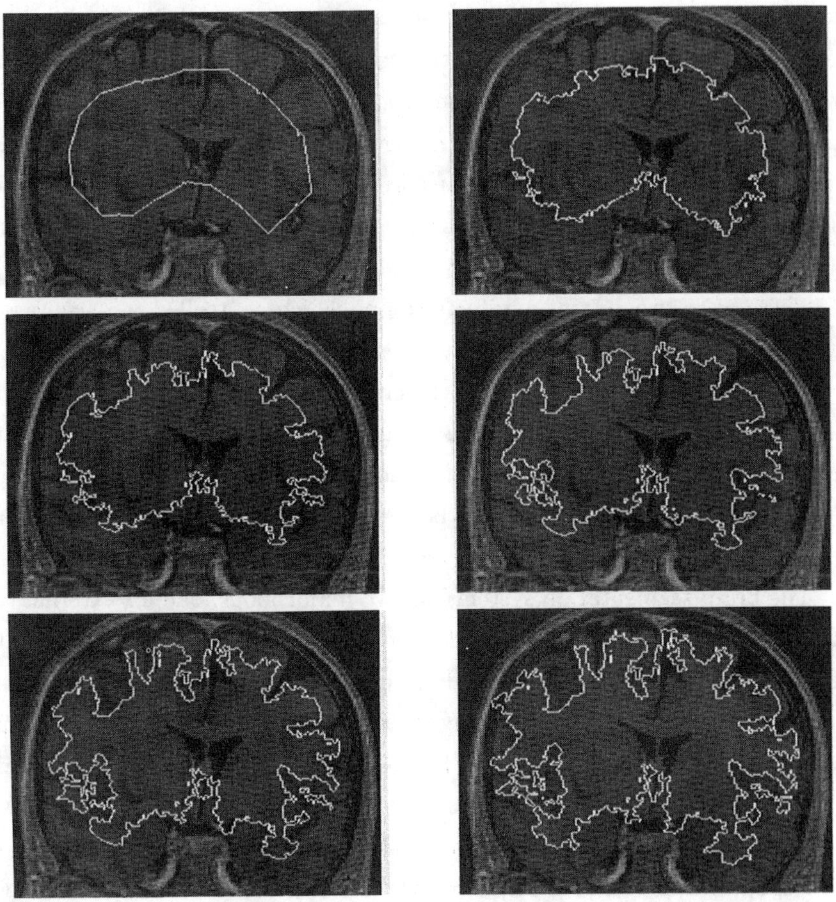

Figure 7.14: The above images show the growth of the zero-level-curve to segment the white matter in the human brain MR images. The narrow band width was 25 pixels on either side of the zero-level-curve, with the land mines as five pixels wide. Note, the deformation process had the ability to move in and out during the growth process.

7.5.3 Numerical Stability, Signed Distance Transformation Computation, Sensitivity of Parameters and Speed Issues

Numerical implementation requires very careful design and all variables should be of type float or double. This is because the finite difference comparisons are done with respect to zero. Also, the re-initialization stage and isocontour extraction depend upon the sign[10] of the level set function which must be tracked well. During the signed distance transform computation, of all of the distances for the inside region were made positive and after computation of all the distances of the grid points, the distances were made negative.

There were two sets of parameters: one which controlled the accuracy of the results and the other which controlled the speed of the segmentation process. The accuracy parameter was the error threshold ϵ_{th} in fuzzy clustering. The smaller the ϵ_{th}, the better the accuracy of classification and crisper the output regions, however, it would take longer to converge. A good value for T_1-weighted MR brain images was between 0.5 to 0.7 with number of classes kept to 4 (WM/GM/CSF/Background).

The brain segmentation system has two major loops, one for external tubing (called the "narrow band") and a second, internal loop for estimating the final field flow in the "narrow band" (see fig. 7.3). These two kinds of iterations were responsible for controlling the speed of the entire system. The outer loop speed was controlled by how fast the re-initialization of the signed distance transformation could be estimated given the zero-level-curve. This was done by the "fast marching method" using Sethian's approach. The second kind of speed was controlled by how fast the "field flow" converged. This was controlled by the weighting factor w_R. Thus the parameters which controlled the speed were: (i) "narrow band width" (W) and land mine width ($\triangle_l$) and (ii) regional term w_R. The larger the narrow band width, the longer it took to compute the "flow field". The range of w_R was kept between 0.1 to 0.5 and the best performance was obtained at 0.25, keeping the level set constants α, γ and ϵ fixed to 0.5, 1.0 and 1.0, respectively for all the experiments of the MR brain data set. We are continuing to explore in more depth the analysis on speed, sensitivity and stability issues as we get different types of pulse sequence

[10] if it is positive or negative

parameters for human brain acquisitions and tissue characterstics.

7.6 Advantages of the Regional Level Set Technique

Overall, the following are the key advantages of this brain segmentation system. (**1**) The greatest advantage of this technique is its high capture range of "field flow". This increases the robustness of the initial contour placement. Regardless of where the contour was placed in the image, it would find the object to segment itself. (**2**) The key characteristic of this system was that it was based on region, so the local noise or edge did not distract the growth process. (**3**) The technique is non-local and thus the local noise does not distract the final placement of the contour or the diffusion growth process. (**4**) The technique is not controlled by elasticity coefficients, unlike the parametric contour methods. There is no need to fit the tangents to the curves and compute the normals at each vertex. In this system, the normals were embedded in the system using the divergence of the field flow. (**5**) The technique is very suitable for medical organ segmentation since it can handle all the cavities, concavities, convolutedness, splitting or merging. (**6**) The issue of finding the local minima, or global minima, unlike the optimization techniques of the parametric snakes, does not arise. (**7**) This technique is less prone to the normal computations error, which is very easily incorporated in the classical balloon force snakes for segmentation. (**8**) It is very easy to extend this model from semi-automatic to completely automatic because the region is determined on the basis of prior information. (**9**) This technique is based on the propagation of curves (just like the propagation of ripples in the tank or propagation of the fire flames) utilizing region statistics. (**10**) This method adjusts automatically to topological changes of the given shape. Diffusion propagation methods employ a very natural framework for handling topological changes (joining and breaking of the curves). (**11**) The technique can be applied to unimodal, bimodal and multi-modal imagery, which means it can have multiple gray level values. (**12**) It implements the "fast marching method" in the "narrow band" for solving the Eikonal equation for computing signed distances. (**13**) One can segment any part of the brain depending upon the membership function of the brain image. (**14**) It is easily extendable to 3-D surface estimation. (**15**) The methodology is very flexible and can easily incorporate other features for controlling the speed of the curve. This is done by adding an extra term to the region, gradient and curvature speed terms. (**16**) The system takes care of the corners easily, unlike the parametric curves, which require special handling at corners of the boundary. (**17**) The technique is extendable to multi-scale resolutions which means that at lower resolutions, one can compute region segmentations. These segmented results can then be used for the higher resolutions. (**18**) The technique is extendable to multi-phase, in which existing multiple level set functions automatically merge and split during the course of the segmentation process.

7.7 Discussions: Comparison with Previous Techniques

This section briefly presents the comparisons between the region-based level sets versus the pervious techniques for cortical segmentation. For comprehensive details on the comparison between different techniques, see the recent state-of-the-art paper by Suri *et al.* [32]. Under the class of 2-D boundary-based techniques (as shown in figure 7.1), the current techniques are based on two approaches, parametric and geometric. These two techniques can be stand alone or fused with region-based techniques (so-called region-based parametric snakes or region-based geometric snakes). This Chapter is a example of region-based geometric snake because the propagation of the active contour is navigated by the regional forces computed using the regional-statistics such as fuzzy clustering. Earlier techniques such as stand alone parametric curves or regional-parametric snakes fail to estimate the deep convolutions of sulci and gyri (see Kapur *et al.* [33],[34]). The main reason being the unstability of the elasticity constants of parametric curves and directionality of the normal computation of the propagating curves. Recently McInerney *et al.* [35] presented his work where the classicial parametric snakes were made topological adaptive, but they did not apply these to the cerebral cortex. In the case of region-based geometric snakes, Leventon *et al.* [36] very recently proposed a fusion of shape model to classical geometric level set snake. This work is close to the work this Chapter presents, the key difference is: we model the shape by statistical fuzzy clustering embedded in the level set snake, while Leventon *et al.* modeled the shape by adding an extra term to the curve evolution equation. A complete pros and cons of this technique appears in Suri *et al.* [32].

7.8 Conclusions and Further Directions

Region-based level set snakes are a very powerful technique for segmenting white matter/gray matter in MR slices of human brain. We showed how one can apply the region-based level set technique for segmenting the brain using fast techniques. First, the Chapter introduced the importance of 2-D brain segmentation in different fields of medicine. Then, we presented a significant amount of level of survey and presented the classification tree of the current state-of-the-art brain segmentation techniques both based on active (supervised) and non-active (unsupervised) contours. We then introduced the level set snake model and incorporation of both regional forces and speed control methods. The core of the Chapter explored fast brain segmentation system implementation, which solves the regional level set function in the "narrow band" using the "fast marching method". Then, we presented the results for the MR brain scan. Then, the Chapter concluded with some critical advantages of the current techniques compared to parametric snakes and non-active contour techniques. Finally, the Chapter discussed the comparison of the suggested technique with other available techniques.

Note, the system used the fuzzy clustering method for computing the fuzzy membership values which were used in the regional speed computation. Recently, the authors have developed a mathematical morphology based speed control function which acts as a regularizer for making the propagation more robust and leak free. It would also be worth exploring how either the neural network or learning models would do in terms of the performance evaluation if clustering was to be replaced. A relationship between learning techniques and active contour models was attempted by Suri *et al.* [31]. The initial results on sagittal, coronal and transverse MR brain slices were very encouraging and need to be explored in three dimensions.

7.8.1 Acknowledgements

Special thanks go to John Patrick, Marconi Medical Systems, Inc., (MMS) for his encouragements during the course of this research. Thanks to IEEE Press for permitting me to reproduce this material from my International Journal of Engineering in Medicine and Biology (EMBS). Thanks are due to Marconi Medical Systems, Inc. for the MR data sets. Thanks to Dr. Sameer Singh, Editor-In-Chief, Pattern Analysis and Applications for his valuable suggestions.

Bibliography

[1] Suri, Jasjit S., Setarehdan, S. K., Singh, S., Book Title: Advanced Algorithmic Approaches to Medical Image Segmentation: State-of-the-Art Applications in Cardiology, Neurology, Mammography and Pathology. Chapter 4: "Advances in Computer Vision, Graphics, Image Processing, and Pattern Recognition Techniques for MR Brain Cortical Segmentation and Reconstruction: A Review Towards fMRI", First Eds. In Press. 2001.

[2] Kass, W., Terzapolous, D., Snakes: Active Contour Models, International J. of Computer Vision, Vol. 1, No. 4, pp. 321-331, 1988.

[3] Suri, Jasjit S., Computer Vision, Image Processing and Pattern Recognition in Left Ventricle Segmentation: Last 50 Years, J. of Pattern Analysis and Applications, Vol. 3, No. 3, pp. 209-244, Sep. 2000.

[4] Osher, S., and Sethian, J.A., Fronts propagating with curvature-dependent speed: algorithms based on Hamiltons-Jacobi formulations, J. Computational Physics, Vol. 79, No. 1, pp. 12-49, 1988.

[5] Sethian, J. A., An Analysis of Flame Propagation, Ph.D. thesis, Department of Mathematics, University of California, Berkeley, CA, 1982.

[6] Malladi, R., Sethian, J.A., A Unified Approach to Noise Removal, Image-Enhancement, and Shape Recovery, IEEE Trans. in Image Processing, Vol. 5, No. 11, pp. 1554-1568, Nov. 1996.

[7] Kichenassamy S., Kumar A., Olver P., Tannenbaum A., Yezzi A., Conformal curvature flows: from phase transitions to active vision, Arch. Rational Mech. Anal., Vol. 134, pp. 275-301, 1996.

[8] Yezzi A., Kichenassamy S., Kumar A., Olver P. and Tannenbaum A., A geometric snake model for segmentation of medical imagery, IEEE Transaction in Medical Imaging, Vol. 16, pp. 199-209, 1997.

[9] Siddiqui, K., Lauriere, Y. B., Tannenbaum, A. and Zucker, S. W., Area and length minimizing flows for shape segmentation, IEEE Trans. in Image processing, Vol. 7, pp. 433-443, 1998.

[10] Suri, Jasjit S., Leaking Prevention in Fast Level Sets Using Fuzzy Models: An Application in MR Brain, International Conference in Information Technology in Biomedicine, Nov. 2000 (To Appear).

[11] Suri, Jasjit S., White Matter/Gray Matter Boundary Segmentation Using Geometric Snakes: A Fuzzy Deformable Model, To appear in Int. conference in Application in Pattern Recognition (ICAPR), Rio de Janeiro, Brazil, 11-14 March, 2001.

[12] Chenyang, X., On the relationship between the parametric and geometric active contours, Internal Tech. report, Johns Hopkins University, 1999.

[13] Caselles, V., Kimmel, R., and Shapiro, G., Geodesic active contours, Int. J. of Computer Vision, Vol. 22, pp. 61-79, 1997.

[14] Rouy, E., and Tourin, A., A viscosity solutions approach to shape-from-shading, SIAM J. of Numerical Analysis, Vol. 23, pp. 867-884, 1992.

[15] Sethian, J.A., A fast marching level set method for monotonically advancing fronts, Proc. Natl. Acad. Science, Applied Mathematics, Vol. 93, pp. 1591-1595, 1996.

[16] Bezdek, J.C., Hall, L.O., Review of MR image segmentation techniques using pattern recognition, Medical Physics, Vol. 20, pp. 1033-1048, March 1993.

[17] Hall, L.O. and Bensaid, A.M., A comparison of neural networks and fuzzy clustering techniques in segmenting MRI of the brain, IEEE Trans. In Neural Networks, Vol. 3, No., pp. 672-682, 1992.

[18] Sheehan, F. H., Haralick, R.M., Suri, J.S., and Shao, Y., US Patent #: 5,734,739, Method for determining the contour of an In Vivo Organ Using Multiple Image Frames of the Organ, March 1998.

[19] Berger, M. J., Local Adaptive Mesh Refinement, Journal of Computational Physics, Vol. 82, pp. 64-84, 1989.

[20] Sethian, J. A., Curvature Flow and Entropy Conditions Applied to Grid Generation, J. Computational Physics, Vol. 115, pp. 440-454, 1994.

[21] Tababai, A. J. and Mitchell O. R., Edge location to subpixel values in digital imagery, IEEE Transactions on PAMI, Vol. 6 (2), pp. 188-201, March 1984.

[22] Huertas and Medioni, G., Detection of intensity changes with subpixel accuracy using Laplacian-gaussian masks, IEEE Transactions in PAMI, Vol. 8 (5): pp. 651-664, Sep. 1986.

[23] Gao, J., Kosaka, A., and Kak, A.C., A deformable model for human organ extraction, Proc. IEEE International Conference on Image Processing (ICIP), Vol.3, pp. 323-327, Chicago, October 1998.

[24] Cao, S., and Greenhalgh, S., Finite-difference solution of the Eikonal equation using an efficient, First-arrival, wavefront tracking scheme, Geophysics, Vol. 59, No. 4, pp. 632-643, April 1994.

[25] Chen, S., Merriman, B., Osher, S., and Smereka, P., A Simple Level Set Method for Solving Stefan Problems, Journal of Computational Physics, Vol. 135, pp. 8-29, 1997.

[26] Sethian, J.A., US Patent #: 6,018,499, Three-dimensional seismic imaging of complex velocity structures, Issued Jan. 25, 2000.

[27] Adalsteinsson, D., and Sethian, J.A., The fast construction of extension velocities in level set methods, J. Computational Physics, Vol. 148, No. 1, pp. 2-22, 1999.

[28] Malladi, R., Sethian, J.A., and Vemuri, B.C., Shape modeling with Front Propagation, Vol. 17, No. 2, pp. 158-175, Feb. 1995.

[29] Suri, Jasjit S., Haralick, R.M., and Sheehan, F.H., Greedy Algorithm for Error Correction in Automatically Produced Boundaries from Low Contrast Ventriculograms, Int. J. of Pattern Applications and Analysis, Vol. 1, No. 1, pp. 39-60, Jan. 2000.

[30] Sedgewick, R., Algorithms in C, Fundamentals, data structures, sorting, searching, Addison-Wesley, ISBN: 0201314525 (v. 1), 1998.

[31] Suri, Jasjit S., Active Contour Vs. Learning: Computer Vision Techniques in CT, MR and X-ray Cardiac Imaging, Proceedings of the Fifth International Conference in Pattern Recognition and Information Processing, ISBN 83-87362-16-6, pp. 273-277, Minsk, Belarus, 1999.

[32] Suri, Jasjit S., Singh, S., and Reden, L., Computer Vision and Pattern Recognition Techniques for 2-D and 3-D MR Cerebral Cortical Segmentation: A State-of-the-Art Review, Accepted for Publication in Journal of Pattern Analysis and Applications, 2001.

[33] Kapur, T., MS Thesis, Brain Segmentation, Artificial Intelligence Lab., Massachusetts Institute of Technology, 1997.

[34] Kapur,T., Grimson, W.E.L., Wells, III, W.M., Kikinis, R., Segmentation of brain tissue from Magnetic Resonance Images, Medical Image Analysis, Vol. 1, No. 2, pp. 109-127, 1996.

[35] McInereney, T., and Terzopoulos, D., Topologically Adaptable Snakes, 5th International Conference in Computer Vision (ICCV), pp. 840-845, 1995.

[36] Leventon, M.E., Grimson, W. Eric L. and Faugeras, O., Statistical Shape Influence in Geodesic Active Contours, Proceedings of the Computer Vision and Pattern Recognition (CVPR), Vol. 1, pp. 316-323, June 2000.

Chapter 8

Subjective Surfaces

Alessandro Sarti [1]

8.1 Introduction

The phenomenon of contours that appear in the absence of physical gradients has aroused considerable interest among psychologists and computer vision scientists. Psychologists suggested a number of images that strongly requires image completion to detect the objects. In Figure 8.1, the solid triangle in the center of the figure appears to have well defined contours, even in completely homogeneous areas. Kanizsa called the contours without gradient "anomalous contours" or "subjective contours" [16], because the missed boundaries are provided by the visual system of the subject.

Subjective contours are not a property of the image alone, but they depends both on the position of the point of view and on the geometric properties of the image. Kanizsa pointed out that "if you fix your gaze on one of these contours , it disappears, yet if you direct your gaze to the entire figure, the contours appear to be real" [16] [17] [18] [19]. It is evident that the perception of spatial patterns is dependent on the location of the gaze and that the breaking of the shift invariance between the observer and the image plays an important role in perceptual organization.

As in [35], we define a segmentation as a piecewise constant graph that varies rapidly across the boundary between different objects and stays flat within it.

In our approach, the segmentation is a piecewise constant approximation of the point of view- or reference surface, while in [35] the segmentation is an

[1] University of Balogna, Balogna, Itlay

PDE & Level Sets: Algorithmic Approaches to Static & Motion Imagery
Edited by Jasjit Suri and Swamy Laxminarayan, Kluwer Academic/Plenum Publishers, 2002

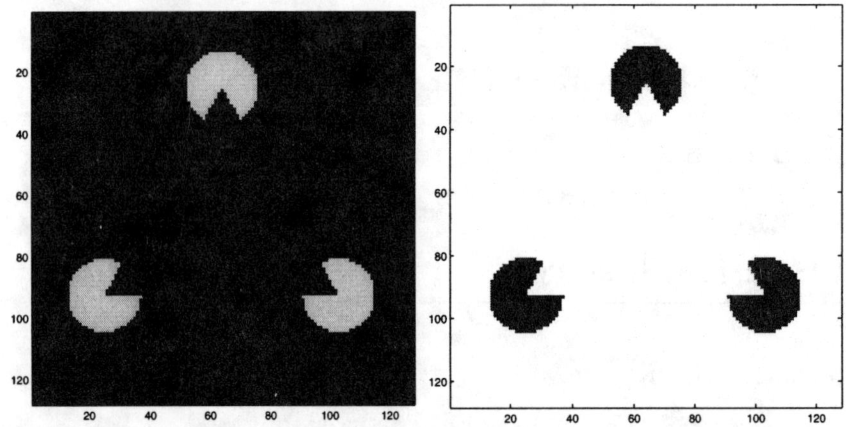

Figure 8.1: A sample set of images with subjective boundaries proposed and analyzed by Gaetano Kanizsa in [16]. The classic triangle of Kanizsa (left) and its brightness inversion (right).

approximation of the image itself. To achieve the piecewise constant graph, an initial surface depending on the point of view is evolved with a mean curvature flow with respect to the Riemannian metric given by the image features. During the evolution, the point-of-view surface is attracted by the existing boundaries and steepens. The surface evolves towards the piecewise constant solution by continuation and closing of the boundary fragments and the filling in the homogeneous regions. A solid object is delineated as a constant surface bounded by existing and recovered shape boundaries. The theoretical basis of the method has been presented in [42] and its extension to 3D image completion has been discussed in [43] and [45]. In [44] we outlined the geometric interpretation of the flow and we proved the basic analytical results about existence, uniqueness and maximum principle of the associated parabolic partial differential equation. In this work we review the main characteristics of the method and analyze in more depth its ability in segmenting figures proposed in classical studies of psychology of the Gestalt [16], [17], [18], [19], [56]. The mathematical model relies on a considerable body of work in front propagation and geometric flows for image analysis. Level set methods, introduced by Osher and Sethian [39], track the evolution of curves and surfaces implicitly defined as zero level set of a higher dimensional function [52]. Malladi, Sethian and Vemuri [31] and Caselles, Catte, Coll, and Dibos in [4] used this technology to

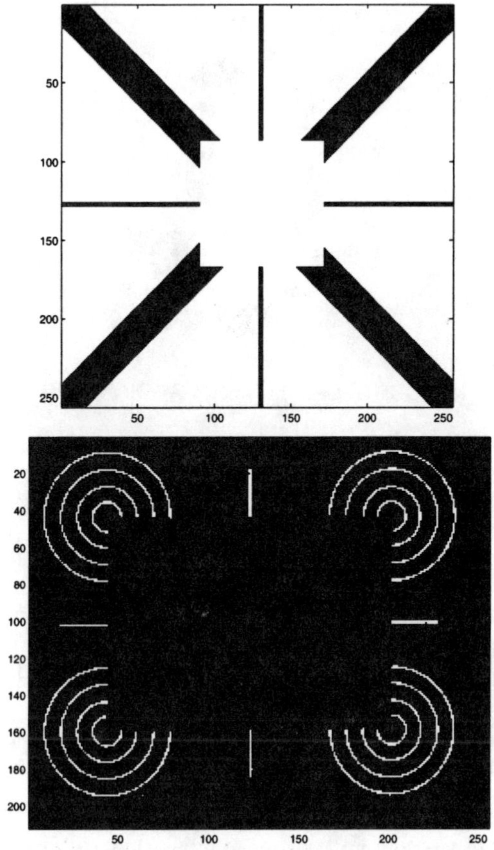

Figure 8.2: Images with termination points. Termination points help the formation of subjective boundaries.

segment images. In [5] a variational geometric interpretation of curve evolution for image segmentation is proposed. In [22], [54], [55] an intrinsic geometric formulation for image filtering as Riemannian surface evolution is presented.

Our approach takes a more general view of the segmentation problem. Rather than follow a particular front or level curve which one attempts to steer to the desired edge we begin with an initial surface, chosen on the basis of a user-supplied reference fixation point. We then flow this *entire surface* under speed law dependent on the image gradient, without regard to any particular level set. Suitably chosen, this flow sharpens the surface around the edges and connects segmented boundaries across the missing information.

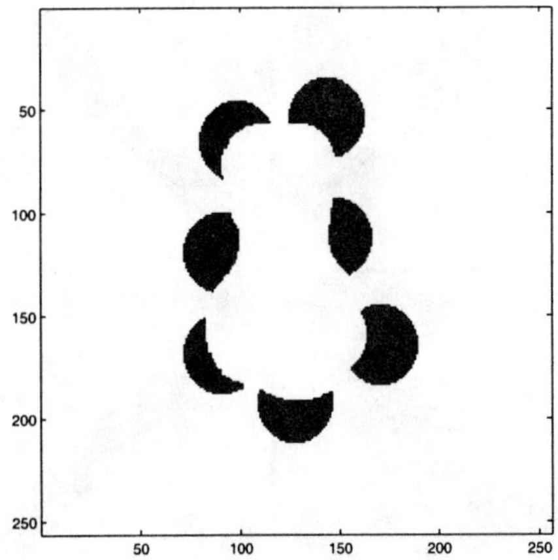

Figure 8.3: Image with amorphous shape. The formation of subjective boundaries is possible without any a priory knowledge.

The Chapter is organized as the following. In Section 7.2 we recall some basic concepts of the phenomenology of Gestalt about modal and amodal boundary completion in perceptual grouping. In Section 7.3 we discuss the mathematical modelling of boundary completion. We describe past work and state of the art in subsection 7.3.1 and introduce the proposed differential model in subsection 7.3.2. In Section 7.4 we deal with proof of existence, uniqueness and maximum principle of the solution of the model equation. Section 7.5 shows how to approximate the main equation with finite difference scheme. In Section 7.6 we produce results of the application of the method to modal and amodal completion in cognitive and medical images. The Appendix contains the Matlab programs utilized to simulate the formation of subjective surfaces.

8.2 Modal and Amodal Completion in Perceptual Organization

Human visual grouping was studied extensively by the Gestalt psychologists in the early part of the century [56]. Along the path going from the surface of the physical object to the observer radiations are completely independent one to the other. The retina is constituted in its turn by a mosaic of histologically separated elements. At the end of this chain during which the unity of the

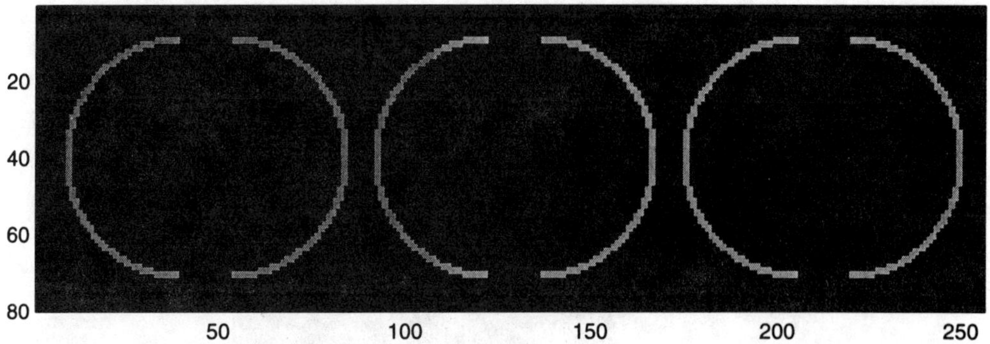

Figure 8.4: 6 fragments with semicircular shape are grouped by the visual system as circles instead of "X", even if in the "X" configuration the fragments are closer then in the circle configuration. Closure wins over proximity.

original object is completely lost, the object shows up again at the perceptual level as a unit. In which way is it possible to reconstruct at the perceptual level the unity of the physical object? This is the central question faced by the Gestalt psychology of the perception. Several factors that lead to human perceptual grouping have been identified: similarity, proximity, continuity, closure, symmetry. Following the Gestalt principles the segmentation problem is considered as a two stage process: first low level cues like gradients, T-junctions, termination points are extracted from the image and second an integration (field) process acts on the cues to construct the perceived objects. A problem that has aroused particular interest at the experimental and theoretical level concerns the emergency in the perceptual field of boundaries without any discontinuity of the stimulus [19]. Indeed, if we look at the set of images of figure 8.1 we perceive phenomenological objects without any physical corresponding one. For example in the first image a solid triangle is perceived even if only 3 white pacman-like inducers are present as physical information. The boundaries of the triangle are called "illusory boundaries" or "subjective boundaries" because they are created by the visual system of the subject by completion of existing boundaries. The analysis of a number of similar situations suggests the definition of a set of common phenomenical characteristics [16], [17], [19]. First, the presence of subjective boundaries always goes with the perception of a subjective surface delimited by boundaries. Kanizsa suggested that bound-

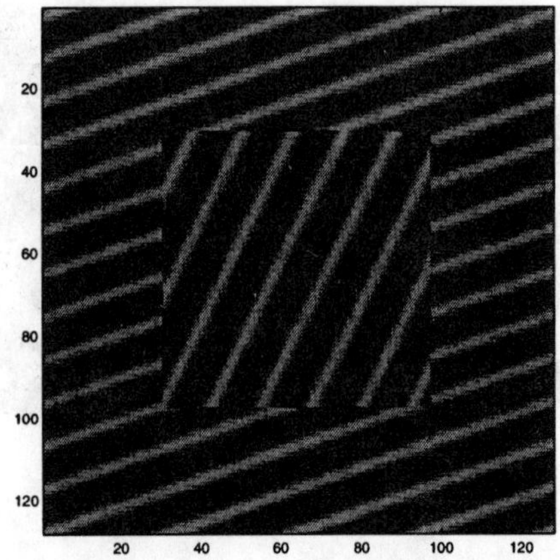

Figure 8.5: Virtual boundaries are produced also by texture images.

aries are a secondary effect generated by the perceptual presence of the illusory surface. The surface seems dislocated in the third dimension an it's perceived over the other figures. About the individuation of factors that determine the formation of such surfaces, a condition is always present. The prerequisite is the existence od irregular parts that need a completion to become regular. After completion such parts are transformed in simpler and more regular shapes. For example figure 8.1 can be described as constituted by three circular sectors, but the preferred perception is given by three black disks partially occluded by a white triangle. The latter perceptual configuration holds the advantage of simplicity and regularity with respect to the first one. The condition needed to this improvement of the overall organization is that the central white region is perceived as a triangle overlapped to the other figures and to the ground. As outlined in [16] the pop up of the triangle is invariant up to the inversion of the brightness function, Fig. 8.1, right. Subjective boundaries are strongly enhanced by the presence of termination points, as depicted in Fig. 8.1. Indeed a black rectangle is perceived in Fig. 8.1 left, even if none of the existing boundaries is aligned with the rectangle. A priory knowledge of the object geometry is not necessary to perform boundary completion. In facts illusory boundaries pop up from completely amorphous figures as illustrated in the image of Fig. 8.1. The subjective boundaries of figure 8.1 are really perceived with the modality of vision therefore the completion process is called "modal completion". In figure 8.1 we perceive the presence of a white square partially

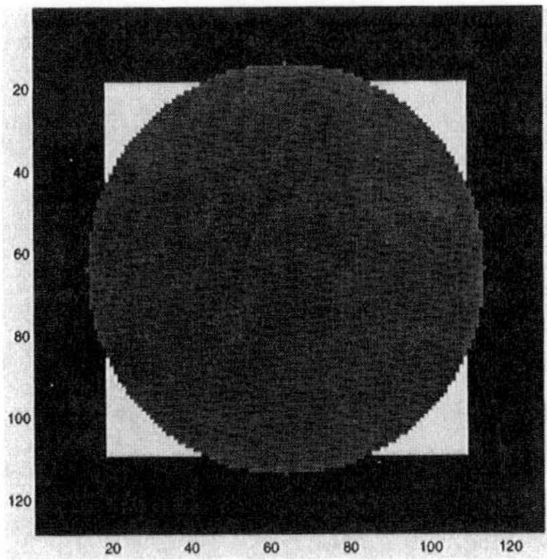

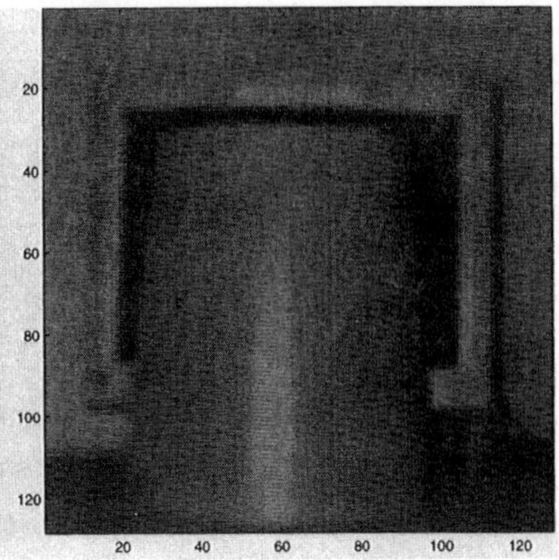

Figure 8.6: Examples of amodal completion. The visual system interpret the image on the left as a gray disk partially occluding a white square. A completion of the square is performed starting from the four white inducers. Similarly the image on the right is understood as a trash can occluding a computer screen. The amodal completion of the screen is performed.

occluded by a gray disk. The occluded contours of the square are only imagined and not really seen with the modality of vision: in this case the completion process is called by psychologists "amodal completion". Amodal completion is always present in every image and it is performed during the process of figure-ground segregation under the perspective that any object is partially occluding the ground [16].

8.3 Mathematical Modelling of Figure Completion

8.3.1 Past Work and Background

In this section, we review some of the other work that has attempted to recover subjective contours. In Mumford [36], the idea was that distribution of subjective contours can be modeled and computed by particles traveling at constant speeds but moving in directions given by Brownian motion. More recently, Williams and Jacobs [57],[58] introduced the notion of a stochastic completion field, the distribution of particle trajectories joining pairs of position and direction constraints, and showed how it could be computed. However, the difficulty with this approach is to consistently choose the main direction of particle motion; in other words, do the particles move parallel (as needed to complete Fig. 8.1, left) or perpendicular (as needed to complete 8.1, center) to the existing boundaries, i.e. edges? In addition, in this approach, what is being computed is a distribution of particles and not an explicit contour/surface, closed or otherwise. In this work, we are interested in recovering explicit shape representations that are reproduce that of the human visual perception, especially in regions with no image-based constraints such as gradient jump or variation in texture.

A combinatorial approach is considered in [50]. A sparse graph is constructed whose nodes are salient visual events such as contrast edges and L-type and T-type junctions of contrast edges, and whose arcs are coincidence and geometric configurational relations among node elements. An interpretation of the scene consists of choices among a small set of labels for graph elements. Any given labelling induces an energy, or cost, associated with physical consistency and figural interpretation. This explanation follows the classical 2 1/2 D sketch of David Marr [34].

A common feature of both completion fields, combinatorial methods, as well as variational segmentation methods [35] is to postulate that the segmentation process is independent of observer's point of focus. On the other hand, methods based on active contours perform a segmentation strongly dependent on the user/observer interaction. Since their introduction in [20], deformable models have been extensively used to integrate boundaries and extract features from images. An implicit shape modelling approach with topological adaptability and significant computational advantages has been introduced in [31], [4], [32]. They use the level set approach [39], [?] to frame curve motion with a curvature dependent speed. These and a host of other related works rely on edge information to construct a shape representation of an object. In the presence of large gaps and missing edge data, the models tend to go astray and away from the required shape boundary. This behavior is due to a constant speed component in the governing equation that helps the curve from getting trapped by isolated spurious edges. On the other hand, if the constant inflation term is switched off, as in [5], [46], [47], the curve has to be initialized close to the final shape for reasonable results. Recently in [6] the authors use geometric curve evolution for segmenting shapes without gradient by imposing a homogeneity constraint, but the method is not suitable for detecting the missing contours shown in Figure 8.1.

The approach in this study relies on the perspective that segmentation, regardless of dimensionality, is a 'view-point' dependent computation. The 'view-point' or the user-defined initial guess to the segmentation algorithm enters our algorithm via the point-of-view surface. Next, we evolve this reference surface according to a feature-indicator function [42], [43], [44], [45]. The shape completion aspect of our work is relies on two components: (1) the evolution of a higher-dimensional function and (2) a flow that combines the effects of level set curve evolution with that of surface evolution. In what follows, we will review the geometric framework that will make this possible. Computing the final segmentation (a contour or surface) is accomplished by merely plotting a particular level set of a higher dimensional function [42], [43], [44], [45].

8.3.2 The Differential Model of Subjective Surfaces

8.3.2.1 The Image Induced Metric

We consider an image $\mathcal{I} : (x_1, x_2) \to I(x_1, x_2)$ as a real positive function defined in a rectangular domain $\Omega \subset \mathbf{R}^2$. The first task in image analysis is to extract the low level information from the image. The result of this stage is a representation of the image corresponding to *the raw primal sketch*, as introduced by David Marr [34], that involves the detection of image gradient, orientation of structures, T-junctions and texture. Several methods have been proposed to compute the raw primal sketch, including multiscale/multiorientation image decomposition with Gabor filtering [11], wavelet transform [26], deformable filter banks [41], textons [?, ?] etc. For the purpose of the present study we consider a simple edge indicator, namely:

$$h(x_1, x_2) = \frac{1}{1 + (|\nabla G_\sigma(x_1, x_2) * I(x_1, x_2)|/\beta)^2}, \tag{8.1}$$

where:

$$G_\sigma(x_1, x_2) = \frac{\exp(-(|(x_1, x_2)|/\sigma)^2)}{\sigma\sqrt{\pi}}.$$

The edge indicator function $h(x_1, x_2)$ is a non-increasing function of $|\nabla G_\sigma(x_1, x_2) * I(x_1, x_2)|$, where $G_\sigma(x_1, x_2)$ is a gaussian kernel and $(*)$ denotes the convolution. The denominator is the gradient magnitude of a smoothed version of the initial image. Thus, the value of h is closer to 1 in flat areas ($|\nabla I| \rightarrow 0$) and closer to 0 in areas with large changes in image intensity, i.e. the local edge features. The minimal size of the details that are detected is related to the size of the kernel, which acts like a scale parameter. By viewing h as a potential function, we note that its minima denotes the position of edges. Also, the gradient of this potential function is a force field that always points towards the local edge; see Figure 8.7.

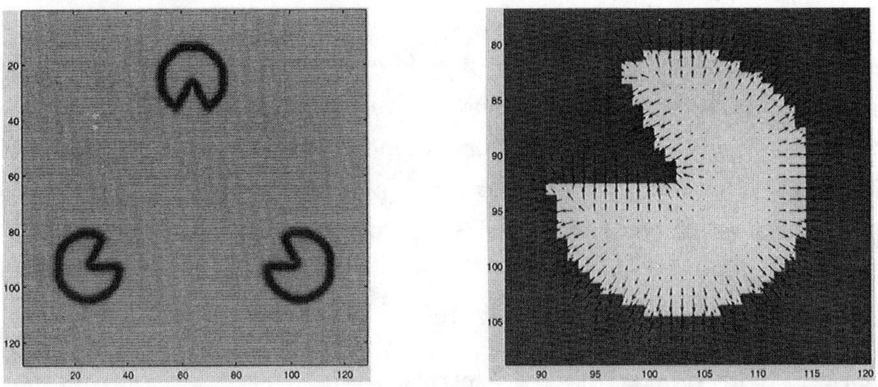

Figure 8.7: Local edge detection: The edge map h and its spatial gradient $-\nabla h$.

We use the edge indicator h to construct a metric in $\mathbf{R}^3$ that will be used as embedding space for the surface evolution. In [42] starting from the edge indicator $h(x_1, x_2)$, a conformal metric $h\delta_{ij}$ i=1,...,3, j=1,...,3 is builded. In the present study we build a more general metric that allows to stretch one direction with respect to the others by a factor $\epsilon > 0$:

$$g = \begin{pmatrix} h & 0 & 0 \\ 0 & h & 0 \\ 0 & 0 & h/\epsilon \end{pmatrix}.$$

The conformal metric proposed in [42] corresponds to the particular case $\epsilon = 1$. The meaning of the stretching factor ϵ and its influence on the boundary completion method will be clarified in the Subsection 7.3.2.4.

8.3.2.2 Riemannian Mean Curvature of Graph

Let us now recall some properties of a Riemannian metric (see example [24]). The scalar product of two vectors X and Y in $(\mathbf{R^3}, \mathbf{g})$ is defined as:

$$< X, Y >_g = X^t g Y,$$

therefore the norm of X with respect to g is:

$$||X||_g = \sqrt{< X, X >_g} = \sqrt{\frac{h}{\epsilon}} \sqrt{\epsilon X_1^2 + \epsilon X_2^2 + X_3^2}.$$

If u is a regular function defined on the set $\Omega \subset \mathbf{R^2}$ with real values, its graph:

$$M = \{(x_1, x_2, u(x_1, x_2)) : (x_1, x_2) \in \Omega\}$$

is a bidimensional submanifold of $(\mathbf{R^3}, \mathbf{g})$, with the natural metric. A basis (e_1, e_2) of the tangent plane at any point is the following:

$$e_1 = (1, 0, \partial_1 u)^t, \quad e_2 = (0, 1, \partial_2 u)^t.$$

It is well known that the mean curvature of the graph of u in the euclidean metric is:

$$H_e = div(\nu_e) = -\partial_i \Big(\frac{\partial_i u}{\sqrt{1 + |\partial_1 u|^2 + |\partial_2 u|^2}} \Big), \tag{8.2}$$

where

$$\nu_e = \frac{(-\partial_1 u, -\partial_2 u, 1)}{\sqrt{1 + |\partial_1 u|^2 + |\partial_2 u|^2}}$$

is a vector of unitary length, orthogonal to M with respect to the euclidean scalar product (see for example [9]).
Similarly, the defnition of mean curvature in a Riemannian space $(\mathbf{R^3}, \mathbf{g})$, is given by

$$H_g = div_g(\nu_g), \tag{8.3}$$

where

$$div_g(\cdot) = -\frac{1}{\sqrt{det(g)}} \partial_i \Big(\sqrt{det(g)} (\cdot)_i \Big) = -\frac{1}{\sqrt{h^3}} \partial_i \Big(\sqrt{h^3} (\cdot)_i \Big)$$

is the Riemannian divergence and the vector

$$\nu_g = \frac{g^{-1} \nu_e}{||g^{-1} \nu_e||_g} = \frac{(-\partial_1 u, -\partial_2 u, \epsilon)}{\sqrt{h} \sqrt{|\partial_1 u|^2 + |\partial_2 u|^2 + \epsilon}} \tag{8.4}$$

is the normal unit vector with respect to the metric g (see [2]).

Finally, the Riemannian mean curvature of the manifold M is given in these notations as:

$$H_g = -\frac{1}{\sqrt{h^3}}\partial_i\Big(h\frac{\partial_i u}{\sqrt{\epsilon+|\partial_1 u|^2+|\partial_2 u|^2}}\Big). \tag{8.5}$$

Remark 8.3.1. Note that the mean curvature of a graph vanishes if and only if it is a critical point of the volume form. If B is the 3×2 matrix (e_1, e_2), this can be computed as:

$$vol(M) = \int_\Omega \sqrt{det(B^t gB)}dx_1 dx_2$$

where $B^t gB$ is the metric induced on the graph (see [24]).

In particular the value of the functional is decreasing along the motion and this property has been used to give an integral definition of mean curvature motion. We recall the following weak approaches to the problem: the definition of motion of varifolds by mean curvature [3], [14], [15], the variational approach of Almgren-Taylor-Wang [1], the definition of minimizing movements of De Giorgi [8].

8.3.2.3 Graph evolution with weighted mean curvature flow

We say that the graph of u evolves by its mean curvature, if each point (x_1, x_2, u) of the graph M moves with speed proportional to H is the direction orthogonal to the graph. (See for example [13] or [10] for mean curvature motion in an euclidean setting and [7], [2], for level sets evolution in a Riemannian, or Finsler manifold).

Following [42] here we requires that each point of the graph moves with speed h^2H_g in the normal direction. In other words, it evolves according to the ODE:

$$(\dot{x_1}(t), \dot{x_2}(t), \dot{u}(t)) = -h^2 H_g \nu_g(x_1(t), x_2(t), u(t)) =$$

$$= -H_g\sqrt{h^3}\frac{(-\partial_1 u, -\partial_2 u, \epsilon)}{\sqrt{|\partial_1 u|^2+|\partial_2 u|^2+\epsilon}}.$$

Since by the chain rule:

$$\dot{u}(t) = \frac{d}{dt}u(x_1(t), x_2(t), t) = \dot{x_1}\partial_1 u + \dot{x_2}\partial_2 u + \partial_t u,$$

we immediately have:

$$\partial_t u = \dot{u}(t) - \dot{x_1}\partial_1 u - \dot{x_2}\partial_2 u = -H_g\sqrt{h^3}\sqrt{|\partial_1 u|^2+|\partial_2 u|^2+\epsilon}.$$

By identity (Eq. 8.5) the motion of the graph u by its weighted mean curvature in the metric g is:

$$\partial_t u = \sqrt{|\partial_1 u|^2 + |\partial_2 u|^2 + \epsilon}\,\partial_i\Big(\frac{h\partial_i u}{\sqrt{\epsilon + |\partial_1 u|^2 + |\partial_2 u|^2}}\Big). \tag{8.6}$$

As ϵ goes to 0, this equation is the Evans-Spruck type regularization of the curvature flow of a single level set. Here, on the contrary, we are interested in the evolution of the whole graph.

8.3.2.4 The Model Equation

The model equation of weighted mean curvature flow of graphs for image segmentation and boundary completion yields:

$$\begin{cases} \partial_t u = h\frac{(\epsilon+(\partial_2 u)^2)\partial_{11}u - \partial_1 u \partial_2 u \partial_{12} u + (\epsilon + (\partial_1 u)^2)\partial_{22} u}{|\partial_1 u|^2 + |\partial_2 u|^2 + \epsilon} + \partial_1 h \partial_1 u + \partial_2 h \partial_2 u & \\ & \textit{in } Q_T = \Omega \times]0, T[\\ u(x,t) = \min(u_0) & \textit{in } S_T = \partial\Omega \times]0, T[\\ u(x,0) = u_0 & \textit{for } x \in \Omega. \end{cases} \tag{8.7}$$

To avoid the asymptotic convergence to the trivial constant solution, we consider the function $\frac{u}{\sup u}$. The indicator function h is computed as in (8.2). The input to the model is a user-defined point-of-view or a reference surface u_0, centered in the object we are interested in segmenting. Different choices exist for the reference surface; as examples, we show two such choices in Fig. (8.8). In the next examples, we use $u_0 = 1/(\mathcal{D} + \epsilon)$, where $\mathcal{D}$ is the distance from the initial point of view. To achieve the image segmentation, the initial surface depending on the point of view is evolved with the weighted curvature flow. During the evolution, the point-of-view surface is attracted by the existing boundaries and steepens. The surface evolves towards the piecewise constant solution by continuation and closing of the boundary fragments and the filling in the homogeneous regions. The set where u attains its maximum, is the segmented figure.

The first term on the right hand side is a parabolic term that evolves the surface in the normal direction under its mean curvature weighted by the edge indicator h. The surface motion is slowed down in the vicinity of edges ($h \to 0$). The second term on the right corresponds to pure passive advection of the surface along the underlying velocity field $-\nabla h$ whose direction and strength depend

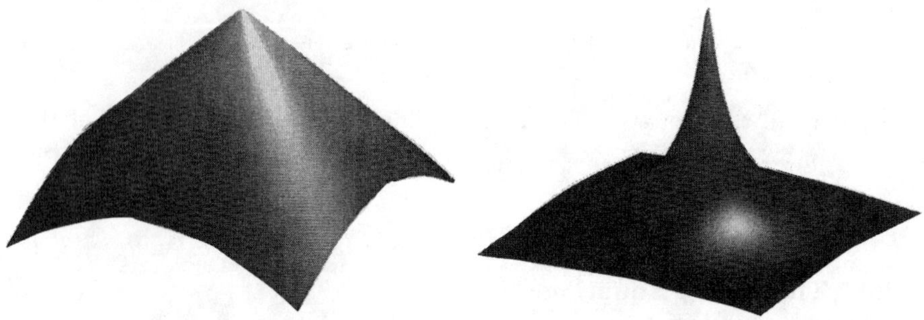

Figure 8.8: Point-of-view surfaces: on the left $u_0 = -\mathcal{D}$, where $\mathcal{D}$ is the distance function from the fixation point, and on the right $u_0 = 1/\mathcal{D}$.

on position. This term pushes/attracts the surface in the direction of the image edges. Note that $h(I(x_1, x_2))$ is not a function of the third coordinate, therefore the vector field $-\nabla h$ lies entirely on the (x_1, x_2) plane.

The following characterizes the behavior of the model Eqn. (8.7) in different regions of the image. In regions of the image where edge information exists, the advection term drives the surface towards the edges. The level sets of the surface also get attracted to the edge and accumulate. Consequently, the spatial gradient increases and the surface begins to develop a discontinuity. Now, when spatial derivatives $|\partial_1 u|, |\partial_2 u| \gg 1$, the Eqn. (8.7) approximates to:

$$\partial_t u \approx h\frac{(\partial_2 u)^2\partial_{11}u - \partial_1 u\partial_2 u\partial_{12}u + (\partial_1 u)^2)\partial_{22}u}{|\partial_1 u|^2 + |\partial_2 u|^2} + \partial_1 h\partial_1 u + \partial_2 h\partial_2 u, \quad (8.8)$$

which is nothing but the geodesic level set flow for shape recovery [5], [21], [33]. In addition, the (parabolic) first term in Eqn. (8.8) is a directional diffusion term in the tangent direction and limits diffusion across the edge itself.

The region inside the objects where $h \to 1, |\nabla h| \to 0$ the surface is driven by the Euclidean mean curvature motion towards a flat surface. In these regions, we observe $|\partial_1 u|, |\partial_2 u| \ll 1$ and equation (8.7) approximates to the non uniform diffusion equation:

$$\partial_t u \approx h(\partial_{11}u + \partial_{22}u) + \partial_1 h\partial_1 u + \partial_2 h\partial_2 u. \quad (8.9)$$

If the image gradient inside the object is actually equal to zero, then $h = 1$ and Eqn. (8.9) becomes a simple linear heat equation and the flow corresponds to linear uniform diffusion.

We now address the regions in the image corresponding to subjective contours. In our view, subjective contours are simply continuation of existing edge fragments. As we explained before, in regions with-well defined edge information, Eqn. (8.7) causes the level curve accumulation thereby causing an increase in the spatial gradient of u. Due to continuity in the surface, this edge fragment information is propagated to complete the missing boundary. The main equation (8.7) is a mixture of two different dynamics, the level set flow (8.8) and non uniform diffusion (8.9) and locally, points on the u surface move according to one of these mechanisms. In the steady-state solution, the points inside the objects are characterized by pure linear diffusion, while points on the boundary are characterized by the level set edge enhancing flow.

Let us outline that ϵ weighted the two dynamics (8.8) and (8.9). If ϵ is large with respect to spatial derivatives, then the behaviour of the flow (8.7) is mostly diffusive. In the opposite, when ϵ is small, the behaviour is mostly like level set plane curve evolution. In other words, the stretching of the metric in the direction x_3 given by the weighting factor ϵ determines how likely geodesic boundaries are formed. In the Results Section, we will present a comparison among the flows (8.7), (8.8) and (8.9) and we will observe the undesirable characteristics of both the extreme dynamics.

Finally, let us note that a similar piecewise constant solution can be achieved with different models. In [48], the authors have used the weighted Perona-Malik model to extract subjective surfaces by anisotropic diffusion in Riemannian space.

8.4 Existence, Uniqueness and Maximum Principle

In the sequel we will denote $(x, t) = (x_1, x_2, t)$ any point in Q_T, $\nabla u = (\partial_1 u, \partial_2 u)$ the spatial gradient of u. We will also denote $Lip(\bar{Q}_T)$ the set of functions Lipschitz continuous on $\bar{Q}_T$, and $C^{21}(Q_T)$ the set of $C^1(Q_T)$ functions, whose second derivatives with respect to the spatial variables are continuous. We will also set:

$$(a_{ij}(x,p)) = \frac{h(x)}{\epsilon + |p_1|^2 + |p_2|^2} \begin{pmatrix} \epsilon + p_2^2 & -p_1 p_2 \\ -p_1 p_2 & \epsilon + p_1^2 \end{pmatrix}, \quad a(x,p) = \partial_i h p_i,$$

so that the equation in (8.7) becomes:

$$Pu := -\partial_t u + a_{ij}(x, \nabla u)\partial_{ij} u + a(x, \nabla u) = 0, \quad in\ Q_T = \Omega \times [0,T]. \quad (8.10)$$

The existence result for the initial boundary problem associated euclidean non parametric mean curvature flow is extremely classic: it is due to Jenkins and Serrin [23] for convex sets and extended to another family of open sets by Serrin [51], and very recently by [37], [38]; general boundary conditions have been studied by Huisken in [13]. In [28] many curvature equations are considered, and several existence results are provided. Our equation does not seem to satisfy these conditions, but we will show that the classical results stated for example in [28], can be applied to it and for every positive ϵ we find a classical solution. When $\epsilon \to 0$, the equation in (8.7) degenerates. Existence of viscosity solutions for the analogous problem on all the space have been proved in [10], [7], [21], [2]. Here, if $\epsilon = 0$, we will prove the existence of a viscosity solution on the bounded set Ω.

Let us first note that, if u is a solution of (8.7) and we set $v = u - \min u_0$, then v is also a solution of (8.7), with initial condition $v_0 = u_0 - \min u_0$, and boundary datum 0. Because of the particular choice of the initial datum, the minimum of initial condition is 0 and it is attained on the boundary of Ω. By simplicity, we will also assume to modify the initial datum in such a way that it is 0 on the boundary of Ω.

As it is well known, the main existence theorem for quasilinear elliptic equations is based on some a priori estimates of the solutions, which are assumptions on the set of the solutions of (8.7).

Theorem 8.4.1. Assume that the initial datum u_0 is of class $Lip(\bar{\Omega})$, and satisfies $u_{0|\partial\Omega} = 0$.

Assume that there exists a constant C only dependent on T, the functions h and u_0 such that any solution $u \in C^{21}(Q_T) \cap Lip(\bar{Q}_T)$ of problem (8.7) satisfies the a priori estimate

$$\sup_{Q_T} |u| + \sup_{Q_T} |\nabla u| \leq C.$$

Then problem (8.7) has a solution of class $C^\infty(Q_T) \cap Lip(\bar{Q}_T)$.

Proof The assertion is a consequence of Theorems 8.3 and 12.10 in [28]. Indeed, by Theorem 12.10 there exists a constant C_1 such that any solution of class $C^{21}(Q_T) \cap Lip(\bar{Q}_T)$ satisfies the condition

$$[Du]_\alpha \leq C_1,$$

for a suitable $\alpha \in]0,1[$, where $[Du]_\alpha$ is the α-Hölder coefficient. Then Theorem 12.10 applies and it ensures the existence of a solution. This is of class $C^\infty(Q_T)$, since the equation is uniformly parabolic.

In the following two subsections we will provide the required a priori bound for u and ∇u.

8.4.1 Comparison and Maximum Principle for Solutions

Proposition 8.4.1. Assume that $u \in C^{21}(Q_T) \cap C(\bar{Q}_T)$ is a solution of (8.7) in a parabolic cylinder Q_T, and that the matrix (a_{ij}) is nonnegative. Also assume that

$$a(x,0) = 0 \ \ in\ \Omega. \tag{8.11}$$

Then

$$\sup_{Q_T} u = \sup_{\Gamma_T} u_0, \quad \inf_{Q_T} u = \inf_{\Gamma_T} u_0,$$

where Q_T is defined in (8.7), and $\Gamma_T = \bar{\Omega} \cup S_T$ is the parabolic boundary of Q_T (see for example Theorem 9.5 in [28] for the proof).

Since condition (8.11) is obviously satisfied, then the maximum principle holds for solutions of our equation. In particular, since $u = 0$ in S_T and $u_0 \geq 0$ in Ω, also $u \geq 0$ in Q_T, and

$$\sup_{Q_T} |u| = \sup_{\Omega} |u_0| = C, \tag{8.12}$$

where the last equality defines C, and it is obviously independent of ϵ.

Proposition 8.4.2. Let P be the operator defined in (8.10), where the coefficients a_{ij} and a are independent of u. If u and v are functions in $C^{21}(Q_T) \cap C(\bar{Q}_T)$ such that $Pu \geq Pv$ in $\bar{Q}_T - \Gamma_T$, and $u \leq v$ on Γ_T, then $u \leq v$ in $\bar{Q}_T$ (see for example Theorem 9.1 in [28] for the proof).

From this theorem, we immediately infer the uniqueness of solutions of problem (8.7). Indeed, if u and v are two solutions, then $Pu = Pv$ in $\bar{Q}_T - \Gamma_T$, and $u = v$ on Γ_T. Thus, they coincide because of the previous theorem.

8.4.2 A Priori Estimate for the Gradient

The estimates for the gradient are classically divided in two steps. First, using the maximum principle, the gradient on all Q_T is estimated in terms of the gradient at the boundary. Since the coefficients a_{ij} are independent of u, and a is linear in p, the classical proof of Bernstein can be applied to the operator P. We refer to [12], where the proof is given under these assumptions:

Theorem 8.4.2. Let $u \in C^{21}(Q_T) \cap Lip(\bar{Q}_T)$ be a solution of (8.7). Then there exists a constant C depending on the coefficient h, and T, and the trace of a_{ij} such that

$$\sup_{Q_T} |\nabla u| \le C \sup_{\Gamma_T} |\nabla u|.$$

The second step is the estimate of the gradient at the parabolic boundary.

Theorem 8.4.3. Assume that Ω is convex, $u \in C^{21}(Q_T) \cap Lip(\bar{Q}_T)$ is a solution of (8.7), and that the initial datum u_0 is of class $C^1(\bar{\Omega})$. Then there exists a constant $C > 0$ dependent on the initial datum u_0, and on the least eigenvalue of (a_{ij}) such that

$$\sup_{\Gamma_T} |\nabla u| \le C.$$

Proof Let $x_0 \in S_T$ be fixed, and let ν be the outer normal in $\mathbf{R}^2$ (with respect to the euclidean metrics) to $\partial\Omega$ at the point x_0. Let

$$v(x) = f(< \nu, x_0 - x >), \tag{8.13}$$

where $< \cdot, \cdot >$ is the standard scalar product in $\mathbf{R}^2$, and f is a real function to be chosen later. Since

$$\partial_i v = -f'(< \nu, x_0 - x >)\nu_i, \quad and \quad \partial_{ij} v = f''(< \nu, x_0 - x >)\nu_i \nu_j,$$

substituting in the operator P defined in (8.10), we get

$$Pv = -\partial_t v + a_{ij}\partial_{ij} v + \partial_i h \partial_i v = f''(< \nu, x_0 - x >) a_{ij}\nu_i\nu_j - \partial_i h f'(< \nu, x_0 - x >)\nu_i \le$$

(if $\sup \left|\frac{\partial h}{\partial \nu}\right| = S$, λ_1 is the least eigenvalue of $a_{ij}(x,p)$, $\lambda_1 = \min_{x,p} \lambda(x,p)$, $f' \ge 0$, and $f'' \le 0$)

$$\le f''(< \nu, x_0 - x >)\lambda_1 + S f'(< \nu, x_0 - x >) = 0. \tag{8.14}$$

If $S \ne 0$ and $f(t) = \frac{C\lambda_1}{S}\left(1 - exp\left(-\frac{S}{\lambda_1} t\right)\right)$. Since Ω is convex, $< \nu, x_0 - x > \ge 0 \ in \ \Omega$. Then it is possible to choose the constant C in such a way that

$v(x) \geq u_0(x)$ in Ω. Besides $v(x) = f(< \nu, x_0 - x >) \geq 0 = u(x,t)$ in S_T. Thus $v(x) \geq u(x)$ in Γ_T, and $Pv \leq 0 = Pu$ in Q_T, by (8.14). By Proposition 8.4.2 $v(x) \geq u(x)$ in Q_T. Since $v(x_0) = u(x_0) = 0$, then for every positive t,

$$\frac{v(x_0 - s\nu) - v(x_0)}{-s} \leq \frac{u(x_0 - s\nu) - u(x_0)}{-s} \leq 0 \tag{8.15}$$

and

$$\frac{\partial v(x_0)}{\partial \nu} \leq \frac{\partial u(x_0)}{\partial \nu} \leq 0.$$

And this gives a bound for the normal derivative: $-C \leq \frac{\partial u(x_0)}{\partial \nu} \leq 0$. The tangential component of ∇u is 0, since u is constant on S_T.

We explicitly remark that the constant in Theorem 8.4.3 depends on the least eigenvalue of a_{ij}, so that it depends on ϵ, while the constants in Proposition 8.4.1 and Theorem 8.4.2 are independent of ϵ. In order to provide an a priori bound independent of ϵ, we can extend h to a new function h_e defined in a neighborhood Ω_e of Ω, in such a way that $\frac{\partial h_e}{\partial \nu} = 0$ at the boundary. Then we prove

Proposition 8.4.3. Assume that Ω_e is a rectangle, and $\frac{\partial h_e}{\partial \nu} = 0$ in a neighborhood of the boundary, $u \in C^{21}(Q_{eT}) \cap Lip(\bar{Q}_{eT})$ is a solution of (8.7), and that the initial datum u_0 is of class $C^1(\bar{\Omega}_e)$. Then there exists a constant $C > 0$ only dependent on the initial datum u_0 and on the trace of (a_{ij}) such that

$$\sup_{\Gamma_T(\Omega_e)} |\nabla u| \leq C.$$

Proof We suitably modify the previous proof. We call

$$\Omega = [a,b] \times [c,d], \quad \Omega_e = [a_e, b_e] \times [c_e, d_e],$$

and we choose a point $x_0 \in \partial\Omega_e$. Assume that $x_0 \in]a_e, b_e[\times \{c_e\}$, and define v as in (8.13). Choosing $f(t) = kt$, where k is constant and $S = \sup_{[a_e,b_e]\times[c_e,c]} \left|\frac{\partial h}{\partial \nu}\right| = 0$, by (8.14) we deduce

$$Pv \leq 0 \quad on\ [a_e, b_e] \times [c_e, c],$$

Choosing k in such a way that $\inf_{[a_e,b_e]\times\{c\}} v \geq \max u_0 \geq \max_{[a_e,b_e]\times\{c\}} u$, we deduce

$$v \geq u \quad on\ \Gamma_T([a_e, b_e] \times [c_e, c]),$$

and by Proposition 8.4.2 $v(x) \geq u(x)$ in $Q_T([a_e, b_e] \times [c_e, c])$, while $u(x_0) = v(x_0)$. Arguing as in (8.15) we conclude the proof.

8.4.3 Existence and Uniqueness of the Solution

We can now conclude the proof of the existence of a solution:

If we make no assumption on the function h, for any fixed $\epsilon > 0$ by Proposition 8.4.1, Theorems 8.4.2 and 8.4.3 we have the estimate:

$$\sup_{Q_T} |u| + \sup_{Q_T} |\nabla u| \leq C, \tag{8.16}$$

with a constant C dependent on ϵ. Hence we can apply Theorem 8.4.1, and we have a C^∞ solution of problem (8.7), which is unique, by Proposition 8.4.2.

If we assume that h is constant on a neighborhood of the boundary of Ω, for every ϵ we find as before an unique solution u_ϵ of class C^∞ of problem (8.7). This time we have a stronger estimate, since the constant C in (8.16) is independent from ϵ, by Proposition 8.4.3. Hence the family u_ϵ is equicontinuous and uniformly converges as ϵ tends to 0 to a viscosity solution of problem (8.7), with $\epsilon = 0$.

8.5 Numerical Scheme

In this section, we show how to approximate Eqn. 8.7 with finite differences. The proof of existence of viscosity solutions (Section 3), provides the theoretical justification to exploit PSC (Propagation of Surfaces by Curvature) numerical schemes introduced in [39]. These schemes approximate the equation of motion of propagating fronts (surfaces), which resembles Hamilton-Jacobi equations with viscosity terms. Then a correct entropy-satisfying approximation of the difference operator is built by exploiting the technology of hyperbolic conservation laws.

Let us consider a rectangular uniform grid in space-time (t, x, y); then the grid consists of the points $(t_n, x_l, y_m) = (n\Delta t, l\Delta x, m\Delta y)$. Following standard notation, we denote by u^n_{lm} the value of the function u at the grid point (t_n, x_l, y_m). We approximate time derivative with a first order forward difference. The first term of Eqn. 8.7 is a parabolic contribution to the equation of motion and we approximate this term with central differences. The second term on the right corresponds to passive advection along an underlying velocity field ∇h whose direction and strength depend on edge position. This term can be approximated using the upwind schemes. In other words, we check the sign of each component of ∇h and construct one-sided difference approximation to the gradient in the appropriate (upwind) direction [39].

With this, we can write the complete first order scheme to approximate equation (8.7) as follows:

$$u_{lm}^{n+1} = u_{lm}^{n} + \Delta t \left\{ \begin{array}{c} \left[h_{lm} \frac{(\epsilon + D_{lm}^{0x^2}) D_{lm}^{0yy} - 2 D_{lm}^{0x} D_{lm}^{0y} D_{lm}^{0xy} + (\epsilon + D_{lm}^{0y^2}) D_{lm}^{0xx}}{\epsilon + D_{lm}^{0x^2} + D_{lm}^{0y^2}} \right] \\ - \left[\begin{array}{c} [\max(h_{lm}^{0x}, 0) D_{lm}^{-x} + \min(h_{lm}^{0x}, 0) D_{lm}^{+x} \\ + \max(h_{lm}^{0y}, 0) D_{lm}^{-y} + \min(h_{lm}^{0y}, 0) D_{lm}^{+y}] \end{array} \right] \end{array} \right\},$$

where D is a finite difference operator on u_{lm}^n, the superscripts $\{-, 0, +\}$ indicate backward, central and forward differences respectively, and the superscripts $\{x, y\}$ indicate the direction of differentiation. We impose Dirichlet boundary conditions by fixing the value on the boundary equal to the minimum value of the point-of-view surface. The time step Δt is upper bounded by the CFL (Courant-Friedrich-Levy) condition that ensures the stability of the evolution [27]. For further detail on the numerical scheme we refer to [39].

8.6 Results

In this section, we present results of several computations aimed at performing both modal and amodal completion of objects with missing boundaries. The approach consists of a user-defined point-of-view or a reference surface and an edge indicator function computed as a function of the image. Different choices exist for the reference surface; we show two of them in Fig. 8.8. In the next examples we use $\Phi_0 = 1/\mathcal{D}$, where $\mathcal{D}$ is the distance from the initial point of view and $\sigma = 0.3$ and $\epsilon = 10^-6$ are the fixed values that we use. First, we consider the classical triangle of Kanizsa (Fig. 8.1) and apply the algorithm in order to perform a modal completion of the missing boundaries. We compute the edge map as shown in the left image of Fig. 8.9 and then choose a reference point approximately at the center of the perceived triangle (center image of Fig. 8.9). The evolution of the surface under the flow induced by Eqn. 8.7 is visualized in Fig. 8.10. The so called subjective surface is the steady state piece-wise linear surface shown at the end of this sequence. The triangle boundary shown in the right image of Fig. 8.9 is found by plotting the level set $\bar{\Phi} = \{max(\Phi) - \epsilon\}$ of the subjective surface. Note that in visualizing the surface, we normalize it with respect to its maximum.

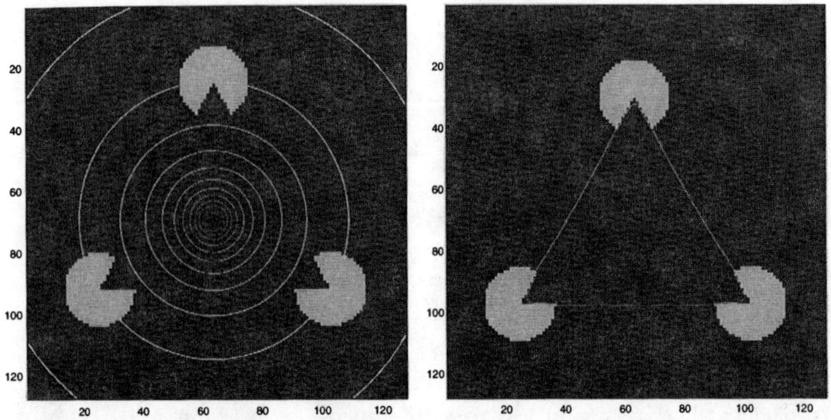

Figure 8.9: Two steps of the boundary completion of the triangle of Kanizsa: on the left a set of equispaced contour lines of the point-of-view surface are drawn and on the right is the level set of the subjective surface that corresponds to the triangle boundary as estimated by the algorithm.

In Subsection 7.3.2.4 we noted that the model equation (Eqn. 8.7) is a combination of two dynamics weighted by the stretching factor ϵ: a geodesic flow for $\epsilon = 0$ and a linear diffusion flow for $\epsilon \to \infty$. In the next experiment, we show what the boundary completion result looks like under these two extremes specially for the case when the user-defined fixation point is a bit off center. In the left image of Fig. 8.11, we consider a slightly off center initial condition. As shown in the right image of Fig. 8.11, the flow under Eqn. 8.7 succeeds in producing a good segmentation of the triangle. If we consider a strongly off center initial condition as in Fig. 8.12, the triangle is still present in the subjective surface, but the closest white inducer becomes predominant. On the other hand, the flows under both Eqn. 8.8 and Eqn. 8.9 fail to produce a good completion even with a slightly off center point of view; see Fig. 8.13. In facts the level set flow (Eqn. 8.8) causes the formation of false surface gradient due to the off center initial condition (Fig. 8.13, left), and the flow under Eqn. 8.9 produces a result that is too diffusive (Fig. 8.13, right).
The PDE based subjective surface model is able to extract the Kanizsa triangle starting from the brightness inversion of the original Kanizsa image, as depicted in Fig. 8.14.

In Fig. 8.15 and 8.16, we show the subjective surface computation from

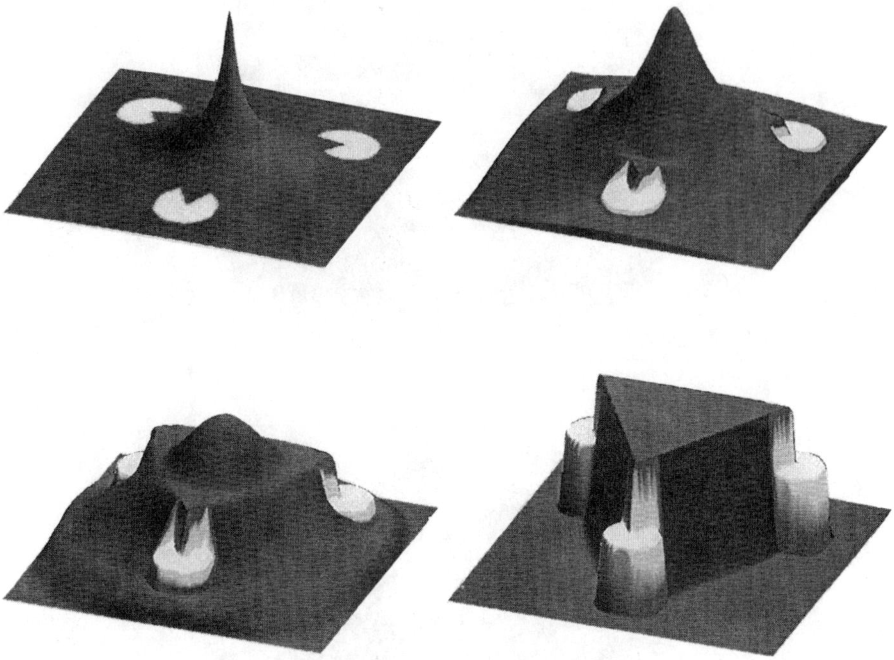

Figure 8.10: Four time frames showing the evolution of the point-of-view surface (upper left) towards the subjective surface (bottom right). In this visualization the original image has been texture mapped onto the surface. *(See color insert)*

images with termination points and little or no (aligned) edge information. We render the perceived square in the final image of Fig. 8.15 and the perceived rectangle in the final image of Fig. 8.16. Segmentation of amorphous shape is visualized in Fig. 8.17. As mentioned in the introductory section, the initial surface can be evolved using any "feature-indicator" and not just under the influence of an edge-indicator function g. In order to perform texture segmentation, we replace the the usual edge-indicator $g(I)$ with the orientation detector $g(|J_v|)$, where J_v is the Jacobian of $\vec{v} = \frac{I_x^2 - I_y^2, 2I_xI_y}{I_x^2+I_y^2}$. The result of this computation is shown in Fig. 8.18.

In Fig. 8.19 we show an example of multiple objects segmentation. Three circles with missing boundaries are present in the image. The fixation point is chosen inside the middle circle and the initial surface is its distance function

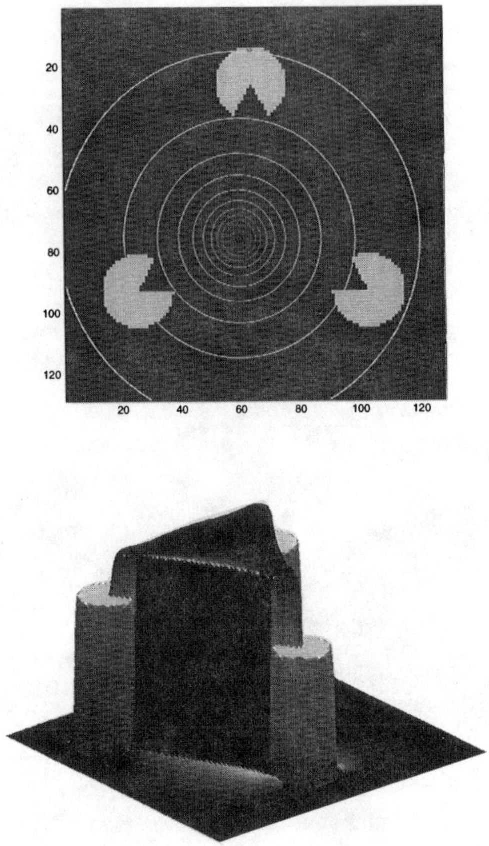

Figure 8.11: A slightly off center fixation point: on the left equispaced contour lines of the point-of-view surface are shown and the computed triangular contour is shown on the right.

(Fig.8.19 upper). When the subjective surface is computed a level set is selected in order to choose the segmented object: for $\bar{u} = \{\max(u) - \varepsilon\}$ only one circle is segmented (Fig.8.19 middle) and for $\bar{u} = \varepsilon$ all the object of the scene are segmented (Fig.8.19 bottom).

Echographic images are difficult candidates for shape recovery because they possess highly noisy structures and large parts of the boundary are often found absent thereby making shape recovery very difficult. We are interested in developing segmentation methods that deal with non-continuous edges in extremely noisy images. In Fig. 8.20, we show one such computation; we use a line

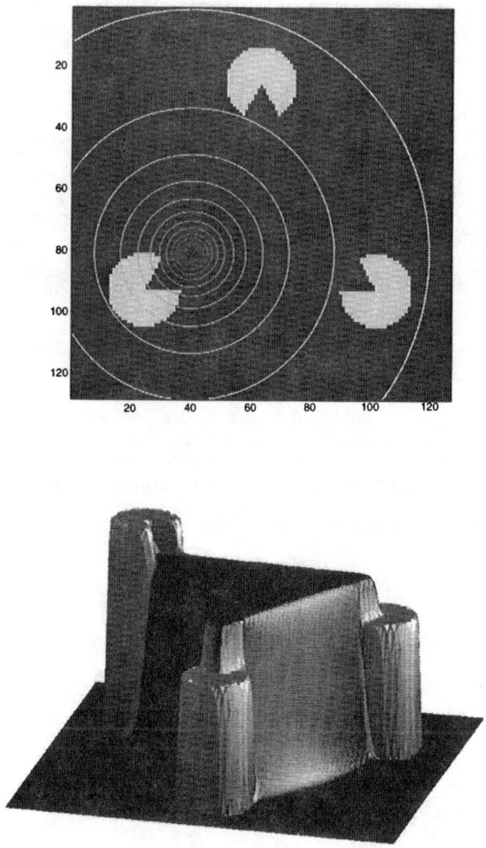

Figure 8.12: A strongly off center fixation point: on the left equispaced contour lines of the point-of-view surface are shown and on the right the subjective surface is visualized.

initialization instead of a fixation point and the point-of-view surface is constructed to be the distance function from this initial line. The final result, a particular level set of the the subjective surface is shown in the right image of Fig. 8.20. In Fig.8.21, we show four stages of the subjective surface evolution, where natural boundary conditions have been imposed.

The subjective contours we have considered so far are called "modal" contours because they are "perceived" in the visual experience. Now we consider "amodal" contours that are present in images with partially occluded shapes. Consider the example of a white square partially occluded by a gray disk as

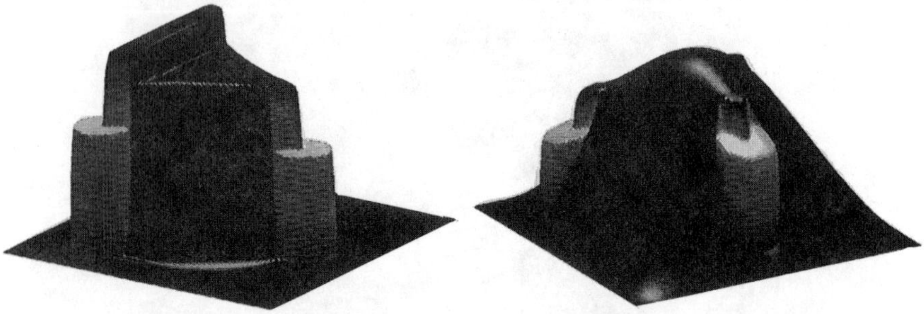

Figure 8.13: Comparison with different metrics: On the left is shown the result of the segmentation with pure level set curve evolution ($\epsilon = 0$). On the right is shown the result of the segmentation with pure nonuniform diffusion. The point of view surface is the same as in Fig.8.11).

shown in Fig. 8.22. Our goal is to recover the shapes of both the square and the disk. We employ a three step procedure: first, we build the edge map g_1 of the image and choose a point of focus inside the disk and perform the segmentation of the grey disk O_{disk}. Second, we build another edge map $g_2 = \begin{cases} 1 & (x,y) \in O_{disk} \\ g_1 & otherwise \end{cases}$ so that all the image features belonging to the first object are inhibited in the new function. As the third step we perform the modal completion of the partially occluded square using the new edge map g_2. Again, the process is completely automatic after the initial point of reference and the entire process is shown in Fig. 8.22. Finally, we present a set of amodal completion results from a real image. As shown in Fig. 8.23 our test image is one of a trash can placed in front of a computer monitor and our goal is to extract the outline of the computer monitor that is partially occluded by the trash can. In the first row left to right of Fig. 8.23 we show the original image, the point-of-view surface, and some of its level curves. So, the initial point of reference is chosen to be inside the trash can region. The first step is to extract the shape of the trash can using the original edge map information; this step is shown in the second row of the figure. Once the trash can shape has been extracted, its edge features are eliminated to produce a new edge indicator function shown in the left image of the third row of Fig. 8.23. Under the

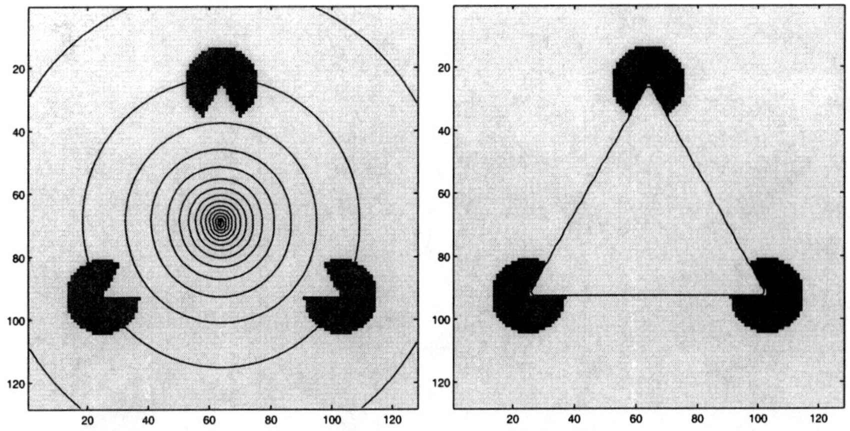

Figure 8.14: Segmentation of the brightness inverted Kanizsa triangle. On the left is shown the initial surface (isolines) and on the right is visualized the level set of the subjective surface corresponding to the triangle boundary as estimated by the algorithm.

influence of this edge function, we succeed in extracting the shape of partially occluded computer screen; see the third row of the figure. We then repeat the process and eliminate the edge features corresponding to the computer screen producing yet another edge function. The flow (Eqn. 8.7) under the edge function shown in the left image of the bottom row produces the subjective surface (bottom center) and the shape of the partially occluded computer monitor (bottom right). More examples of subjective surface segmentation applied to texture and photographic images can be found in [49].

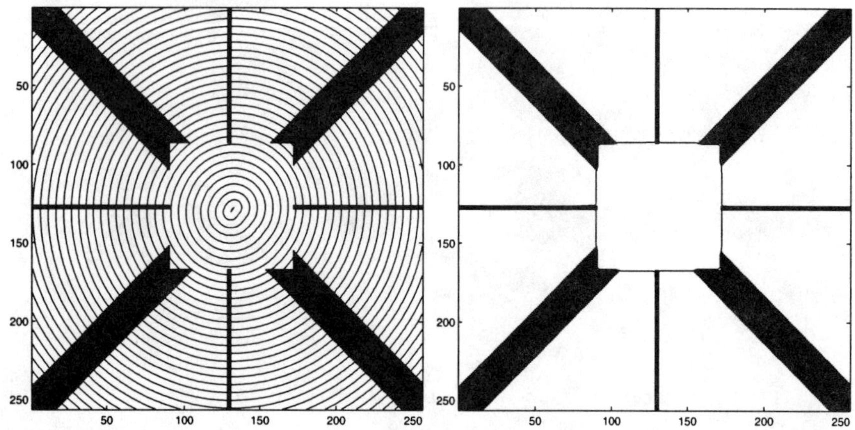

Figure 8.15: Modal completion of a figure with termination points.

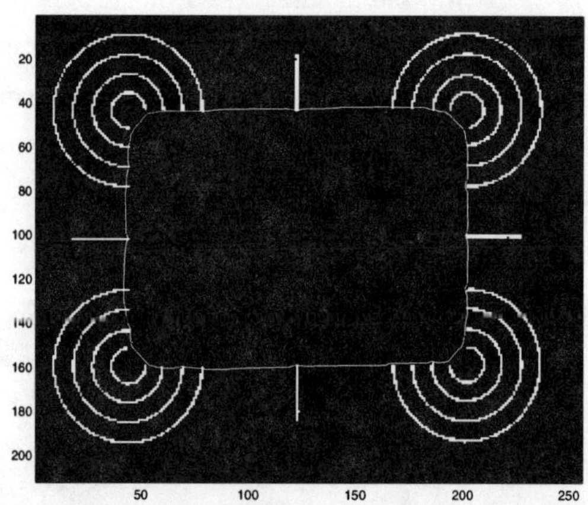

Figure 8.16: Modal completion of a figure with little or no aligned edge information.

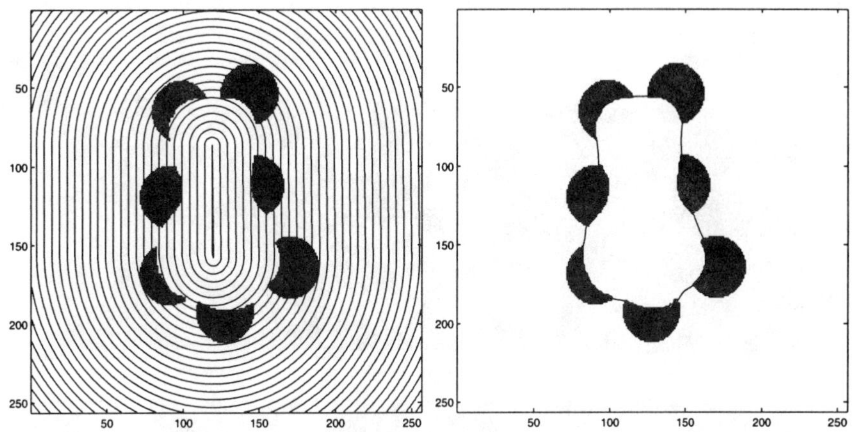

Figure 8.17: Segmentation of amorphous shape

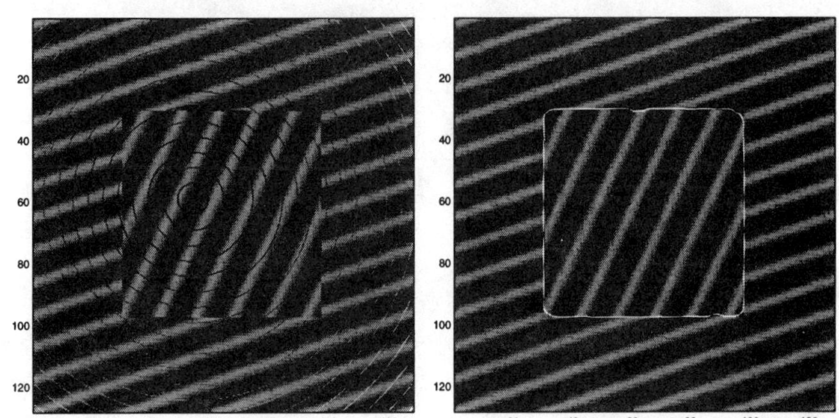

Figure 8.18: Segmentation of a texture image

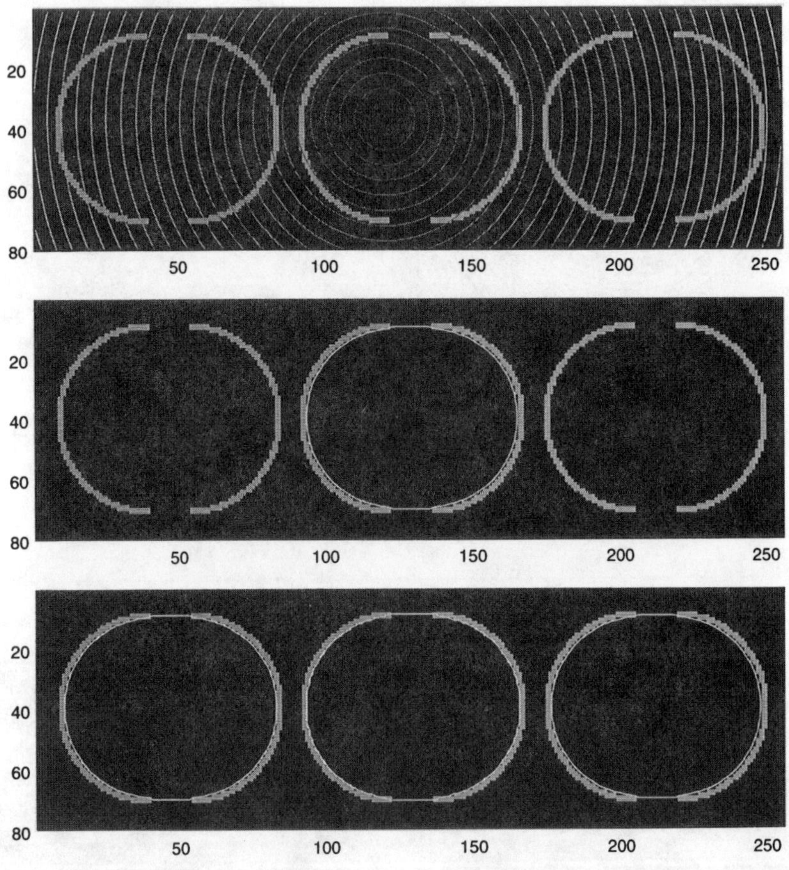

Figure 8.19: Boundary completion of figure 8.1. Level curves of the point of view surface (upper), level curve $\bar{u} = \{\max(u) - \varepsilon\}$ of the subjective surface (middle) and level curve $\bar{u} = \varepsilon$ of the subjective surface segmenting all the circles together (bottom).

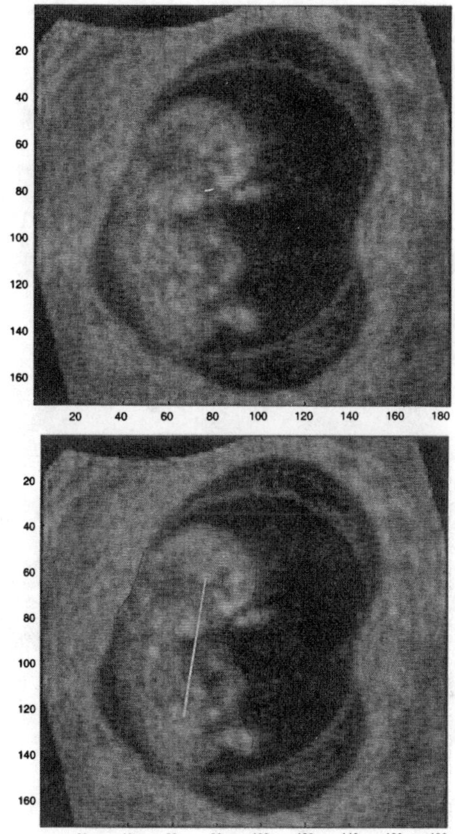

Figure 8.20: Fetal echography presenting the shape of a baby (left) and segmentation of the baby with the level set $\bar{u} = \{\max(u) - \varepsilon\}$ of the subjective surface (right). *(See color insert)*

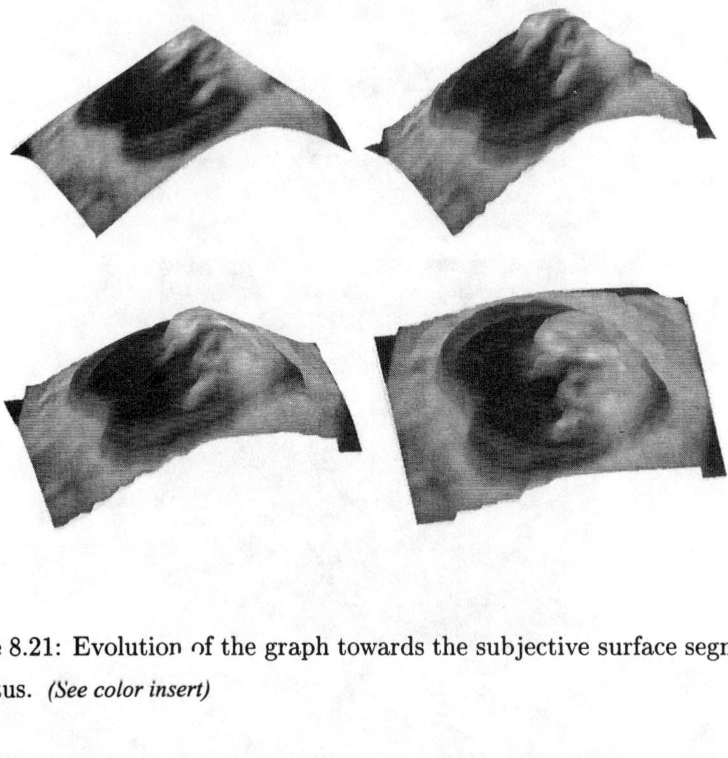

Figure 8.21: Evolution of the graph towards the subjective surface segmenting the fetus. *(See color insert)*

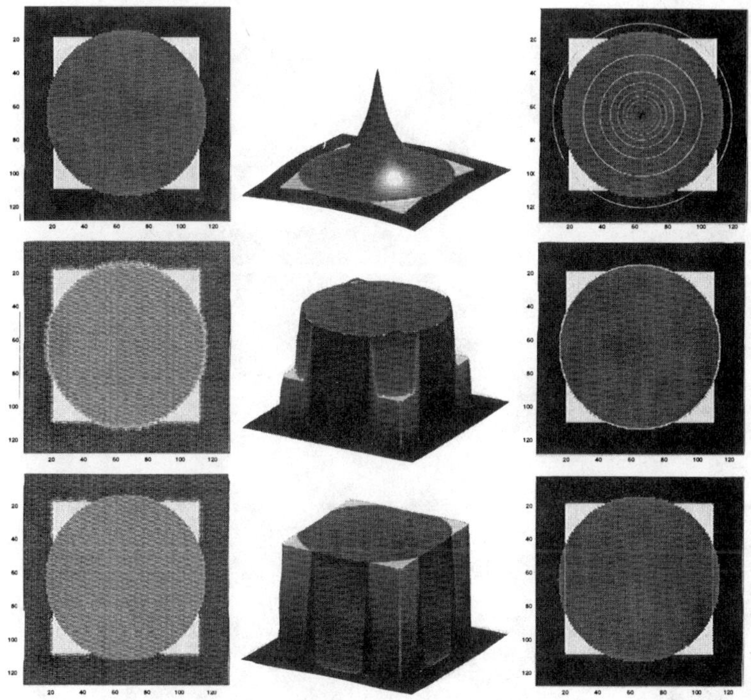

Figure 8.22: Amodal completion of the white square partially occluded by the gray disk. In the first row the original image (left) and the point-of-view surface (center, right) are shown. In the second row, the edge map g_1 (left), the subjective surface (center), and the occluding disk boundary (right) are shown. The amodal completion of the square is shown in the third row. The new edge map g_2 (left) is obtained from the previous one by simply removing the features corresponding to the occluding object (disk). This new edge map allows the formation of a new subjective contour (center) and the square boundary (right). We use the value $\beta = 0.3$ in the edge indicator.

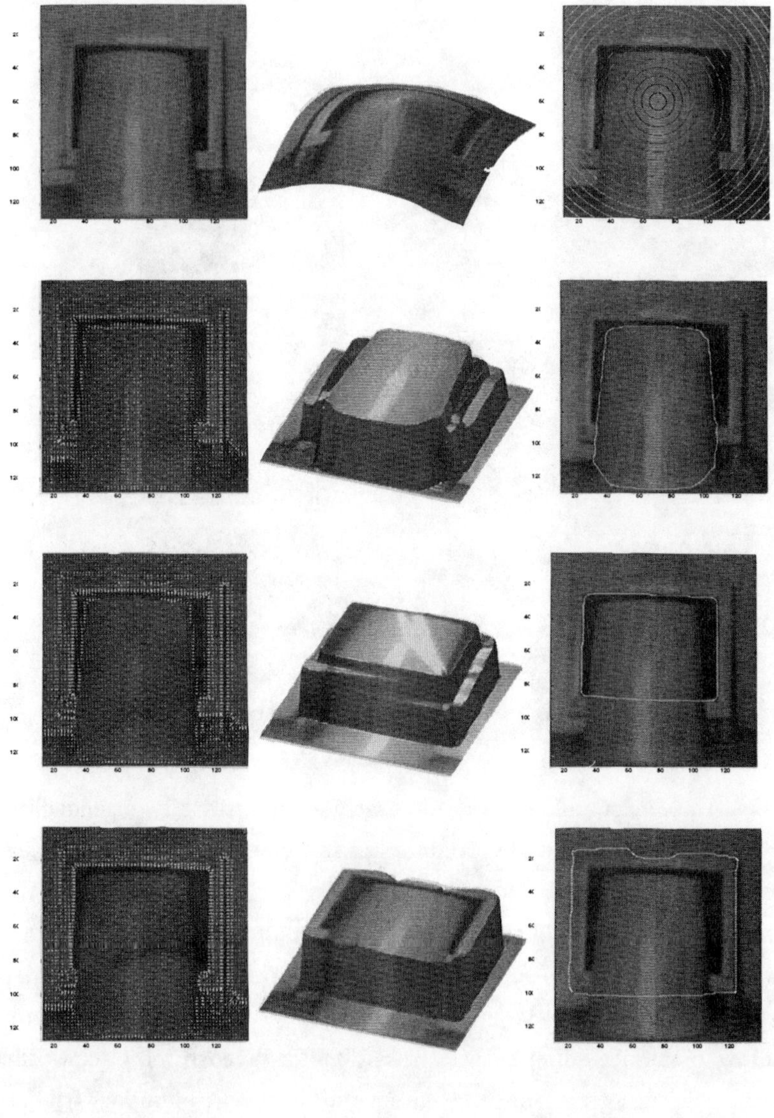

Figure 8.23: Extraction of partially occluded shapes. The computer screen and the computer monitor are amodally completed.

Bibliography

[1] Almgren, F., Taylor, J. E. and Wang, L., Curvature-driven flows: a variational approach, SIAM J. Control Optim., Vol. 31, pp. 387-437, 1993.

[2] Bellettini, G. and Paolini, M., Anisotropic motion by mean curvature in the context of Finsler geometry, Hokkaido Math. J., Vol. 25, No. 3, pp. 537-566, 1996.

[3] Brakke, K. A., The Motion of a Surface by its Mean Curvature, Princeton University Press, Princeton, 1978.

[4] Caselles, V., Catte, F., Coll, T. and Dibos, F., A Geometric Model for Active Contours, Numerische Mathematik, Vol. 66, pp. 1-31, 1993.

[5] Caselles, V., Kimmel, R. and Sapiro, G., Geodesic active contours, IJCV, Vol. 22, No. 1, pp. 61-79, 1997.

[6] Chan, T. F. and Vese, L. A., Active Contours without Edges, CAM Report 98-53, UCLA Dept. of Mathematics, Dec. 1998.

[7] Chen, Y. G., Giga, Y. and Goto, S., Uniqueness and existence of viscosity solutions of generalized mean curvature flow equations, SIAM J. of nonlinear analysis, Vol. 29, No. 1, pp. 182-193, 1992.

[8] De Giorgi, E., New Problems on Minimizing Movements, in Boundary Value Problems for Partial Differential Equations and Applications, Vol. 29, (Lions, J. L. and Baiocchi C., eds.), Masson, Paris, 1993.

[9] Do Carmo, M. P., Differential Geometry of Curves and Surfaces, Prentice Hall, 1976.

[10] Evans, L. C. and Spruck, J., Motion of level sets by mean curvature, J. Diff. Geom., Vol. 33, pp. 635-681, 1991.

[11] Gabor, D., Theory of Communication, J. Inst. Elect. Eng., Vol. 93, pp. 429-457, 1946.

[12] Gilbarg, D. and Trudinger, N. S., Elliptic Partial differential equations of second order, Springer-Verlag, Berlin, 1983.

[13] Huisken, G., Non parametric mean curvature evolution with boundary conditions, J. Diff. Eq., Vol. 77, pp. 369-378, 1989.

[14] Ilmanen, T., Generalized flow of sets by mean curvature on a manifold, Indiana Univ. Math. J., Vol. 41, No. 3, pp. 671-705, 1992.

[15] Ilmanen, T., Convergence of the Allen Cahn equation to Brakke's motion by mean curvature, J. Diff. Geom., Vol. 38, pp. 417-461, 1993.

[16] Kanizsa, G., Subjective Contours, Scientific American, pp. 48-52, April 1976.

[17] Kanizsa, G., Organization in Vision, Hardcover, 1979.

[18] Kanizsa, G., Grammatica del vedere, Il Mulino, 1980.

[19] Kanizsa, G., Margini quasi percettivi in campi con stimolazione omogenea, Rivista di Psicologia, Vol. XLIX, No. 1, pp.7-30, 1955.

[20] Kass, M., Witkin, A. and Terzopoulos, D., *Snakes: Active Contours Models*, IJCV, Vol. 1, No. 4, pp. 321-331, 1988.

[21] Kichenassamy, S., Kumar, A., Olver, P., Tennabaum, A. and Yezzi, A., Conformal curvature flow: from fase transiction to active vision, Arch. Rat. Mech. Anal, Vol. 134, pp. 275-301, 1996.

[22] Kimmel, R., Malladi, R. and Sochen, N., Images as embedded maps and minimal surfaces: Movies, Color, Texture, and Medical Images, to appear in International Journal of Computer Vision, 2001.

[23] Jenkins, H. and Serrin, J., The Dirichlet problem for the minimal surface equation in hyger dimensions, J. Reine Angew. Math., Vol. 299, pp. 170-187, 1968.

[24] Jost, J., Riemannian geometry and geometric analysis, Springer, Berlin, 1995.

[25] Julesz, B., Textons, the elements of texture perception, and their interactions, Nature, Vol. 91, No. 7, pp. 91-97, 1981.

[26] Lee, T. S., Image representation using 2D Gabor-wavelets, IEEE Transaction on Pattern Analysis and Machine Intelligence, Vol. 18, No. 10, pp. 959-971, 1996.

[27] Le Veque, R. J., Numerical Method for Conservation Laws, Birkhauser, Boston, MA, 1992.

[28] Liebermann, G. M., Second order parabolic differential equations, World Scientific, Singapore, 1996.

[29] Malik, J., Belongie, S., Leung, T. and Shi, J., Contour and Texture Analysis for Image Segmentation, in Perceptual Organization for Artificial Vision Systems, Boyer, K. L. and Sarkar, S., editors, Kluwer Academic Publishers, 2000.

[30] Malik, J., Belongie, S., Shi, J. and Leung, T., Textons, Contours and Regions: Cue Combination in Image Segmentation, Int. Conf. Computer Vision, Corfu, Greece, Sept. 1999.

[31] Malladi, R., Sethian, J. A. and Vemuri, B., Topology independent shape modeling scheme, SPIE Proceedings on Geometric Methods in Computer Vision II, San Diego, pp. 246-258, 1993.

[32] Malladi, R., Sethian, J. A., Vemuri, B. C., Shape Modeling with Front Propagation: A Level Set Approach, IEEE Transactions on Pattern Analysis and Machine Intelligence, Vol. 17, No. 2, 1995.

[33] Malladi, R. and Sethian, J. A., A real-time algorithm for medical shape recovery, in Proceedings of ICCV'98, pp. 304-310, Mumbai, India, January 1998.

[34] Marr, D., Vision, W. H. Freeman & Co., San Francisco, 1982.

[35] Mumford, D. and Shah, J., Optimal Approximations by Piecewise Smooth Functions and Associated Variational Problems, Communications on Pure and Applied Mathematics, Vol. XLII, pp. 577-685, 1989.

[36] Mumford, D., Elastica and Computer Vision, Algebraic Geometry and Its Applications, Chandrajit Bajaj (ed.), Springer-Verlag, New York, 1994.

[37] Oliker, V. I. and Uraltseva, N. N., Evolution of nonparametric surfaces with speed depending on Curvature, The Mean Curvature Case, Commun. Pure Appl. Math., Vol. 46, No. 1, pp. 97-135, 1993.

[38] Oliker, V. I. and Uraltseva, N. N., Evolution of nonparametric surfaces with speed depending on curvature. Some remarks on Mean curvature and anisotropic flows., in Ni, Wei-Ming (ed.) et al., Degenerate diffusions. Proceedings of the IMA workshop, held at the University of Minnesota, MN, USA, from May 13 to May 18, 1991. New York: Springer-Verlag. IMA Vol. Math. Appl., Vol. 47, pp. 141-156,1993.

[39] Osher, S. and Sethian, J. A., Front Propagating with Curvature Dependent Speed: Algorithms Based on Hamilton Jacobi Formulation, Journal of Computational Physics, Vol. 79, pp. 12-49, 1988.

[40] Perona, P. and Malik, J., Scale space and edge detection using anisotropic diffusion, In Proc. IEEE Computer Society Workshop on Computer Vision (1987).

[41] Perona, P., Deformable kernels for early vision, IEEE Transactions on Pattern Analysis and Machine Intelligence, Vol. 17, No. 5, pp. 488-499, 1995.

[42] Sarti, A., Malladi, R. and Sethian, J. A., Subjective Surfaces: A Method for Completion of Missing Boundaries, Proceedings of the National Academy of Sciences of the United States of America, Vol. 12, No. 97, pp. 6258-6263, 2000.
Published online before print May 23, 2000: http://www.pnas.org/cgi/content/full/110135797

[43] Sarti, A., Malladi, R. and Sethian, J. A., Subjective Surfaces: A Method for Completing Missing Boundaries, LBNL-45302, University of California, Berkeley, 2000.

[44] Sarti, A. and Citti, G., Subjective Surfaces and Riemannian Mean Curvaure Flow of Graphs, to appear in Acta Mathematica Universitatis Comenianae, 2001.

[45] Sarti, A., Malladi, R. and Sethian, J. A., Subjective Surfaces: A Geometric Model for Boundary Completion, to appear in International Journal of Computer Vision, 2001.

[46] Sarti, A. and Malladi, R., A geometric level set model for Ultrasound image analysis, LBNL-44442, Lawrence Berkeley National Laboratory, October 1999; to appear in Geometric Methods in Bio-Medical Image Processing, Ed. Malladi, R., Springer Verlag, 2001.

[47] Sarti, A., Ortiz, C., Locket, S. and Malladi, R., A unified geometric model for 3D confocal image analysis in cytology, IEEE Transactions on Biomedical Engineering, Vol. 47, No. 12, pp. 1600-1610, 2000.

[48] Sarti, A. and Citti, G., Subjective Surfaces by Riemannian Perona-Malik, private communication.

[49] http://math.lbl.gov/ ~asarti

[50] Saund, E., Perceptual Organization of Occluding Contours Generated by Opaque Surfaces, CVPR, 1999.

[51] Serrin, J., The problem of Dirichlet for quasilinear elliptic differential equations with many independent variables, Philos. Trans. Roy. Soc. London Ser. A, Vol. 264, pp. 413-496, 1969.

[52] Sethian, J. A., Curvature and the Evolution of Fronts, Comm. Math. Phys., Vol. 101, pp. 487-499, 1985.

[53] Sethian, J. A., Level Set Methods and Fast Marching Methods, Cambridge University Press, 1999.

[54] Sochen, N., Kimmel, R. and Malladi, R., A General Framework for Low Level Vision, IEEE Transactions on Image Processing, Vol. 7, No. 3, March 1998.

[55] Sochen, N. and Zeevi, Y. Y., Images as Manifolds Embedded in a Spatial-Feature Non-Euclidean Space, Submitted to IEEE Transactions on Pattern Analysis and Machine Intelligence.

[56] Wertheimer, M., Laws of Organization in Perceptual Forms, London: Harcourt (Brace and Jovanovich), 1938.

[57] Williams, L. R. and Jacobs, D. W., Stochastic Completion Fields: A Neural Model of Illusory Contour Shape and Salience, Neural Computation, Vol. 9, No. 4, pp. 837-858, 1997.

[58] Williams, L. R. and Jacobs, D. W., Local Parallel Computation of Stochastic Completion Fields, Neural Computation, Vol. 9, No. 4, pp. 859-881, 1997.

8.7 Acknowledgements

The work was supported in part by the Director, Office of Science, Office of Advanced Scientific Computing Research, Mathematical Information, and Computational Science Division of the U.S. Department of Energy under contract No. DE-AC03-76SF00098, and the Office of Naval Research under grant FDN00014-96-1-0381. The study has been also partially supported by University of Bologna under Funds for Selected Research Topics.

The software is not copyrighted. The author grants permission to use, copy, modify and distribute this software only for research purpose.

8.8 APPENDIX

SUBJECTIVE SURFACES
MATLAB MAIN PROGRAM

Alessandro Sarti
DEIS, University of Bologna and
Department of Mathematics
LBNL, University of California
Berkeley

KANIZSA TRIANGLE

```
[X0 Y0]=meshgrid(1:128,1:128); R=45; r=12; x0=R.*cos(0)+54;
y0=R.*sin(0)+25; x1=R.*cos(120/360*2*pi)+54;
y1=R.*sin(120/360*2*pi)+25; x2=R.*cos(240/360*2*pi)+54;
y2=R.*sin(240/360*2*pi)+25; c0=((X0-x0).*(X0-x0)+(Y0-y0-39).*(Y0-y0-39))¡(r.*r);
c1=((X0-x1).*(X0-x1)+(Y0-y1-39).*(Y0-y1-39))¡(r.*r);
c2=((X0-x2).*(X0-x2)+(Y0-y2-39).*(Y0-y2-39))¡(r.*r);
```

```
l1=((X0-x0)./(x1-x0))¿ ((Y0-y1)./(y1-y0)); l2=((X0-x1)./(x2-x1))¡
((Y0-y2)./(y2-y1)); l3=((X0-x2)./(x0-x2))¡ ((Y0-y0)./(y0-y2));
I0=170.*(c0+c1+c2).*(1-l1.*l2.*l3)+40; I0=rot90(I0);
I0([10:120],:)=I0([15:125],:);
[nx ny]=size(I0); I0=double(I0)/255.; I00=I0;

VISUALIZE
colormap(gray); image(I0.*70,'EraseMode','None'); axis image;
drawnow; hold on;
[X Y] =meshgrid(0:nx-1,0:ny-1);
INITIAL CONDITION [x, y]=ginput;
I=sqrt((X-x(1)).*(X-x(1))+(Y-y(1)).*(Y-y(1)));
Imax=max(max(I))

COMPUTE THE METRIC g
beta=0.000001; g=1./(1+(G(I0)./beta));
figure(5) colormap gray image(I00.*70+10,'EraseMode','None'); axis image;
drawnow; hold on; quiver(-Dy(g),-Dx(g),'k'); pause

SOLVE PDE
dt =0.1; Iter=3000; for i = 1:Iter,
i
I= I + dt.*(g.*(KG(I)) + Adv(I,Dx(g),Dy(g)));
if (mod(i,10)==1) figure(2); colordef black; surf(-I,I0); shading interp;
light; view(30,30); drawnow; end
I([1:nx],1)=Imax;
I([1:nx],ny)=Imax;
I(1,[1:ny])=Imax;
I(nx,[1:ny])=Imax;
end
```

SUBJECTIVE SURFACES
MATLAB FUNCTIONS

Alessandro Sarti
DEIS, University of Bologna and

Department of Mathematics
LBNL, University of California
Berkeley

```
% Centered X derivative
% Use: f = Dx(Matrix)
function f = Dx(Mat)
[m n] = size(Mat);
f = (Mat([2:m m],1:n) - Mat([1 1:m-1],1:n))./2;

% Centered Y derivative
% Use: f = Dy(Matrix)
function f = Dy(Mat)
[m n] = size(Mat);
f = (Mat(1:m,[2:n n]) - Mat(1:m,[1 1:n-1]))./2;

% Forward X derivative
% Use: f = Dpx(Matrix)
function f = Dpx(Mat)
[m n] = size(Mat);
f = Mat([2:m m],1:n) - Mat;

% Forward Y derivative
% Use: f = Dpy(Matrix)
function f = Dpy(Mat)
[m n] = size(Mat);
f = Mat(1:m,[2:n n]) - Mat;

% Backward X derivative
% Use: f = Dmx(Matrix)
function f = Dmx(Mat)
[m n] = size(Mat);
f = Mat - Mat([1 1:m-1],1:n);

% Backward Y derivative
% Use: f = Dmy(Matrix) function f = Dmy(Mat)
```

```
[m n] = size(Mat);
f = Mat - Mat(1:m,[1 1:n-1]);

% XX derivative
% Use: f = Dxx(Matrix)
function f = Dxx(Mat)
[m n] = size(Mat);
f = Mat([2:m m],1:n) - 2.* Mat + Mat([1 1:m-1],1:n);

% YY derivative
%Use: f = Dyy(Matrix)
function f = Dyy(Mat)
[m n] = size(Mat);
f = Mat(1:m,[2:n n]) - 2.*Mat + Mat(1:m,[1 1:n-1]);

% Module of the gradient
% Use: f = G(Matrix)
function f = G(Mat)
[m n] = size(Mat);
f = sqrt(Dx(Mat).*Dx(Mat)+Dy(Mat).*Dy(Mat));

% Euclidean mean curvature
% Use: f = KG(Matrix)
function f = KG(M)
[m n] = size(M);
eps=0.000001;
f=(Dxx(M).*(eps+Dy(M).*Dy(M))-2.*Dy(M).*Dx(M).*Dx(Dy(M))+Dyy(M).
*(eps+Dx(M).*Dx(M)))./((Dx(M).*Dx(M)+Dy(M).*Dy(M))+eps);

% Advection term with upwinding
% Use: f = Adv(I,Fx,Fy)
function f = Adv(I,Fx,Fy)
f=((Fx>0).*Dpx(I) +(Fx<0).*Dmx(I)).*Fx +((Fy>0).*Dpy(I)+(Fy<0).*Dmy(I)).*Fy
;
```

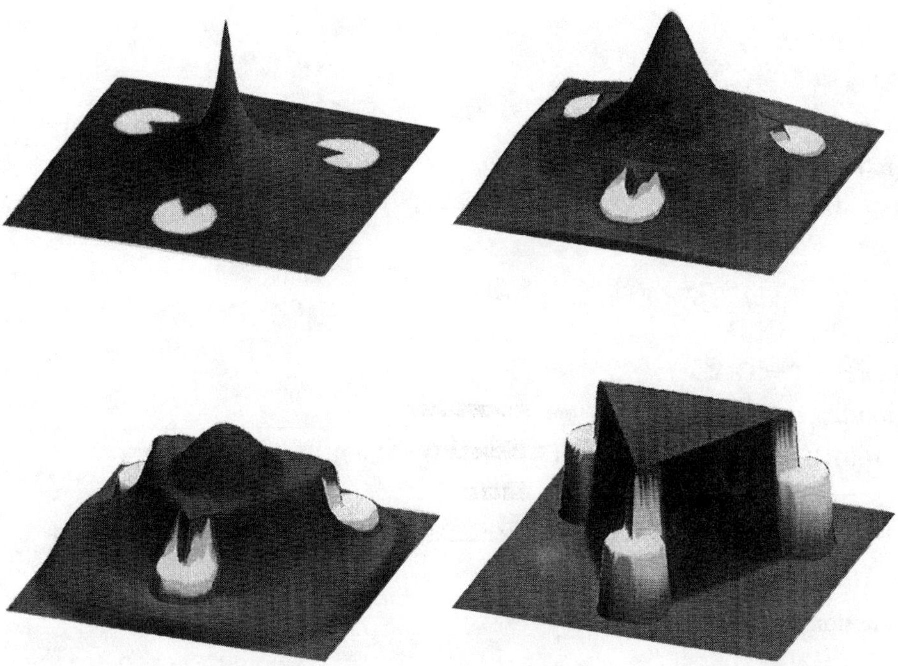

Figure 8.24: COLOR PLATES. Four time frames showing the evolution of the point-of-view surface (upper left) towards the subjective surface (bottom right). In this visualization the original image has been texture mapped onto the surface. *(See color insert)*

Chapter 9

The Future of PDEs and Level Sets

Jasjit S. Suri[1], *David Chopp*[2], *Alessandro Sarti*[3] *and Swamy Laxminarayan*[4]

9.1 Introduction

We have seen that the field of level sets and PDE has opened doors for not only theoretical mathematicians but a very large community of engineering and non-engineering fields. The field of levels sets and PDEs has emerged more than previously thought because of its ability to solve very difficult problems in image processing and graphics. Level sets have made a tremendous impact on medical imagery due to its ability to perform topology preservation and fast shape recovery. This has dominated the binary, grayscale and color imaging frameworks, which the eye can perceive. It has the ability to find boundaries and surfaces deep seated in 2-D and 3-D volumes, respectively. It has also demonstrated its ability to find solutions for completion of cognitive objects with missing boundaries. This field of applied mathematics has penetrated into more than 30 fields of engineering/non-engineering and seems to be expanding more and more each day. The book would be incomplete if we did not discuss the future on PDE and level sets. This chapter is focused on the future aspects of the level sets and PDEs. Some of this work can be seen by Suri *et al.* [1].

[1]Marconi Medical Systems, Inc., Cleveland, OH, USA
[2]Northwestern University, Evanston, IL, USA
[3]University of Balogna, Balogna, Itlay
[4]New Jersey Institute of Technology, Newark, NJ, USA

PDE & Level Sets: Algorithmic Approaches to Static & Motion Imagery
Edited by Jasjit Suri and Swamy Laxminarayan, Kluwer Academic/Plenum Publishers, 2002

We have seen in Chapter 1 the basic introduction on PDEs and level sets. Chapter 2 presented the basic level set and its extentions. The same chapter presented a brief survey the modern implementation of the level set method beginning with its roots in hyperbolic conseravtion laws and Hamilton-Jacobi equations. The same chapter also discussed the extentions to the level set method to solve a broad range of interface motion problems such as reinitialization, velocity extensions, and coupling with finite element methods. Regularizers in level set framework was discussed in Chapter 3. It is here the concept of fusion of frameworks was framed. The application of PDEs in shown in Chapter 4. This chapter was like a review on the level sets and PDEs.

In Chapter 5, the authors described a new algorithm for color image segmentation and a novel approach for image sequence segmentation using PDE framework. The color image segmentation algorithm was used for image sequence intra-frame segmentation, and that gave accurate region boundaries. Because this method produced accurate boundaries, the accuracy of motion boundaries of the image sequence segmentation algorithms was improved when it was integrated in the sequence segmentation framework. The authors implemented this in a multi-resolution framework along with a narrow banding framework, which is significantly faster than both single resolution and traditional multi-resolution methods. As a color image segmentation technique, it is unsupervised, and its segmentation is accurate at the object boundaries. Since it uses the Markov Random Field (MRF) and mean field theory, the segmentation results are smooth and robust. Examples were shown using dermatoscopic images and image sequence frames. The Chapter then presented a new approach to the image sequence segmentation that contained three parts: (i) global motion compensation, (ii) robust frame differencing and (iii) curve evolution. In the global motion compensation, we used a fast technique, where we needed only a sparse set of pixels evenly distributed in the image frames. Block-matching and regression were used to classify the sparse set of pixels into inliers and outliers according to the affine model. With the regression, the inliers of the sparse set, which are related to the global motion, were determined iteratively. For the robust frame differencing, the method used a local structure tensor field, which robustly represented the object motion characteristics. With the level set curve evolution, the algorithm detected all the moving objects and spotted out the objects' outside contours. The approach discussed in Chapter 5 is computationally efficient, and does not require a dense motion field and is insensitive to global/background motion and noise. Its efficacy is demonstrated on both TV and surveillance video.

In Chapter 6, the authors described a novel approach to image sequence segmentation and its real-time implementation. This approach used the 3-D structure tensor to produce a more robust frame difference and used curve evolution to extract whole (moving) objects.

In Chapter 7, the authors presented a fast region-based level set approach for extraction of white matter, gray matter, and cerebrospinal fluid boundaries from two dimensional magnetic resonance slices of the human brain. This is a classical example of fusion of two different frameworks, which made the level sets more powerful than ever. The forces applied in the level set framework utilized three kinds of speed control functions based on region, edge and curvature. Regional speed functions were determined based on a fuzzy membership function computed using the fuzzy clustering technique while edge and curvature speed functions were based on gradient and signed distance transform functions. The level set algorithm was implemented to run in the "narrow band" using a "fast marching method".

In Chapter 8, a geometric model for segmentation of images with missing boundaries was presented. Some classical problems of boundary completion in cognitive images, like the pop-up of subjective contours in the famous triangle of Kanizsa, were framed from a surface evolution framework. The method was based on the mean curvature evolution of a graph with respect to the Riemannian metric induced by the image. Existence, uniqueness and maximum principle of the parabolic PDE were proved. A numerical scheme introduced by Osher and Sethian for evolution of fronts by curvature motion was adopted. Results were presented for modal completion of cognitive objects with missing boundaries.

Having discussed the different aspects of PDE and level set frameworks for static and motion imagery using a combination of different frameworks, this chapter bascially puts forward some of the challenges in the level set and PDE frameworks applied to medical and non-medical imaging fields. Section 9.2 presents the medical imaging perspective and section 9.3 presents the medical imaging covering the mathematical and non-medical imaging perspective. In section 9.4 we discuss the future on subjective surfaces.

9.2 Medical Imaging Perspective: Unsolved Problems

The class of differential geometry, also called PDE in conjunction with level sets, was shown to dominate image processing, in particular to medical imaging, in a major way. We still need to understand how the regularization terms can be integrated into the level sets to improve segmentation schemes. Even though the application of level sets has gone well in the fields of medical imaging, biomedicine, fluid mechanics, combustion, solidification, CAD/CAM, object tracking/image sequence analysis and device fabrication, we are still far away from achieving stable 3-D volumes and a standard segmentation in real-time. By standard, we mean that which can segment the 3-D volume with a wide variation in pulse sequence parameters. We will probably see in the near future the modeling of front propagation that takes into account the physical constraints of the problem, for example, minimization of variation geodesic distances, rather than simple distance transforms. We will probably also see more incorporation of likelihood functions and adaptive fuzzy models to prevent leaking of the curves/surfaces. A good example of integration of the low level processes into the evolution process could be given as: $\frac{\partial \phi}{\partial t} = L(x,y)\,(\beta_0 - \beta_1 \kappa)\,|\nabla\, \phi|$, where $L(x,y) = 1 - max(S_1, S_2, S_i, ..., S_n)$, where S_i is the low level process from edge detection, optical flow, stereo disparity, texture, etc. The better the $S_i(x,y)$, the more robust could be the level set segmentation process. We also hope to see more papers on level sets where the segmentation step does require a re-initialization stage. It would also, however, be helpful if we could incorporate a faster triangulation algorithm for isosurface extraction in 3-D segmentation methods.

We will see a massive effort by the computer vision community to integrate regularization terms to improve the robustness and accuracy of the 3-D segmentation techniques. In earlier chapters of this book, we have shown the role of PDE and level set method for image smoothing, image diffusion and image denoising. Also shown was how curve/surface propagation hypersurfaces based on differential geometry are used for the segmentation of objects in still imagery. We have also shown the relationship between the parametric deformable models and curve evolution framework; incorporation of clamping/stopping forces to improve the robustness of these topologically independent curves/surfaces.

We have discussed considerably the segmentation of an object in motion imagery based on PDE and the level set framework. In this Chapter, we have also presented research in the area of coupled PDEs for edge preservation and smoothing. Some coverage has also been given on PDE in miscellaneous applications. This Chapter concludes with the advantages and the disadvantages of segmentation modeling via geometric deformable models (GDM), PDE and level sets.

9.2.1 Challenges in Medical Imaging

Some of the challenges in medical imaging are:

1. *Bleeding prevention:* Bleeding pervention during the tracking process of the blood vessels. This is particularly a difficult process where we have to detect and track the blood vessels in black blood angiography data sets. Figure 9.1 shows the vessels detected using the scale-space techniques, which need to be tracked in 3-D using level sets.

2. *Interface extraction:* 2-D Interface extraction during the brain segmentation of white matter/gray matter. This involves the extraction of the white/gray matter during the level set propagation scheme.

3. *3-D level sets:* Three dimensional level sets in medical imaging. This is a new area and has started to draw much attention. Due to the robustness and speed of the geometric snakes and surfaces, 3-D level sets have dominated the 3-D medical imaging in a big way. This is indeed challenging for thin and thick structures.

4. *Optimization of volume segmentation:* Optimization issues on the medical imaging volume segmentation. 3-D level sets involves computing the 3-D Eikonal equation (see Chapter 2). In medical imaging, when the volumes are large ($256 \times 256 \times 256$), the Eikonal equation can take large times. One possible method was the fast marching method suggested by Sethian. Another possible way is the narrow banding approaches. We still need more faster methods for the above volumes, and this is one of the challenging areas.

5. *Integration of scale-spaces and level sets in angiography:* This is a new and challenging field which is emerging. 3-D segmentation of blood vessels is

important in the following areas:

> (**1**) neuro-surgical planning, interventional procedures and treatments; (**2**) time saving for performing 3-D segmentation; (**3**) distinguishing between the veins and arteries; (**4**) relative placement of the anatomical structures with respect to vasculature; (**5**) blood flow process and hemodynamics; (**6**) stenosis and aneurysm assessment/quantification; (**7**) disease monitoring/remission, and (**8**) quantification of vascular structures.

For all the above motivating areas of research, we need tracking of the blood vessels. The tracking in the noisy data is a one of the very difficult problems. We present that one way to attempt this is to fuse scale-space framework with level set framework. Scale-space has been demonstated by Suri *et al.* [2] for vessel detection in white and black blood angiography. The appendix (see section 9.6) presented a brief algorithm for vessel detection using the scale-space framework. These vessels are very thin (from 1 mm to 10 mm) and need a very careful design for the white and black blood angiography volumes. The algorithm discussed in appendix helps in this process.

6. *Numerical stability:* Another area of challenge is the numerical stability of the algorithms which is a very critical component in segmentation of the medical data sets.

7. *Numerical methods for solving PDE*: The challenging problem lies in solving the PDE in higher dimensional space. For example, if we have a 10 dimensional space, and if we use Finite Element Method, the number of nodes increases exponentionally.

9.3 Non-Medical Imaging Perspective: Unsolved Issues in Level Sets

The level set method has made a dramatic impact in a broad range of applications, and will continue to expand in the future. Even applications which do not at first appear to be related to interface motion, for example robotic

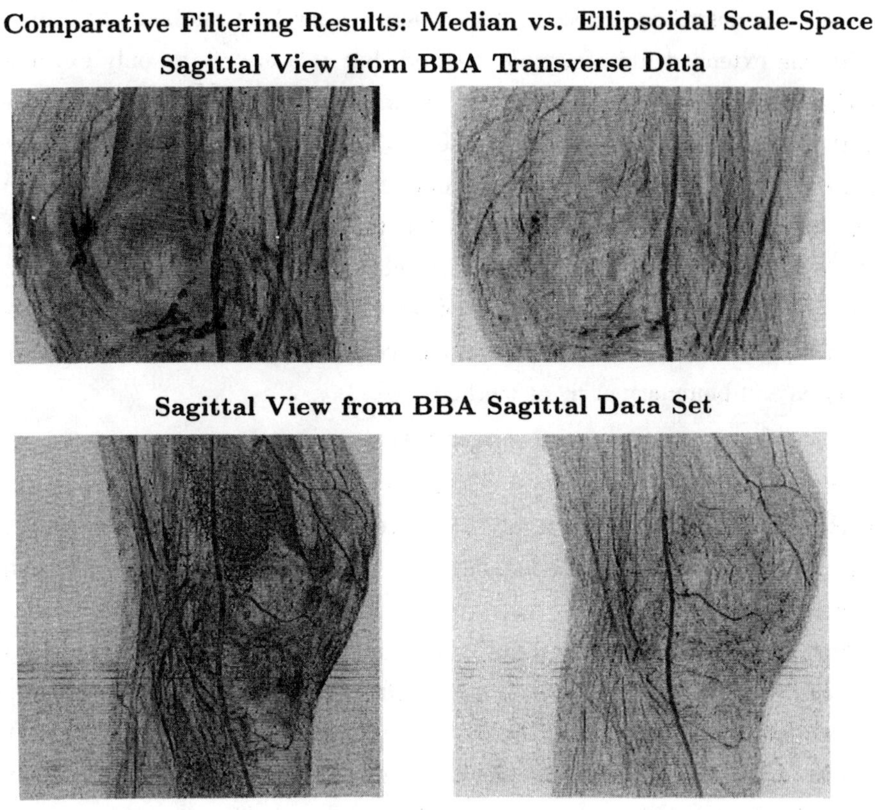

Figure 9.1: Challenging black blood data set showing the vessels. As seen the original data is very noisy and we need robust level set techniques for tracking such data sets. Here, we see the comparison between 3-D median filtering vs. ellipsoidal scale-space filtering algorithm. **Left Column**: 3-D median filtering. **Right Column**: 3-D ellipsoidal filtering. **TopRow**: sagittal views from the transverse acquired data set. **BottomRow**: sagittal views from the sagittal acquired data set.

path planning [11], have had aspects of the level set and fast marching methods applied to them with great success.

The future of the level set method is now headed toward the coupling of the level set method with other established numerical methods. One example of this was described in section 2.4.4 where the level set method was coupled with the extended finite element method, but this is not the only example. Other examples include coupling with the immersed interface method [10], and with the popular volume of fluid method [15]. The coupling with the immersed interface method brings the second order accuracy of solving elliptic equations with jump discontinuities to the level set method which identifies the location of those discontinuities. The coupling with the volume of fluid method brings the careful mass conservation properties of the volume of fluid method to the level set method. Other possible combinations could be established with boundary integral and boundary element methods.

Another possible combination which is yet to be explored is coupling the level set method with the very method it was intended to replace: the marker particle method. While this combination seems counter-intuitive, it may prove worthy of consideration. Even though the marker particle method has some serious drawbacks, it is very fast. For some applications, for example surface diffusion which involves a fourth order non-linear differential operator, the level set method is very expensive. Often, surface diffusion is only one part of a larger simulation, yet can be the most computationally intensive. Turning to marker particle methods to handle short-time surface diffusion may prove to be an intelligent solution, especially in light of the recent improvements in the reinitialization process described in section 2.2.3.1.

Another area that is not fully explored is new representations for more complex interfaces. In section 2.5.4, simple line and planar cracks are represented by multiple level set functions. However, this becomes unwieldy when considering a compound crack with multiple branches, for example the spider web shaped cracks in a broken window. What is needed is a way to capture endpoints more precisely without whole additional level set functions to identify a few individual points such as a crack tip.

A similar example is the case of trying to model foam. In a model for foam it might be possible to use the level set method to follow the motion of the many interfaces. The many triple junctions can be handled using the techniques described in section 2.4.3.1, but there still remain several significant challenges to be overcome. First, there is the representation of perhaps hundreds of bubbles. In the method of section 2.4.3.1, each of the bubbles would require its own level set function. This would mean a huge computational cost. A second challenge in this problem is how to handle spontaneous interface breaking. In a real foam, the interface between two bubbles may become too thin and break so that the two bubbles become one. Resolving the thickness of the films along with the larger foam structure is computationally too expensive to be practical, so it would be helpful if some way of tracking this information on top of the level set representation would be good.

Moving towards the fast marching method, it may be possible to use the fast marching method to overcome the time step restriction of the level set method imposed by the Courant-Friedrichs-Levy condition. In this technique, the fast marching method is used to compute the evolution of the interface for an indefinite amount of time using a single pass through the mesh. This approach was used in [14, 13] to advance the moving crack tip. To illustrate this method, consider the following algorithm:

- Set the speed function F at all nodes, using the velocity extension method if necessary.
- Use 2.21 to determine the time of first crossing map. The level curve $\phi = \Delta t$ of this map represents the location of the interface at time Δt.
- To take a time step of size Δt, simply subtract Δt from every grid point of ϕ. This will leave $\phi = 0$ as the new interface at time $t + \Delta t$.

This algorithm circumvents the time step restriction. If the velocity field is static, then there is nothing new to be solved, but if the velocity field should be time dependent, then the interface can be moved using a Δt much larger than would otherwise be allowed.

There are two open questions that concern this approach. First, the standard velocity extension idea is not designed for larger values of Δt. A look at the characteristics reveals that while the characteristics are normal to the interface initially, they need not remain that way as is assumed by the velocity extension method. The fast marching method will have to be modified to take this into account before this algorithm can be successfully employed. For present implementations of the velocity extension, this is not an issue because

Δt is effectively taken small steps, but it will become an issue when it is used to take larger time steps.

The second open question is related to the fast marching method. Can the fast marching method be improved so that the restriction that the speed function F assigned if a same sign be removed ? The difficulty with this problem is the fact that a single point on the mesh could be assigned two values, one from the part of the front with a positive speed and one from the part of the front with a negative speed. Which value that point should take is not clear, but must be resolved in order to solve this problem. It may be that solving this problem is related to solving a more general static Hamilton-Jacobi equation where the Hamiltonian is non-convex. This question is addressed next.

Without a doubt, the most rapid expansion of applications in the future will involve implementation of single-pass algorithms such as the fast marching method. These methods offer the ability to solve static Hamilton-Jacobi equations rapidly, assuming certain restrictions on the Hamiltonian. Consider a more general static Hamilton-Jacobi equation given by

$$H(\nabla\phi, \mathbf{x}) = 0 \tag{9.1}$$

(compare with 2.10). The fast marching method can be used to solve 9.1 provided that H is isotropic, i.e. independent of the direction of $\nabla\phi$.

However, there are many static Hamilton-Jacobi equations for which this condition does not hold. For example, suppose we wish to compute the time of first arrival map of driving from Chicago. If we are considering air travel, then the speed of the aircraft would be essentially the same independent of which direction it is travelling, in other words, the Hamiltonian is independent of direction. In this situation, the time of first arrival map would be a circular cone with vertex at Chicago, and the shortest path between Chicago and Los Angeles is traced out by a straight line between the two cities. In this case, the Hamiltonian is called isotropic.

However, if we restrict the travel to driving, there are intervening mountains, highways, and other features which make the shortest path much less than a straight line. This crooked path is the result of a Hamiltonian which is direction dependent. For example, from a point on a highway, is it faster to drive parallel with traffic, or orthogonal? Clearly, the speed at which the vehicle will travel depends heavily on which direction the vehicle is pointed. In this case, the time of first arrival map would be distorted according to the terrain, and the Hamiltonian is called anisotropic. See Figure 9.2 for the effect of a road being added to an otherwise featureless landscape.

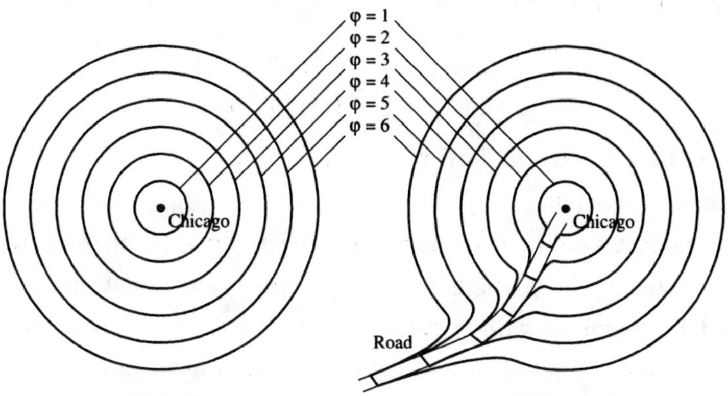

Figure 9.2: Examples of isotropic and anisotropic time of first crossing maps

Recent work of Sethian and Vladimirsky [12] solved the case of for a convex anisotropic Hamiltonian where the Hamiltonian is written in the form

$$F\left(\frac{\nabla\phi}{||\nabla\phi||},\mathbf{x}\right)||\nabla\phi|| = 1 \tag{9.2}$$

for some direction depedendent speed function $F \geq 0$. The Hamiltonian is convex if at every point $\mathbf{x}$, the function F sweeps out a convex region, see Figure 9.3. The method proposed in [12] is called the ordered upwind method,

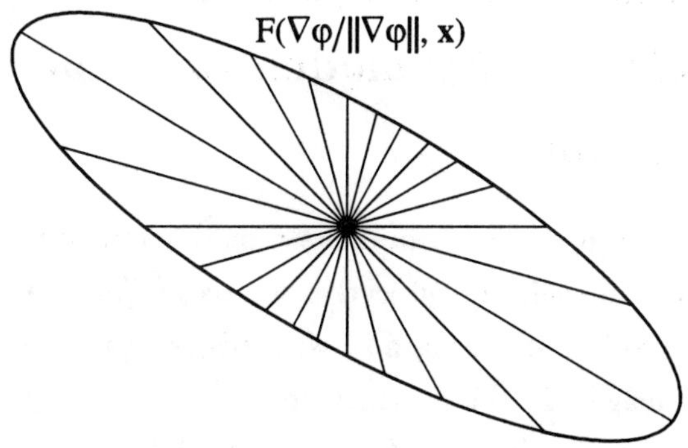

Figure 9.3: Example of a convex Hamiltonian

and works very similar to the fast marching method. The key difference is in how the update process works. For the isotropic case, the value of the solution at a grid point depended only on the neighboring grid points. In the anisotropic case, the solution at a given grid point may depend upon points much farther away. How far depends upon the severity of the anisotropy measured by the ratio

$$R = \frac{\max_{\nabla\phi/\|\nabla\phi\|} F(\nabla\phi/\|\nabla\phi\|, \mathbf{x})}{\min_{\nabla\phi/\|\nabla\phi\|} F(\nabla\phi/\|\nabla\phi\|, \mathbf{x})}. \tag{9.3}$$

The larger the ratio R, the larger the region of grid points in which a given grid point may depend.

Both the fast marching method, and the more general ordered upwind method, are examples of single-pass algorithms. The equations which they solve used to be solved with iterative procedures that required many passes through the mesh. These new methods now solve the same equations with a single pass through the mesh. The difference in speed can be dramatic, and can be important in many applications relevant to image processing, for example in such areas as robotic vision and path planning.

While the ordered upwind method does increase the number of problems that can be solved using this single-pass technology, there still remains the challenging problem of solving an arbitrary static Hamilton-Jacobi equation with a possibly non-convex Hamiltonian using a single-pass method. This problem is difficult due to the complex behavior of the characteristic curves. Next, we will discuss the future of the concept of the subjective surfaces.

9.4 The Future on Subjective Surfaces: Wet models and dry models of visual perception

The study discussed in this book presents a mathematical model and a computational method to build up subjective surfaces. The subjective surface is obtained with an area minimizing flow with respect to a Riemannian metric induced by the image. In this method first we compute the image induced metric and second we evolve a surface with its Riemannian mean curvature towards the minimal surface.

In the future we plan to investigate the link between oscillatory neural models, expressed by a phase difference equation and Riemannian mean curvature flow of graphs, i.e. the subjective surface model. We plan to establish a relationship between "wet models" (neurophysiological models) and "dry models" (Mumford Shah functional, mean curvature flows). In particularly we will look for a formal link between the Euler Lagrange functional associated to the phase equation, and the Mumford-Shah functional, embedded in specific geometry which can be either a riemannian one, or the subriemannian one of the primary visual cortex. Accordingly a relationship will be established between the difference equation and the flow of the Mumford and Shah, or *curvature equations in riemannian and subriemannian setting.* Preliminary results have been presented in [17, 21].

From the neurological point of view there is a large amount of experimental evidence that grouping is represented in the brain with a temporal coding, meaning that semantically homogeneous areas in the image would be encoded in the synchronization (phase locking) of oscillatory neural responses. The visual cortex is then modelled by [22] as a collection of oscillators coupled with long range sparse interactions, represented by a difference equation. In dimension one and with uniform connections its ability to reach phase locking solutions and to present phase discontinuities has already been outlined.

In [17, 21] we consider the same equation in the n-dimensional space and with space variant anisotropic connections, and prove a relationship between this equation and the variational models. This provides a preliminary biological justification for these models, and in particular to the subjective surface model [20].

Indeed, several neuro-physiological studies show that the association field between cortical columns are space variant and strongly anisotropic. Then we denote $|\eta|_g$ the norm with respect to the riemannian metric g, and $D^{\epsilon}_{g\eta}u(x)$ the difference quotient with respect to the metric.

The resulting equation is then

$$\partial_t u(t) = \int_{\mathbf{R^n}} D^{-\epsilon}_{\eta}\left(\frac{|\eta|}{|\eta|_g} e^{-|\eta|_g} \phi_{\epsilon|\eta|_g}\left(D^{-\epsilon}_{g\eta} u\right)\sqrt{g}\right) d\eta, \tag{9.4}$$

for a periodic and odd function $\phi_{\epsilon|\xi|}(z)$. The Euler Lagrange functional associated to equation (9.4) is

$$\hat{F}_{\epsilon}(u) = \int_{\mathbf{R^n}} \left(\int_{\mathbf{R^n}} e^{-|\eta|_g} \varphi_{\epsilon|\eta|_g}\left(D^{\epsilon}_{g|\eta|} u\right)\sqrt{g}dx\right) d\eta,$$

where $\varphi_{\epsilon|\xi|}$ is a primitive of $\phi_{\epsilon|\xi|}$.

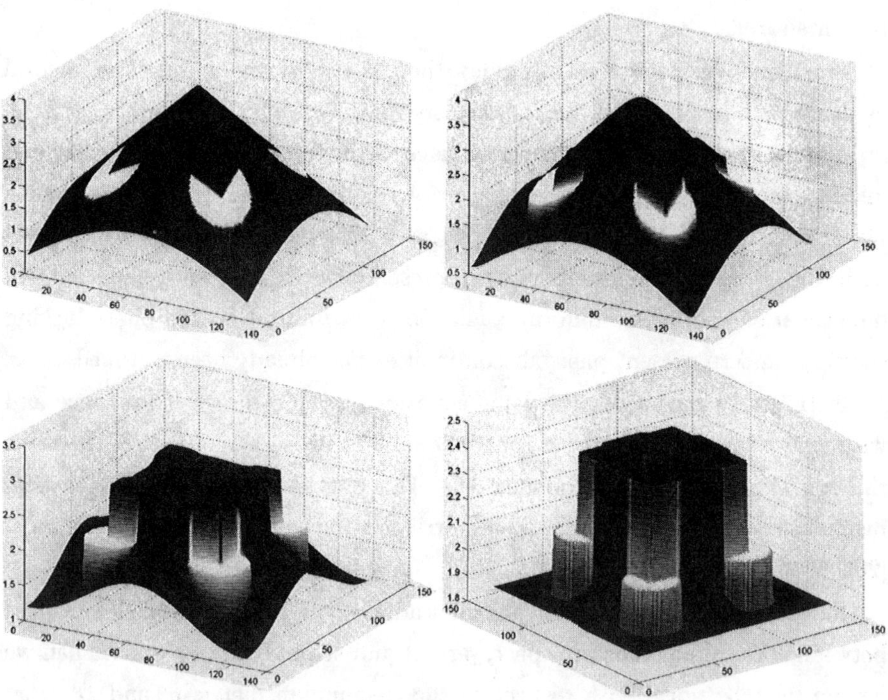

Figure 9.4: Evolution of a surface with the phase equation of neural oscillators Eqation (9.4). See [17] for details.

We are presently proving that the family F_ϵ Γ-converges as ϵ goes to 0 to the Mumford-Shah functional in a Riemannian space. If g^{ij} is the inverse the metric, the norm of the riemannian gradient is $|\nabla_g u|_g^p = (g^{ij}\partial_i u \partial_j u)^{p/2}$, and the natural functional is:

$$MS(u, \mathbf{R^n}) = \int_{\mathbf{R^n}} |\nabla_\mathbf{g} \mathbf{u}|_\mathbf{g}^\mathbf{p} \sqrt{\mathbf{g}} \mathbf{dx} + \int_{\mathbf{S(u)}} |\nu_\mathbf{g}|_\mathbf{g} \sqrt{\mathbf{g}} \mathbf{dH^{n-1}},$$

where $S(u)$ is the jump set of u, and ν_u its normal. The technique we use is a refinement of the proof of Braides [16], for the isotropic case.

Finally we plan to study the flow (u_ϵ) associated to equation (9.4). For $p = 1$ the associated flow is the motion by curvature in a Riemannian setting, as studied in the context of subjective surfaces method.

9.5 Research Sites Working on Level Sets/PDE

The list of web sites working in the area of level sets and PDE applied to imaging sciences is as under:

```
http://www.math.ucla.edu/~imagers/htmls/reports.html
http://www.ceremade.dauphine.fr/~cohen/
http://www.math.ucla.edu/~hzhao/
http://www-sop.inria.fr/epidaure/
http://graphics.stanford.edu/~fedkiw/
http://www.math.uci.edu/~zhao/research/image/image.html
http://www.math.uci.edu/~zhao/publication/publication.html
http://www.cim.mcgill.ca/
http://www.bic.mni.mcgill.ca/users/maudette/homepro.html
http://iacl.ece.jhu.edu/projects/gvf/
http://www.acm.caltech.edu/~seanm/software/cpt/cpt.html
http://www.gg.caltech.edu/~david/3D_scan_conv.html
http://www.irisa.fr/vista/
http://www.csd.uch.gr/~tziritas/pina/publications.html
http://www.comp.leeds.ac.uk/drm/
http://www.comp.leeds.ac.uk/andyb/welcome_in_frame.html
http://www.iie.edu.uy/investigacion/grupos/gti/investigacion.php3
```

```
http://vis-www.cs.umass.edu/~dima/umassmed/
http://www.cise.ufl.edu/~vemuri/
http://www.math-info.univ-paris5.fr/~gk/thierry/curri.html
http://dali.eng.tau.ac.il/~nk/
http://www.cs.technion.ac.il/~ron/
http://www.esam.northwestern.edu/~chopp/index.html
http://www.ms.uky.edu/~math/MAreport/
http://www.ms.uky.edu/~skim/ImageProcessing/
http://www.cmis.csiro.au/ismm2002/numerical_geometry_tutorial.htm
http://www.imm.dtu.dk/image/people.htm
http://www.imm.dtu.dk/~jab/
http://www.gg.caltech.edu/~david/
```

9.6 Appendix

Consider an image I and its Taylor expansion in the neighborhood of a point $\mathbf{x}_0$ as:

$$I(\mathbf{x}_0 + \delta\mathbf{x}_0, \sigma) = \underbrace{I(\mathbf{x}_0, \sigma)}_{0^{th}-order} + \underbrace{\delta\mathbf{x}_0{}^T \nabla_{0,\sigma}}_{1^{st}-order} + \underbrace{\delta\mathbf{x}_0{}^T \mathcal{H}_{0,\sigma}\, \delta\mathbf{x}_0}_{2^{nd}-order} + \ldots. \tag{9.5}$$

This expansion approximates the structure of the image up to the second order. $\nabla_{0,\sigma}$ and $\mathcal{H}_{0,\sigma}$ are the gradient vector and Hessian matrix of the image computed at $\mathbf{x}_0$ at scale σ. To calculate the differential operators I, the scale-space framework is adapted. In this framework, the differentiation is defined as a convolution with Derivative of Gaussian (DoG). This is given as:

$$\frac{\partial}{\partial x} L(\mathbf{x}, \sigma) = \sigma^{\gamma}\, I(\mathbf{x}) \otimes \frac{\partial G}{\partial \mathbf{x}}(\mathbf{x}, \sigma), \tag{9.6}$$

where $G(\mathbf{x}, \sigma)$ is the 3-D Gaussian kernel defined as:

$$G(\mathbf{x}, \sigma) = \frac{1}{(2\pi\sigma^2)^{\frac{D}{2}}} e^{\frac{||\mathbf{x}||^2}{2\sigma^2}}, \tag{9.7}$$

where $D = 3$, due to three dimensional processing. The parameter γ was introduced by Lindeberg[5] (see Lindeberg [3]-[9]). This was used to define a family of normalized derivatives. This normalization was particularly important for a fair comparison of the response of differential operators at multiple

[5]known as the Lindeberg Constant (LC)

scales. With no scales used, the LC=1.0. The second order information (called Hessian) has an intuitive justification in the context of the tubular structure detection. The second derivative of a Gaussian kernel at scale σ generates a probe kernel that measures the contrast between the regions inside and outside the range (-σ, σ). This can be seen in Fig. 9.5 (left), shown below. The third

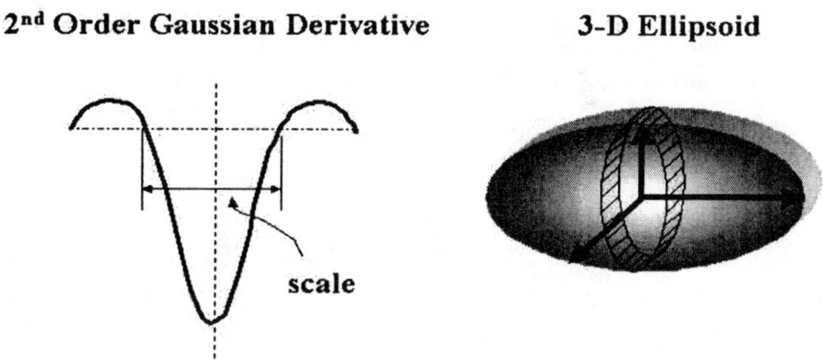

Figure 9.5: Concept of second order Gaussian derivative for edge estimation and ellipsoidal concept for direction estimation. **Left**: 2nd-order Gaussian derivative. **Right**: 3-D ellipsoid.

term in Eq. (9.6) gives the second order directional derivative:

$$\delta \mathbf{x}_0{}^T \mathcal{H}_{0,\sigma}\, \delta \mathbf{x}_0 = (\frac{\partial}{\partial \delta \mathbf{x}_0})(\frac{\partial}{\partial \delta \mathbf{x}_0}) I(\mathbf{x}_0, \sigma) \,. \tag{9.8}$$

The main concept behind the eigenvalue of the Hessian is to extract the principal directions in which the local second order structure of the image can be decomposed. Since this directly gives the direction of the smallest curvature (along the direction of the vessel), application of several filters in multiple orientations is avoided. This latter approach is computationally more expensive and requires a discretization of the orientation space. If $\lambda_{\sigma,k}$ is the eigenvalue corresponding to the kth normalized eigenvector $\mathbf{u}_{\sigma,k}$ of the Hessian $\mathcal{H}_{0,\sigma}$ computed at scale σ, then from the definition of the eigenvalues:

$$\mathcal{H}_{o,\sigma}\,\hat{\mathbf{u}}_{\sigma,k} = \lambda_{\sigma,k}\hat{\mathbf{u}}_{\sigma,k}\,. \tag{9.9}$$

The above equation has the following geometric interpretation. The eigenvalue decomposition extracts three orthonormal directions which are invariant up to a scaling factor when mapped by the Hessian matrix. In particular, a spherical neighborhood centered at $\mathbf{x}_0$ having a radius of unity will be mapped by $\mathcal{H}_0$ onto an ellipsoid whose axes are along the directions given by the eigenvectors of the Hessian and the corresponding axis semi-lengths are the magnitudes of the respective eigenvalues. This ellipsoid locally describes the second order structure of the image (see Fig. 9.5, right). Thus the problem comes down to the estimation of the eigenvalues and eigenvectors at each voxel location in the 3-D volume. The algorithm for filtering is framed in the next sub-section.

9.6.1 Algorithmic Steps for Ellipsoidal Filtering

The algorithm consists of the following steps and is in the spirit of Frangi *et al.*'s approach [23]. The algorithmic steps are given below:

1. *Pre-processing of the MRA Data Sets:* This consists of changing the anisotropic voxels to isotropic voxels. We used trilinear interpolation for this conversion. The second step in this pre-processing is the image resizing primarily for speed concerns. We used the standard wavelet transform method to down sample the volume in order to preserve the high frequency components of the lumen edges.

2. *Edge Volume Generation:* Here the convolution is performed between the image volume with the higher order Gaussian derivative operators. The computation of the second derivatives of Gaussian in the Hessian matrix is implemented using three separate convolutions with 1-D kernels, given as:

$$I_{x^iy^jz^k}(\mathbf{x},\sigma_f) = \underbrace{\frac{d^i}{d\mathbf{x}^i}G(\mathbf{x},\sigma_f)\otimes\{\underbrace{\frac{d^j}{d\mathbf{y}^j}G(\mathbf{y},\sigma_f)\otimes\{\underbrace{\frac{d^k}{d\mathbf{z}^k}G(\mathbf{z},\sigma_f)\otimes I(\mathbf{x})\}}_{convolution-1}\}}_{convolution-2}}_{convolution-3}, \tag{9.10}$$

where $I(\mathbf{x})$ is the interpolated gray scale volume, i, j and k are the non-negative integers satisfying $i+j+k=2$ and $3\ \sigma$ was used as the radius of the kernel. G is the Gaussian kernel in the x, y and z directions. $\frac{d^k}{d\mathbf{z}^k}G(\mathbf{z}, \sigma_f) \otimes I(\mathbf{x})$ is the convolution of the Gaussian kernel with a standard deviation of σ_f. Note that three sets of convolutions are done to obtain the scale-space representation of the gray scale volume rather than one convolution in 3-D. A similar example of 3-D convolution in MRA can be seen by Sato *et al.* [24].

3. *Hessian Analysis:* Running the directional processor for computing the eigenvalues, which is computed using Jacobi's method (see Press *et al.* [25]).

4. *Non-vascular Removal:* Here, the computation of the vessel score is performed to distinguish between the vessels from non-vessels using the eigenvalues based on connectivity, scale and contrast. This can be computed using the combination of components which are computed using the geometry of the shape which in turn is a function of the eigenvalues, λ_1, λ_2 and λ_3,

$$\mathcal{V}(\sigma, \gamma) = \begin{cases} 0 \ if \ |\lambda_2| > 0 \ or \ |\lambda_3| > 0 \\ (1 - exp(-\frac{\mathcal{R}_A^2}{2\alpha^2})) \ exp(-\frac{\mathcal{R}_B^2}{2\beta^2}) \ (1 - exp(-\frac{\mathcal{S}^2}{2\epsilon^2})), \end{cases} \tag{9.11}$$

where γ is the Lindeberg constant and α, β and ϵ are the thresholds which control the sensitivity of the filter for the measurements of features of the image such as area, blobness and distinguishing property given by notations $\mathcal{R}_A^2$, $\mathcal{R}_B^2$ and $\mathcal{S}^2$. The first two geometric ratios are gray-level invariants. This means they remain constant under intensity rescaling. The geometrical meaning of $\mathcal{R}_B^2$ is the derivation from a blob-like structure, but cannot distinguish between a line and a plate-like pattern. The $\mathcal{R}_B^2$ is computed as the ratio of the volume of the ellipsoid to the largest cross-section area, which came out to be a fraction $\frac{|\lambda_1|}{\sqrt{|\lambda_2 \lambda_3|}}$. The "blob-term" is at a maximum for a blob-like structure and is close to zero if λ_1, or λ_1 and λ_2, tend to vanish. $\mathcal{R}_A^2$ referred to the largest area of the cross-section of the ellipsoid in the plane, which was perpendicular to the vessel direction (the least eigenvalue direction). It is computed as the ratio of the two largest second order derivatives. This ratio is basically distinguishing between the plate and line-like structures. Mathematically, it is given as as $\frac{|\lambda_2|}{|\lambda_3|}$. The third term helps in distinguishing the vessel and non-vessel structures. This term is computed as the magnitude of the derivatives, which is the magnitude of the eigenvalues. It is computed using the norm of the Hessian. Frobenius matrix norm[6] was used, since it was straightforward in terms of the three eigenvalues and was given as: $\mathcal{S} = \sqrt{{\lambda_1}^2 + {\lambda_2}^2, \lambda_3^2}$.

5. *Iteration for All Scales:* Repeating the steps 2, 3 and 4 from the starting scale, σ_{min}, to the ending scale, σ_{max}.

6. *Compositing Volumes:* Scale optimization to remove the non-vascular and background structures. The filter optimization was done by finding the best scale σ. This is computed as: $\mathcal{V}(\gamma) = \max_{\sigma_{min} \leq \sigma \leq \sigma_{max}} \mathcal{V}(\sigma, \gamma)$. The volume corresponding to the best scale σ_{opt} is the filtered volume.

9.6.2 Acknowledgements

Dr. Suri would like to thank Dr. Chopp and Dr. Sarti for their contributions on the future aspects of level sets, PDE and subjective surfaces covering medical and non-medical applications. Thanks to Nancy Fitch for proof reading this chapter. Special to Marconi Medical Systems, Inc., previously known as Picker International for the MR data sets.

[6]Frobenius matrix of a given matrix, say **A**, is the rational canonical form of **A** and is mathematically equivalent to $\mathbf{Q}^{-1}\mathbf{A}\mathbf{Q}$, where **Q** is the transformation matrix.

Bibliography

[1] Suri, J. S., Liu, K., Laxminarayan, S., Singh, S., Reden, L., Shape Recovery Algorithms Using Level Sets in 2-D/3-D Medical Imagery: A State-of-the-Art Review, IEEE Trans. in Information Techonology in Biomedicine, March 2002.

[2] Suri, J. S., Liu, K., Laxminarayan, S., Reden, L., Ellipsodial scale-space filtering of white and black blood angiography, To Appear in IEEE Trans. in Information Techonology in Biomedicine, 2002.

[3] Lindeberg, T., Scale-space for discrete signals, IEEE Pattern Analysis and Machine Intelligence, Vol. 12, No. 3, pp. 234-254, 1990.

[4] Lindeberg, T., On scale selection for differential operators, Proceedings of the 8th Scandinavian Conference on Image Analysis (SCIA), pp. 857-866, 1993.

[5] Lindeberg, T., Detecting salient blob-like image structures and their scales with a scale-space primal sketch: A method for focus of attention, Int. J. of Computer Vision, Vol. 11, No. 3, pp. 283-318, 1993.

[6] Lindeberg, T., Edge detection and ridge detection with automatic scale selection, in Proc. of Computer Vision and Pattern Recognition, pp. 465-470, 1996.

[7] Lindeberg, T., Feature detection with automatic scale-space selection, Int. Journal of Computer Vision, Vol. 30, No. 2, pp. 79-116, 1998.

[8] Lindeberg, T., Scale-space Theory in Computer Vision, Kluwer Academic Publishers, 1994.

[9] Lindeberg, T., Discrete Derivative Approximations with Scale-Space Properties: A Basis for Low-Level Feature Extraction, J. of Mathematical Imaging and Vision, Vol. 3, No. 4, pp. 349-376, 1993.

[10] T. Y. Hou, Z. L. Li, S. Osher, and H. K. Zhao. A hybrid method for moving interface problems with application to the Hele-Shaw flow. *Journal of Computational Physics*, 134(2):236–252, 1997.

[11] R. Kimmel and J. A. Sethian. Optimal algorithm for shape from shading and path planning. *J. Math Imaging and Vision*, 14(3):237–244, 2001.

[12] J. A. Sethian and A. Vladimirsky. Ordered upwind methods for static Hamilton-Jacobi equations. *Proceedings of the National Academy of Sciences*, 98(20):11069–11074, 2001.

[13] N. Sukumar, D. L. Chopp, N. Moës, and T. Belytschko. Modeling holes and inclusions by level sets in the extended finite element method. *Computer Methods in Applied Mechanics and Engineering*, 190(46–47):6183–6200, 2001.

[14] N. Sukumar, D. L. Chopp, and B. Moran. Extended finite element method and fast marching method for three-dimensional fatigue crack propagation. *Engineering Fracture Mechanics*, 2001. to appear.

[15] M. Sussman and E. G. Puckett. A coupled level set and volume-of-fluid method for computing 3d and axisymmetric incompressible two-phase flows. *Journal of Computational Physics*, 162:301–337, 2000.

[16] A. Braides. Approximation of Free-Discontinuity Problems Lecture Notes in Mathematics No. 1694, Springer Verlag, Berlin, 1998.

[17] G. Citti, M.Manfredini, A. Sarti, "Neuronal Oscillations in the Visual Cortex: $\Gamma-$convergence to the Riemannian Mumford-Shah Functional", in preparation.

[18] Kanizsa, G., Organization in Vision, Hardcover, 1979.

[19] Petitot, J., Tondut, Y., Vers une Neuro-geometrie. Fibrations corticales, structures de contact et contours subjectifs modaux, Mathmatiques, Informatique et Sciences Humaines, EHESS, Paris, N.145, pp. 5-101, 1998.

[20] Sarti, A., Malladi, R., Sethian, J.A., Subjective surfaces: A Method for Completion of Missing Boundaries, Proceedings of the National Academy of Sciences of the United States of America, Vol 12, N.97, pag. 6258-6263, 2000.

Published online before print May 23, 2000: http://www.pnas.org/cgi/content/full/110135797

[21] Sarti, A., Citti, G., Manfredini, M., From Neural Oscillations to Variational Problems in the Visual Cortex, invited paper to Journal of Physiology Paris, Special Isuue on Geomatry and Cognition, J. Petitot ed.

[22] Schuster, H.G., Wagner P., A model for neuronal oscillators in the visual cortex. I: Mean field theory and derivation of the phase equations.", Biol. Cybern., Vol.64, N.1, pp.77-82,1990.

[23] Frangi, A. F., Niessen, W. J., Vincken, K. L. and Viergever, M. A., Multiscale vessel enhancement filtering, in Proc. Medical Image Computing and Computer-Assisted Intervention (MICCAI), Vol. 1496, pp. 130-137, 1998.

[24] Sato, Y., Nakajima, S., Shiraga, N., Atsumi, H., Yoshida, S., Koller, T., Gerig, G. and Kikinis, R., Three-dimensional multi-scale line filter for segmentation and visualization of curvilinear structures in medical images (see web site: http://www.spl.harvard.edu:8000/pages/papers/yoshi/cr.html), Med. Image Anal. (MIA), Vol. 2, No. 2, pp. 143-168, 1998.

[25] Press, W. H, *et al*, Numerical recipes in C : the art of scientific computing, Cambridge University Press, 1988.

Index